DERMATOLOGY
PRINCIPLES AND PRACTICE

Edited by

Elena Dinkollari

ALLIED HEALTH PRESS

Dermatology: Principles and Practice

Editor: **Elena Dinkollari**

Allied Health Press
4164 Lakeshore Road
Burlington ON L7L 1A4
Canada
www.alliedhealthpress.com
Email: orders@arclereducation.com

ISBN: 978-1-77956-244-9

ABOUT THE EDITOR

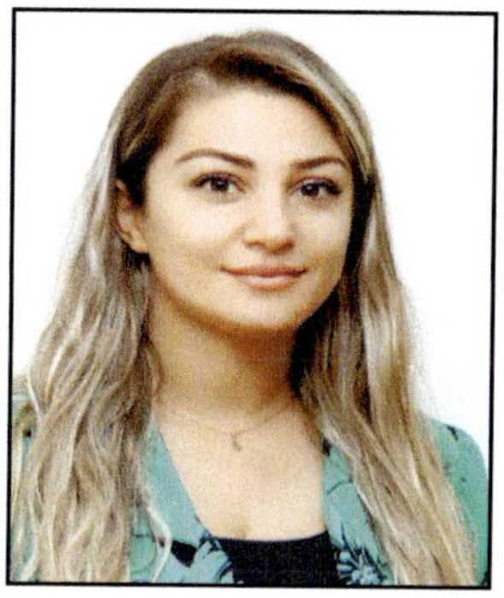

Elena Dinkollari is a highly skilled professional with over 8 years of experience in the field of dermatology and skincare. She graduated from the University of Medicine in Tirana as a Medical Laboratory Technician and later specialized in General Dermatology through a four-year program at Healthcert Education - Bond University. Additionally, she is a certified Organic Formulator by Albania Craftsman Education. Elena runs her private clinic, where she has built a successful practice focusing on organic skincare, haircare, and body care. She has also launched her own brand, which has gained recognition in Albania for its effectiveness and commitment to natural ingredients. Throughout her career, Elena has participated in numerous training programs both in Albania and internationally, further honing her expertise in treating various skin conditions. In 2023, she was honored as one of the most successful professionals in the "40 under 40" magazine.

Word Roots, Prefixes, and Suffixes by Chapter

Chapter 1 Anatomy and Physiology of the Skin

derm/o-, skin
erythemat/o-, redness
dermat/o-, skin
melan/o-, black
-osis, condition / disease
-cyte, cell
cutane-, skin

Chapter 2 Inflammatory Skin Diseases

-itis, inflammation
psor-, itching
hemo/hemat, blood
angi/o-, vessel
-ology, study of

Chapter 3 Infectious Skin Diseases

-oma, tumor
vesic/o-, bladder, sac
dys-, abnormal; difficult
hyper-, excess or over
-algia, pain
fasci-, refers to fascia

Chapter 4 Disorders of Pigmentation

abdomin-, of or relating to the abdomen
angi-, blood vessel
-plasia, development, growth, condition of formation
-rrhea, flow
-sis, state of

Chapter 5 Dermatoses of Pregnancy

-ology, branch of knowledge or science
-ologist, specialist in the study of
-edema, swelling
-iasis, pathological condition or state
-trophy, nourishment, growth

Chapter 6 Skin Cancer

lympho-, relating to the lymphatic system
-oma, tumors or cancers
-genic, creating / causing
carcin-, cancer
onco-, mass / tumor

Chapter 7 Pediatric Dermatology

Pedi-, care or treatment of children or childhood diseases
card-, cardi-, cardio-, heart
entero-, intestine; gut
hepa-, the liver
-cele, hernia, swelling

Chapter 8 Plasma Dermatology: Skin Therapy Using Cold Atmospheric Plasma

-ancy, state or condition
-ical, pertaining to, related to
anti-, against or opposed to
fung-, fungus
onych-, nail
myc-, mykes, fungus.

Chapter 9 Low-Level Laser (Light) Therapy (LLLT) In Skin: Stimulating, Healing, and Restoring

bio-, bios, life
-trop, turned toward, with an orientation toward
aden/o, gland
-amine, nitrogen compound

Chapter 10 Advanced Technologies in Dermatology

capill-, of or pertaining to hair
cyt(o)-, cell
fibr(o), fiber
homo-, denotes something as 'the same' as another, alike, or common
nephr(o)-, of or pertaining to the kidney

Table of Contents

LIST OF FIGURES

LIST OF TABLES

PREFACE

Dermatology has experienced notable advancements recently, particularly in understanding the underlying pathophysiological mechanisms of chronic diseases and developing high-performance imaging techniques such as dermoscopy, confocal microscopy, and optical coherence tomography (OCT), which have greatly improved the diagnosis and management of skin tumors. Additionally, there has been a more refined therapeutic approach to various disorders, including psoriasis, atopic dermatitis, vitiligo, hidradenitis suppurativa, and chronic urticaria.

The pathogenic mechanisms of common immune diseases have been a research focus, revealing the roles of innate and acquired immunity, as well as their products, such as chemokines and pro- and anti-inflammatory cytokines. These insights have led to innovative therapeutic strategies, particularly in biological therapy. However, despite these advancements, many aspects of the main pathophysiological processes underlying these conditions remain unknown, presenting challenges in treatment approaches, especially in conditions like psoriasis and atopic dermatitis.

Psoriasis, characterized by cellular immunity, has shown positive responses to therapies involving monoclonal antibodies or fusion proteins, leading to lesion clearance. Despite the presence of lymphocytes that stimulate keratinocytes in psoriasis, questions remain as to why cell biological therapy targeting these lymphocytes directly is not utilized, instead of focusing on reducing the effectors (cytokines and chemokines) of these cells. One plausible explanation could be current limitations in scientific understanding, which prevent the effective distribution of large cellular structures like lymphocytes to the blood or skin, despite the presence of specific surface markers that could aid in their identification.

While scientific research in dermatology has made significant strides, challenges remain in effectively targeting and eliminating pro-inflammatory cytokine- and chemokine-producing cells in psoriasis. Furthermore, advancements in dermatology aim to enhance the sensitivity of in vivo diagnostic methods to mimic the accuracy of in vitro methods, providing more reliable and accurate diagnostic results for improved patient care and treatment outcomes.

This comprehensive guide aims to provide a thorough understanding of dermatology, covering fundamental principles, diagnostic techniques, common skin conditions, and advanced treatment modalities. It seeks to bridge the gap between basic dermatological knowledge and clinical practice, offering a blend of theoretical concepts and practical insights. By incorporating the latest research and clinical guidelines, it aims to be a valuable resource for dermatologists, dermatology residents, medical students, and healthcare professionals interested in skin health. The book also strives to enhance dermatological education and promote a deeper appreciation for the field by offering engaging content and case studies that illustrate key concepts.

This book serves as a comprehensive reference guide for dermatologists at all stages of their careers, providing up-to-date information on diagnosis, treatment, and management of skin diseases. Students studying dermatology will find this book a valuable resource for understanding the principles and practices of dermatology, helping them develop a solid foundation in the field.

Chapter

ANATOMY AND PHYSIOLOGY OF THE SKIN

1

Contents

Introduction

The skin makes up around 15% of an adult's total body weight, making it the largest organ in the body. It carries out a multitude of essential tasks, such as preventing the body from losing too much water and aiding in thermoregulation, in addition to providing defense against external physical, chemical, and biological threats. The mucous membranes that line the body's surface are a continuous layer of skin (Kanitakis, 2002).

The skin and structures derived from it make up the integumentary system. The epidermis, dermis, and subcutaneous tissue are the three layers that make up the skin. The outermost layer, the epidermis, is made up of a particular group of cells called keratinocytes, which are responsible for producing the protective protein keratin, which is a long, thread-like strand. Collagen, a fibrillar structural protein, is the main component of the dermis, the middle layer. The dermis is located on the panniculus, or subcutaneous tissue, which is made up of tiny fat cell lobes called lipocytes. Depending on where in the body's anatomy they are located, these layers vary greatly in thickness. The epidermal layer on the eyelid, for instance, is the thinnest at less than 0.1 nm, while the epidermal layer on the palms and soles of the feet is the thickest, measuring about 1.5 μm. The back has the thickest dermis, which is 30–40 times thicker than the epidermis that covers it.

Orientation and Directional Terms

Term	Definition	Illustration
Integumentary system	The integumentary system is the body's largest organ, which protects the internal organs and systems from the external environment. It's made up of the skin, hair, nails, and associated glands. The word "integumentary" means the body's outer covering.	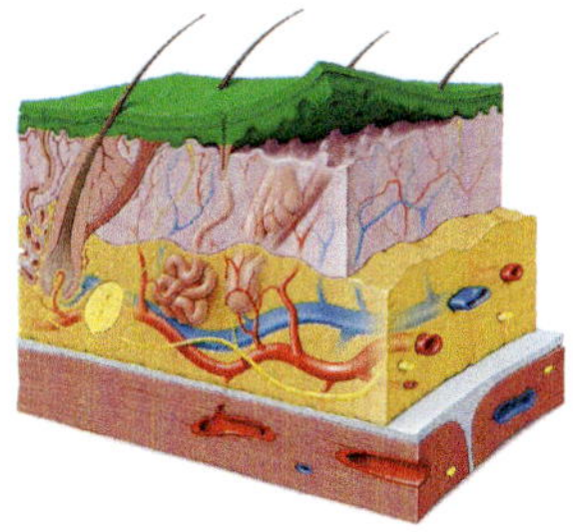
Epidermis	The epidermis, the skin's outermost layer, is composed of several strata and various cell types crucial for its function. Layers of the epidermis: From the deepest to the most superficial, the epidermal layers are the stratum basale, stratum spinosum, stratum granulosum, stratum lucidum, and stratum corneum.	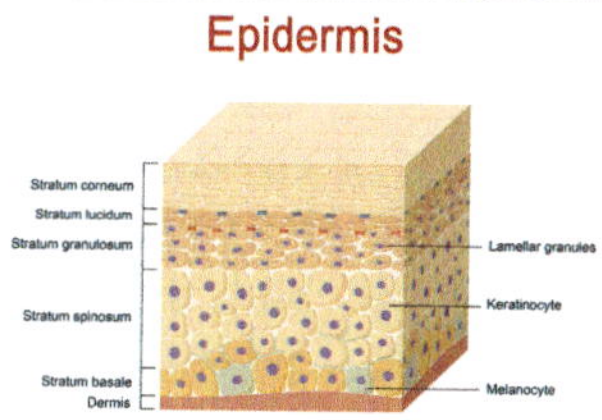
Langerhans cell	A Langerhans cell (LC) is a tissue-resident macrophage of the skin once thought to be a resident dendritic cell. These cells contain organelles called Birbeck granules.	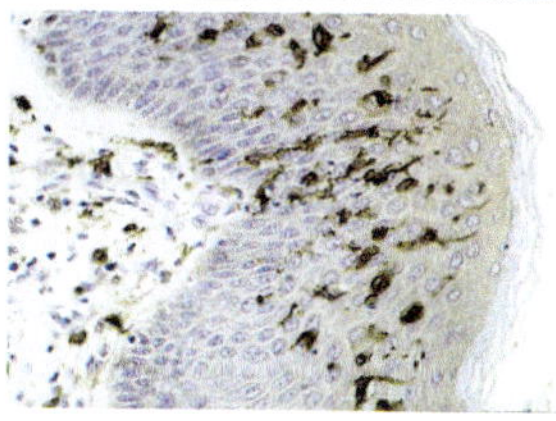
Melanocyte	Melanocyte is specialized skin cell that produces the protective skin-darkening pigment melanin. Birds and mammals possess these pigment cells, which are found mainly in the epidermis, though they occur elsewhere—e.g., in the matrix of the hair. Melanocytes are branched, or dendritic, and their dendrites are used to transfer pigment granules to adjacent epidermal cells.	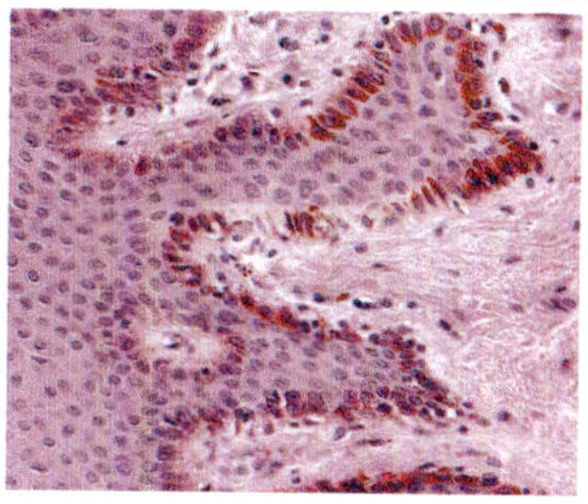
Hair follicle	The hair follicle is an organ found in mammalian skin. It resides in the dermal layer of the skin and is made up of 20 different cell types, each with distinct functions. The hair follicle regulates hair growth via a complex interaction between hormones, neuropeptides, and immune cells.	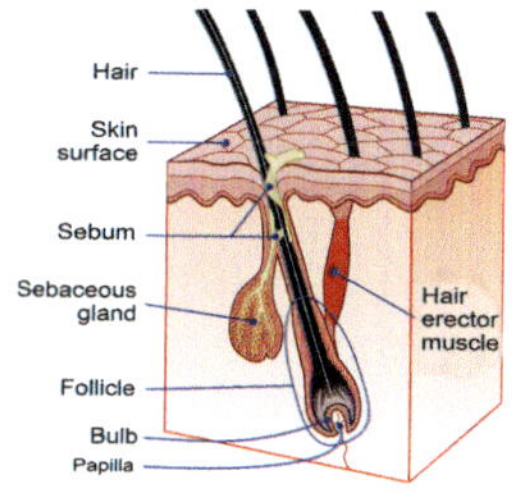

1.1. Epidermis

The two main cell types that make up the stratified, squamous epithelium layer known as the epidermis are dendritic and keratinocytes. The keratinocytes have a lot of stainable cytoplasm and intercellular bridges, which set them apart from the "clear" dendritic cells. Although the keratinocyte cell type makes up the vast majority of the cells in the epidermis, other cell populations such as melanocytes, Langerhans cells, and Merkel cells are also present. The basal cell layer (stratum germinativum), the squamous cell layer (stratum spinosum), the granular cell layer (stratum granulosum), and the cornified or horny cell layer (stratum corneum) are the four layers into which the epidermis is typically divided based on the morphology and position of keratinocytes as they differentiate into horny cells. The terms stratum malpighii and rete malpighii are occasionally used to refer to the lower three layers that make up the living, nucleated cells of the epidermis.

The epidermis is a layer that regenerates continuously and gives rise to derivative structures like sweat glands, nails, and pilosebaceous apparatuses. The epidermis's basal cells go through cycles of proliferation that allow the outer epidermis to regenerate. The epidermis is a dynamic tissue where cells are always moving in an unsynchronized manner. As they approach the skin's surface, various individual cell populations pass not only one another but also melanocytes and Langerhans cells.

1.1.1. Keratinocytes

The main cell type present in the epidermis, the skin's outermost layer, is keratinocytes. They make up 90% of the skin cells in the epidermis of humans. Sometimes, basal keratinocytes are used to refer to basal cells in the stratum basale, or basal layer, of the skin. To protect the environment from harmful bacteria, fungi, viruses, UV light, heat, and water loss, keratinocytes form a barrier. Numerous lipids, enzymes, structural proteins, and antimicrobial peptides support the preservation of the skin's crucial barrier function. Every 40 to 56 days in humans, keratinocytes—which originated from epidermal stem cells in the lower epidermis—migrate towards the surface, differentiate into corneocytes, and ultimately shed (Figure 1.1).

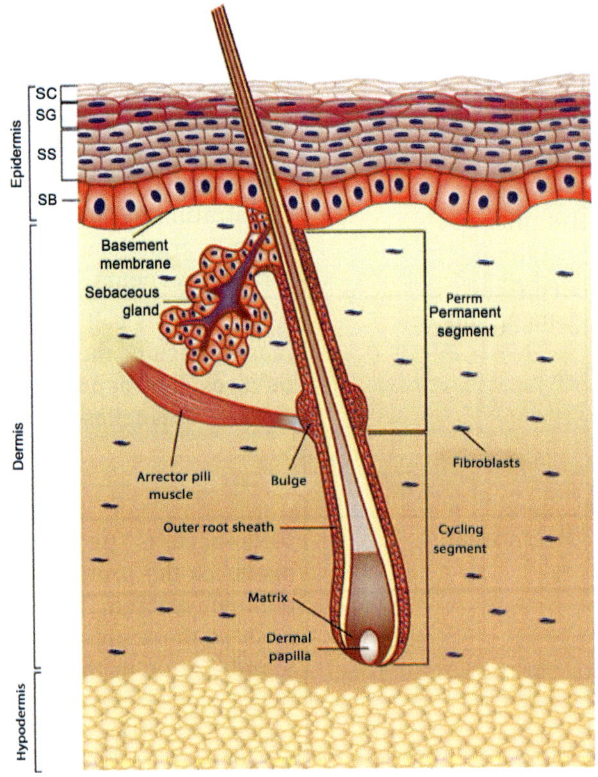

Figure 1.1. *Skin epidermis with keratinocyte and melanocyte cells.*

Source: https://commons.wikimedia.org/wiki/File:Anatomy_of_the_skin.jpg.

1.1.1.1. Function

Keratinocytes mainly serve to create a protective barrier that shields the skin from harm caused by heat, UV rays, dryness, harmful microbes, and viruses.

When pathogens invade the outer layers of the epidermis, keratinocytes can release proinflammatory mediators, especially chemokines like CXCL10 and CCL2 (MCP-1), which draw dendritic cells, monocytes, T lymphocytes, and natural killer cells to the infection site.

1.1.1.2. Structure

The crucial barrier function of the skin is maintained by a variety of structural proteins (filaggrin, keratin), enzymes (such as proteases), lipids, and antimicrobial peptides (defensins). Keratinization is a process in which keratinocytes undergo terminal differentiation and produce an increasing amount of keratin as part of the physical barrier formation, also known as cornification. The outermost layer's fully cornified keratinocytes are continually shedding their cells and being replaced by new ones.

1.1.1.3. Cell Differentiation

Hemidesmosomes connect epidermal stem cells, which are found in the stratum basale, the lowermost layer of the epidermis, to the basement membrane. Random division of epidermal stem cells produces either more stem cells or transit amplifying cells. A portion of the transit amplifying cells keep multiplying, decide to differentiate, and move in the direction of the epidermal surface. The differentiated offspring of those stem cells are arranged into columns known as epidermal proliferation units.

In the course of this differentiation process, keratinocytes move suprabasally to join the stratum spinosum, stratum granulosum, and ultimately the stratum corneum as corneocytes. They also permanently exit the cell cycle and begin to express markers of epidermal differentiation.

Keratinocytes that have finished their differentiation process and lost their cytoplasmic organelles and nucleus are known as corneocytes. Desquamation is the process by which corneocytes eventually shed off to make room for new ones.

Specific keratins, such as keratin 1, keratin 5, keratin 10, and keratin 14, are expressed by keratinocytes at each stage of differentiation, along with additional markers like involucrin, loricrin, transglutaminase, filaggrin, and caspase 14.

It is estimated that the turnover time of keratinocytes in humans is estimated to be 40–56 days, while in mice it is estimated to be 8–10 days.

Factors promoting keratinocyte differentiation are:

- There is a calcium gradient present in the skin, with the lowest concentration found in the stratum basale and increasing concentrations up to the outer stratum granulosum. The highest concentration of calcium is in the stratum corneum due to the cells being dry and unable to dissolve the ions. The elevated extracellular calcium concentrations lead to an increase in intracellular free calcium levels in keratinocytes. This increase is a result of calcium being released from intracellular stores and calcium influx through calcium-sensitive chloride channels and voltage-independent cation channels that are permeable to calcium. Additionally, it is believed that an extracellular calcium-sensing receptor, known as CaSR, also plays a role in the increase in intracellular calcium concentration.
- Cholecalciferol, or vitamin D3, controls the expression of genes involved in keratinocyte differentiation and calcium concentrations, which in turn controls keratinocyte proliferation and differentiation. The complete vitamin

D metabolic pathway, from vitamin D synthesis to catabolism and vitamin D receptor expression, is only present in keratinocytes.

- Cathepsin E.
- TALE homeodomain transcription factors.
- Hydrocortisone.
- Factors that encourage keratinocyte proliferation should be viewed as preventing differentiation since keratinocyte differentiation inhibits keratinocyte proliferation. These factors include:
- The transcription factor p63, which stops the differentiation of epidermal stem cells into keratinocytes. The p63 DNA-binding domain mutations are linked to cleft lip/palate (EEC) syndrome, ectodermal dysplasia, and ectrodactyly. The normal epidermal cell identity was not maintained by the transcriptome of keratinocytes with p63 mutations.
- Vitamin A and its analogs.
- Epidermal growth factor.
- Transforming growth factor-alpha (TGF-α).
- Cholera toxin.

1.1.1.4. Interaction with Other Cells

Melanocytes and Langerhans cells, among other cell types, are linked to keratinocytes in the epidermis. Langerhans cells and intradermal lymphocytes are held in place within the epidermis by keratinocytes, which create tight junctions with the skin's nerves. In addition to producing the chemokines and antimicrobial peptides mentioned above, keratinocytes are also strong producers of anti-inflammatory mediators like TGF-β and IL-10 that influence the immune system. When they become active, they can secrete TNFα and IL-1β, which can cause cutaneous inflammation and activate Langerhans cells.

By absorbing melanosomes—vesicles that contain the endogenous photoprotectant melanin—from epidermal melanocytes, keratinocytes help shield the body from ultraviolet radiation (UVR). Numerous dendrites extend from each melanocyte in the epidermis to connect it to numerous keratinocytes. After that, melanin is stored as supranuclear "caps" within keratinocytes and melanocytes in the perinuclear region, where it shields DNA from UVR-induced oxidative damage.

1.1.1.5. Role in Wound Healing

Keratinocyte migration to fill in the gaps left by wounds is a part of the skin's healing process. The hair follicle's bulge region produces the first group of keratinocytes involved in that repair, which will only last momentarily. Keratinocytes derived from the epidermis will take their place within the healed epidermis.

On the other hand, during the healing of large wounds, epidermal keratinocytes may aid in the formation of new hair follicles. Tympanic perforation healing requires functional keratinocytes.

1.1.1.6. Sunburn Cells

A sunburned cell is a keratinocyte that develops after being exposed to UVA in the presence of psoralens, UVB radiation, or both. It has a pyknotic nucleus and an eosinophilic cytoplasm. It has been said to be an illustration of apoptosis and exhibits early and aberrant keratinization.

1.1.1.7. Aging

Tissue homeostasis deteriorates with age, in part due to stem/progenitor cells' inability to differentiate or self-renew. Epidermal stem cell aging may be largely attributed to DNA damage brought on by reactive oxygen species (ROS) exposure of stem/progenitor cells. Normally, mitochondrial superoxide dismutase (SOD2) guards against reactive oxygen species. A portion of keratinocytes had their proliferation irreversibly stopped by cellular senescence brought on by SOD2 loss in mouse epidermal cells. SOD2 deficiency decreased epidermal thickness and delayed wound closure in older mice.

1.1.1.8. Civatte Body

A damaged basal keratinocyte that has undergone apoptosis is known as a "Civatte body," named after the French dermatologist Achille Civatte (1877–1956). These bodies are almost always covered in immunoglobulins, primarily IgM. Civatte bodies are typically observed in skin lesions associated with a variety of dermatoses, especially discoid lupus erythematosus and lichen planus. Additionally, they may be present in the following conditions: erythema multiforme, bullous pemphigoid, eczema, lichen planopilaris, febrile neutrophilic dermatosis, toxic epidermal necrolysis, varicella-zoster lesions, dermatitis herpetiformis, porphyria cutanea tarda, sarcoidosis, subcorneal pustular dermatosis, transient acantholytic dermatosis, and epidermolytic hyperkeratosis.

1.1.2. Basal Layer

Column-shaped keratinocytes, with their long axis perpendicular to the dermis, adhere to the basement membrane zone in the basal layer, also referred to as the stratum basale. Through desmosomal junctions, these basal cells cling to more superficial squamous cells and form a single layer. The dark-staining oval or elongated nuclei of the basal cells, as well as the presence of melanin pigment transferred from nearby melanocytes, are additional characteristics that set them apart.

The majority of mitotically active epidermal cells that give rise to outer epidermal layer cells are found in the basal layer. Not every basal cell, though, has the capacity to proliferate. Under normal circumstances, the long-lived clonogenic epidermal stem cells in the basal layer move very slowly through the cell cycle. Wounds and other hyperplasiogenic conditions can promote stem cell division, which in turn increases the number of cycling cells in the epidermis. Carcinogenic agents can damage DNA, which can alter the machinery involved in cell proliferation and slow down the rate at which cells divide. In humans, it takes at least 14 days for a basal cell to migrate from the basal layer to the cornified layer, and an additional 14 days are needed for the cell to travel through the cornified layer and reach the outermost epidermis.

1.1.2.1. Cellular Composition and Function

The keratinocyte, which is the main cell type in the stratum basale, is responsible for producing the protein keratin, which is an essential part of the skin's protective barrier. Merkel cells, which are linked to sensory perception, and melanocytes, which generate melanin, the pigment responsible for skin color, are also found in this layer.

1.1.2.2. Role in Skin Regeneration

The Stratum Basale's cells undergo mitosis at a high rate. Older cells are forced toward the surface by their division, where they ultimately desquamate. This turnover is essential for the skin's surface to constantly renew itself and is crucial for wound healing.

1.1.3. Squamous Cell Layer

The squamous cell layer, also referred to as the stratum spinosum, is a layer of the epidermis that lies on top of the basal cell layer and is 5–10 cells thick. Depending on where they are located, the shape, structure, and subcellular characteristics of the various cells that make up the squamous layer vary. For example, cells of the upper spinous layers are usually larger, become flatter as they are pushed toward the skin's surface, and contain lamellar granules. In contrast, suprabasal spinous cells are polyhedral in shape and have a rounded nucleus. Membrane-bound glycoproteins, glycolipids, phospholipids, free sterols, and several acid hydrolases, such as lipases, proteases, acid phosphatases, and glycosidases, are found in lamellar granules. The hydrolytic enzyme abundance suggests that the lamellar granules are a particular kind of lysosome. While the lamellar granules are mainly involved in the function of cells at the interface of the granular and cornified layers, they also play a role in the delivery of stratum corneum lipid precursors into the intercellular space in cells of the upper spinous layer.

Desmosomes, which are widely distributed and facilitate mechanical coupling between epidermal cells, bridge the intercellular spaces between spinous cells and confer resistance against external stresses. Keratin filaments in the cytoplasm are arranged concentrically around the nucleus. At one end, they are attached to desmosomal plaques, but at the end that is closest to the nucleus, they are free. Six polypeptides on the cytoplasmic side of the cell membrane, which are crucial for controlling the calcium needed for desmosomal assembly and maintenance, make up the desmosomal plaques. The name "stratum spinosum" comes from the way the many desmosomes along cell borders resemble spines (Chu, 2008).

An additional kind of connection between epidermal cells is known as a gap junction. These junctions, which essentially create an intercellular pore, enable chemical signals to carry out physiologic communication, which is essential for controlling cell growth, differentiation, and metabolism.

1.1.4. Granular Layer

The stratum granulosum, also known as the granular layer, is the outermost layer of the epidermis that contains living cells. It is made up of flattened cells that have a large number of keratohyaline granules inside of them. The additional synthesis and alteration of the proteins involved in keratinization is carried out by these cells. The thickness of the granular layer varies proportionally to the thickness of the horny cell layer that covers it. For instance, the granular layer beneath thin cornified layer areas might only be 1–3 cell layers thick, but it might be 10 times thicker beneath the palms of the hands and soles of the feet. Extensive parakeratosis, in which keratinocyte nuclei remain after the cells migrate into the stratum corneum, can be caused by a very thin or nonexistent granular layer, ultimately leading to psoriasis.

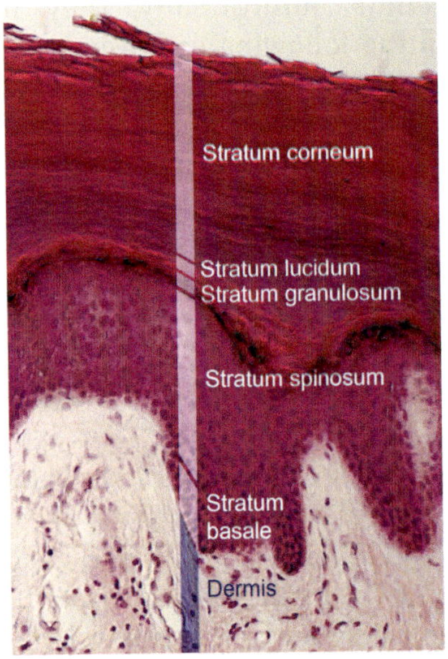

Figure 1.2. *Histologic image showing a section of the epidermis. Stratum granulosum is labeled near the center.*

Source: https://upload.wikimedia.org/wikipedia/commons/e/e4/Epidermal_layers.png.

Cells release lamellar bodies (which contain lipids and proteins) into the extracellular space as this layer transitions into the stratum corneum. As a result, the hydrophobic lipid envelope that gives skin its barrier qualities is formed. Cells simultaneously lose their organelles and nuclei (Figure 1.2).

The formation of the interfibrillary matrix, which holds keratin filaments together, and the inner lining of horny cells both depend on the deeply basophilic, irregularly shaped granules known as keratohyaline granules. Keratin filaments are periodically cut by the keratohyaline granules' enzymatic action, which produces "soft" keratin in the epidermis. On the other hand, keratohyaline granules are absent from the hair and nails, and the tonofibril filaments that travel through the cytoplasm of the cell will solidify due to the addition of disulfide bonds, resulting in "hard" keratin in those structures.

Because the granular layer is a keratogenous zone of the epidermis, lysosomal enzymes that are present in small amounts in the stratum basalis and stratum spinosum are found at high levels in the stratum granulosum. As the granular layer cells abruptly differentiate into horny cornified layer cells, the dissolution of cellular organelles is prepared in this instance.

1.1.5. Cornified Layer

The cornified layer's horny cells, or corneocytes, act as a barrier to stop water loss and foreign material invasion in addition to providing mechanical protection for the underlying epidermis. Surrounding the low-lipid, high-protein corneocytes is an extracellular lipid matrix that is continuous. Technically, the large, flat, polyhedral-shaped horny cells are thought to be dead because they have lost their nuclei during terminal differentiation. To encourage desquamation that moves outward, the physical and biochemical characteristics of the cells in the cornified layer change depending on their location. For example, because the cytoplasm of middle layer cells contains a high concentration of free amino acids, middle layer cells have a much higher capacity for water binding than the deeper layers. In comparison to the more superficial layers, the deep cells are also more densely packed and exhibit a wider variety of intercellular attachments. As the cells divide, desmosomes are broken down by proteases, which helps cause corneocytes to shed during desquamation.

1.2. The Regulation of Epidermal Proliferation and Differentiation

The epidermis is a tissue that regenerates continuously, so it needs to keep its cell count relatively constant and control how epidermal cells interact with one another. As cells migrate during development and throughout life, it is necessary to regulate adhesions between keratinocytes, the interactions between keratinocytes and immigrant cells, the adhesion between the basal lamina and the underlying dermis, and the process of terminal differentiation to produce corneocytes. The dermis beneath the epidermis regulates both epidermal morphogenesis and differentiation. The dermis is essential for maintaining postnatal structure and function. Another important location for the development of epidermal appendages is the epidermal-dermal interface.

The ability of epidermal cells to undergo apoptosis, or programmed cell death, is one of the intrinsic properties that contribute to the maintenance of a constant epidermal thickness. Unlike necrosis, which frequently causes damage to nearby cells, apoptosis results in cell death through an orderly pattern of morphologic and biochemical changes. A variety of cellular signaling molecules, such as hormones, growth factors, and cytokines, control this important homeostatic process. Apoptosis plays a crucial role in the skin's developmental remodeling, cell number regulation, and defense against damaged, mutated, or virus-infected cells. A sort of apoptosis called terminal differentiation evolved to change the keratinocyte into the protective corneocyte. Skin tumors frequently exhibit dysregulation of apoptosis, while conditions like psoriasis can arise from the disruption of dynamic equilibrium maintaining constant epidermal thickness (Kerr, Wyllie, and Currie, 1972).

1.3. Nonkeratinocyte Cells of the Epidermis

1.3.1. Melanocytes

The human body's melanocytes are a diverse group of cells. Even though they are all derived from neural crest cells (NCC), which are embryonic cells with the capacity to produce melanin, their specific roles in all target locations go far beyond this synthesis of melanin. The presence of melanocytes in the human body is not limited to the iris, hair, and epidermis, which contributes to the color of these structures. Melanocytes have also been discovered in the heart, nervous system, and inner ear, and these are probably not the only organ systems in which these cells can be found. It is important to emphasize that other cells, such as cells, can also produce melanin in addition to melanocytes g cells of the ciliary body of the eye, the iris, the retina, and some neurons as well as adipocytes.

The differentiation of melanoblasts into melanocytes, their migration and proliferation, their differentiation into mature melanocytes (producing melanin in special organelles called melanosomes, which have dendritic morphology), their maturation (transporting mature melanosomes to keratinocytes), and their eventual cell death are the various stages that make up the life cycle of melanocytes. Skin melanocytes are produced by multiple neural crest cell populations, including the cranial, dorsal trunk, and ventral trunk. Hair and epidermal melanocytes share the same embryonic ancestry, but they develop differently. There is ongoing discussion regarding the location of melanocyte stem cells in adult skin. The results of experiments unequivocally demonstrate that the trunk NCC that migrates via a ventral pathway may continue to reside in the cutaneous nerves' myelin sheath and, in certain circumstances, produce melanoblasts. Melanocyte development in the embryo offers a chance to gain a better understanding of skin conditions like vitiligo and melanoma and its heterogeneity. Thus, the biology and development of epidermal and hair melanocytes are described in this review.

1.3.1.1. Melanocyte in the Skin as the Epidermal Melanin Unit Element

Melanocytes can be identified by specific proteins such as tyrosinase (TYR), tyrosinase-related protein 1 and 2 (TYRP1, TYRP2/DCT), melanosomal matrix proteins (Pmel17, MART-1), and microphthalmia transcription factor (MITF). These cells are smaller than keratinocytes and have a distinct oval or fusiform shape. Melanocytes contain melanosomes, which are specialized organelles that produce melanin. They are located in the basal layer of the epidermis and form melanin units with about 30–40 keratinocytes. The ratio of melanocytes to keratinocytes is 1:10 in this layer, with around 1200 melanocytes per mm^2 of skin. Adhesion molecules like E- and P-cadherins are involved in creating cell-cell connections. The transfer of melanin from melanocytes to keratinocytes is crucial for determining skin color and providing photoprotection. The accumulation of melanin granules above the keratinocyte nucleus is eventually shed with the outer layer of the skin. The mechanisms behind this melanosome transfer are still being studied.

Recently, Ando et al. proposed a model of melanosomes' transport via the shedding vesicle system through the following stages:

- Surrounded by the membrane pigment globules (PG) containing multiple melanosomes and a few mitochondria are formed in the filopodia of melanocyte dendrites,
- PG are released from different areas of the dendrites into extracellular space,
- PG are captured by microvilli of keratinocytes, which incorporate them in a protease-activated receptor-2 (PAR-2)-dependent way,
- membrane-surrounded PG is degraded,
- single melanosomes are released in a keratinocyte cytosol and reach the perinuclear area.

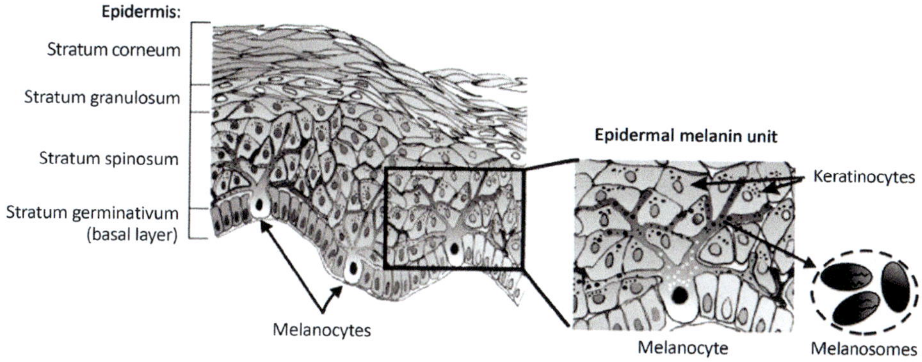

Figure 1.3. *Scheme of the epidermis structure. Melanocytes reside between the basal layer cells and through dendritic processes communicate with about 30–40 keratinocytes in the epidermal melanin unit. Melanocyte synthesizes melanins in melanosomes transported into keratinocytes to protect them from UV radiation.*

Source: https://www.ncbi.nlm.nih.gov/pmc/articles/PMC3834696/#:~:text=Melanocyte%20is%20a%20highly%20differentiated,cell%20loses%20the%20proliferative%20potential.

Regardless of race, epidermal melanin units are similar in size, though they differ in different body parts. Melanocytic dendritic arrangement and melanogenesis intensity are two areas where racial differences are evident.

The specific mechanisms that regulate the organization and quantity of melanocytes in the epidermis remain unknown. Melanocytes, keratinocytes, and dermal fibroblasts communicate through secreted factors and cell-to-cell interactions. Keratinocytes play a role in the growth and function of melanocytes by releasing growth factors and using cell adhesion molecules. Additionally, melanocytes, and keratinocytes produce hormones that control melanocyte growth, melanin production, and the formation of melanocytic dendrites. The communication between keratinocytes and melanocytes through different signaling pathways is crucial for maintaining skin balance. In the presence of ultraviolet radiation, keratinocytes can increase the release of factors that impact various biological activities of melanocytes as detailed in Table 1.1.

Table 1.1. The Paracrine Factors Secreted by Keratinocytes After UV Radiation That Influence Melanocyte Biology

The Factors Derived From Keratinocytes	The Effects on Melanocyte
bFGF	↑ Proliferation
ET-1	↓ Proliferation, ↑ dendricity, ↓ melanogenesis
IL-1α/1β	↑ Proliferation, ↑ melanogenesis, ↑ survival
ACTH	↑ Proliferation, ↑ dendricity, ↑ melanogenesis, ↑ survival
α-MSH	↑ Dendricity, ↑ melanogenesis, ↑ melanosomal transfer
$PGE_2/PGF_{2\alpha}$	↑ Proliferation, ↑ melanogenesis
GM-CSF	↑ Melanogenesis
NO	↓ Melanogenesis
TNF-α	↑ Dendricity, ↑ survival
NGF	↓ Melanogenesis
BMP-4	↑ Proliferation, ↑ dendricity, ↑ melanogenesis

Source: https://www.ncbi.nlm.nih.gov/pmc/articles/PMC3834696/table/T0001/?report=objectonly.

The biology of melanocytes is also regulated by substances secreted by dermal fibroblasts, such as neuregulin 1 (NRG1) and stem cell factor (SCF). These cytokines affect the shape, dendricity, mobility, adhesive qualities, and growth and pigmentation of melanocytes. The melanocyte, a highly active component of the epidermal melanin unit, secretes several signal molecules that target skin immune system cells in addition to keratinocytes. Among the substances released by stimulated melanocytes are proinflammatory cytokines (IL-1α, IL-2, IL-3, IL-6, IL-10, and TNF-α), chemokines (IL-8, CCL2), transforming growth factor (TGF-β), catecholamines, eicosanoids, serotonin, melanocyte stimulating factor (α-MSH), and nitric oxide (NO). Secreted substances also function as autocrine factors. For example, eicosanoids, and α-MSH stimulate melanin synthesis, while IL-1, IL-6, and TNF-α inhibit melanogenesis. Thus, in the epidermis, melanocytes, and collaborating keratinocytes form orderly units. Melanocytes, which have a long lifespan while keratinocytes shed and die, are the stable components of each unit. The duration of melanocyte life in human skin is unknown.

1.3.1.2. Hair Follicle Melanocytes

Melanocytes can be found in the sebaceous gland or in the proximal bulb of each hair follicle, which are both close to the hair. The apex of the dermal papilla is home to the bulbar melanocyte bodies. Between the cortical and medullar keratinocytes, melanocyte dendrites penetrate. Melanocytes to keratinocytes are distributed in a 1:5 ratio, making them denser than the epidermis. The structural and functional interactions of dermal papilla fibroblasts, matrix keratinocytes, and follicular melanocytes result in follicular pigmentation. The term "hair melanin unit" or "follicular melanin unit" refers to this tripartite system. The creation of pigmented hair shafts, the transfer of melanin granules into keratinocytes, and the melanogenic activity of follicular melanocytes are all components of the pigmentation process of hair. The epidermal phagocytosis of melanosomes mediated by receptor PAR2 on keratinocytes is thought to be analogous to the transport of melanin granules to keratinocytes in the growing hair shaft. However, variations relate to melanosome quality and degradation. Compared to epidermal melanocytes, hair melanocytes primarily consist of larger mature Stage IV melanosomes (more on melanogenesis and melanosome stages later in this work), as well as an enlarged Golgi apparatus and rough endoplasmatic reticulum (RER). Compared to epidermal pigment cells, these are bigger and more dendritic. Furthermore, the differentiating keratinocytes in the epidermis degrade nearly all transported melanin, whereas the pigment granules in the hair cortex are only slightly broken down by these keratinocytes. The amount and ratio of yellow-red pheomelanin and brown-black eumelanin are the primary causes of variation in hair color.

The products secreted by nearby cells such as keratinocytes, fibroblasts, and endothelial cells regulate the synthesis of melanin in the hair. These mechanisms can be autocrine or paracrine, and they can be influenced by hormonal signals. Melanocortin receptor 1 (MCR1) and its α-MSH, adrenocorticotropic hormone (ACTH), receptor c-Kit and its ligand SCF, endothelins, various neurotransmitters, cytokines, growth factor, and other regulators similar to those controlling epidermal melanogenesis control pigmentation, which determines hair color. The epidermis follows the same biochemical pathway for the formation of pigment and melanosomes; however, it should be noted that hair follicle melanocytes are more susceptible to the effects of aging than epidermal melanocytes, which leads to the graying of hair. It appears that the dermal papilla-derived fibroblast factors insulin growth factor (IGF-1), keratinocyte growth factor (KGF), noggin, and stem cell factor (SCF) play a unique role in regulating the proliferation and activity of melanocytes and keratinocytes in the hair matrix during hair growth.

While hair melanocytes expire at the end of the hair cycle, which lasts three to eight years, epidermal melanocytes are long-living cells. Only in the anagen stage (growing phase) of the hair growth cycle does the melanogenesis process occur; in the catagen stage (regressing phase) and the telogen stage (resting phase), pigment formation is stopped. Furthermore, it is noted that melanoblasts living in the hair bulge produce new melanocytes during catagen, while fully differentiated bulbar melanocytes perish through apoptosis. In summary, melanocyte survival, proliferation, and differentiation are controlled by the hair follicle microenvironment.

1.3.1.3. Melanocyte Biology

1.3.1.3.1. Melanogenesis

The biochemical process called melanogenesis is in charge of the synthesis of melanin. It occurs in distinct cytoplasmic organelles called melanosomes found in melanocytes. Pheomelanin and eumelanin are the two main forms of melanin that are produced. Their synthesis methods and colors are different. Melanin's many health-promoting qualities include its ability to absorb and scatter UV light, scavenge free radicals, facilitate coupled oxidation-reduction reactions, and store ions. The types of melanins produced depend on the availability of substrates and the activity of the enzymes involved in melanogenesis. Tyrosine is hydroxylated by tyrosinase (TYR) to

L-3,4-dihydroxyphenylalanine (DOPA), which is then quickly oxidized to produce DOPAquinone. When cysteine is present, DOPAquinone reacts with it to produce 3- or 5-cysteinylDOPAs, which oxidize and polymerize to produce pheomelanin, a yellow-red soluble melanin. Brown-black eumelanin is produced when any of the thiols—cysteine, glutathione, or thioredoxin—are absent. DOPAquinone cyclizes spontaneously to produce DOPAchrome. After the DOPAchrome spontaneously loses its carboxylic acid, 5,6-dihydroxyindole (DHI) is produced. DHI-melanin is an insoluble dark brown to black substance that quickly oxidizes and polymerizes. On the other hand, DOPAchrome will produce DHI-2-carboxylic acid (DHICA) in the presence of DOPAchrome tautomerase (TYRP2/DCT). TYRP1 and tyrosinase catalyze additional conversions that result in DHICA-melanin, which is ultimately lighter brown in color.

All forms of melanin are present in human skin, and the ratio of those types influences visible pigmentation. The preservation of skin pigmentation diversity among various ethnic groups is contingent upon the content of eumelanin. The proportion of eumelanin to total melanin determines the color of the skin. Pheomelanin is found in both light and dark skin types in comparable amounts, suggesting that it is not correlated with skin pigmentation. The ratio of eumelanin to pheomelanin determines the color of hair. When it comes to photoprotective qualities, eumelanin outperforms pheomelanin due to its increased resistance to degradation and capacity to neutralize reactive oxygen species (ROS). When it comes to photoprotection, eumelanins are thought to be more effective than reddish pheomelanins. Because of this, lighter skin has a 30–40 times higher risk of developing skin cancer than darker skin. Melanogenesis-related gene products have effects on subcellular, cellular, tissue, and environmental levels. Quinones and hydrogen peroxide, two cytotoxic molecules, are produced as intermediate products during melanogenesis. As a result, melanocytes defend themselves by increasing the amount of the antiapoptotic protein Bcl-2 and dividing the melanogenesis-related regions of melanosomes.

1.3.1.3.2. Melanocytes' Ability of Proliferation and Age-Related Changes

Although keratinocytes may interact with melanocytes via growth factors, cell surface molecules, or other factors related to epidermis proliferation and differentiation, the exact mechanisms governing the organization and quantity of melanocytes in the epidermis remain unknown. Melanocytes are highly differentiated cells found inside melanosomes that produce the pigment melanin. This cell is shaped like a dendritic and dark. The primary function of a melanocyte is to produce melanin. This cell's capacity for proliferation is lost during the differentiation process. It is believed that epidermal melanocytes are a very stable population that rarely proliferates in normal conditions.

While hair melanocytes live for the duration of the hair cycle (median3–5 years), epidermal melanocytes are long-living cells. The environment, particularly UV radiation, and substances released by fibroblasts and keratinocytes affect the density of melanocytes in the skin. 10 to 20% of epidermal melanocytes are lost every 10 years after the age of 30. In addition to having fewer melanocytes overall, older individuals also have larger, more dendritic melanocytes and lower tyrosinase activity. It has been noted that there are connections between aging and melanocyte proliferation. Adult melanocytes proliferate less frequently *in vitro* than melanocytes from fetuses and newborns. Additionally, the proliferative potential of melanocytes in patients with premature aging disorders is diminished.

1.3.1.4. Embryonic Origin of Skin Melanocytes

1.3.1.4.1. More Than One Population of Neural Crest Cells is the Source of Skin Melanocytes

A class of cells known as neural crest cells originates from the ectoderm, the layer of embryonic germ. The center region of the embryonic disc differentiates into neuroectoderm under the inductive influence of the notochord, which manifests as a neural plate in a 4-week-old human embryo. The neural tube and the eventual brain and spinal cord are formed when this plate folds and transforms into the neural tube. A group of cells from the neural plate's margins (known as crests) split off during this process, which is known as neurulation, change from being epithelial to mesenchyme, and migrate out of the neuroepithelium. Neural crest cells, or NCCs, are these neuroectodermal cells that are migrating to various parts of the developing embryo's body. The developmental potential of neural crest cells gradually narrows to become lineage-restricted from their initial multipotent state. Anatomical localization along the cranial-caudal axis determines this potential. For example, cranial NCCs can differentiate into neurons, glial cells, chondrocytes, osteocytes, and muscle cells, while trunk NCCs form endocrine cells and neurons and glial cells in the peripheral nervous system. As these cells multiply, they begin to express different molecular markers.

1.3.1.4.2. Basic Molecular Elements of Embryonic/Fetal Melanocyte Development

Experiments have not been able to determine when NCC begins to exhibit characteristics of melanoblasts, which are precursors to melanocytes. There is disagreement regarding a set of molecular markers for this early stage of melanocyte development in human development. Melanoblasts share characteristics with melanocytes but do not produce melanin. Tyrosine kinase receptor KIT (c-kit); transcription factors like MITF, SOX10, Pax 3, and melanogenic enzyme tyrosinase-related protein (TYRP-2) are the most frequently mentioned molecular markers for the precursors of melanocytes. The precise mechanisms behind melanoblast migration remain unclear, despite the involvement of adhesion molecules like cadherins, integrins, and extracellular matrix components. Melanoblast migration along ephrin and endothelin-3-containing extracellular matrix is made possible by the ephrin receptor (EphR) and the endothelin receptor (EDNRB2).

Endothelins, SCF stem cell factor, Wnt proteins, and neuregulin-1 are key growth factors that regulate melanocyte development from neural crest cells. These regulatory mechanisms have been extensively described in other research studies.

The stem cell factor (SCF), which is secreted by dermal cells, is bound by the c-Kit receptor. This binding activates the pathway, preventing apoptosis and promoting melanoblast proliferation. Melanoblast/melanocyte development requires the Wnt/Frizzled protein/β-catenin-signaling pathway, the Notch pathway, and the MAPK-signaling pathway. The induction of melanocyte fate appears to require components of the Wnt/β-catenin signaling pathway, according to studies conducted in multiple model organisms. Particular significance is given to the Notch signaling pathway during the embryonic stage. Because the ligand for the Notch receptor is a plasma membrane protein (such as Delta), the receptor needs to come into contact with another cell. Because of the involvement of BRAF in the development of melanoma, the MAPK-signaling pathway Ras/Raf/Mek/Erk has drawn particular attention.

The MITF protein, which is a master regulator of melanocyte proliferation, differentiation, and survival, is expressed in response to several of the previously mentioned factors. To stop migrating cells from undergoing apoptosis and to promote the production of melanin, the MITF activates the genes involved in skin migration.

1.3.1.5. Stem Cells for Human Melanocytes in Adults

Melanocytes usually do not proliferate often, but some instances suggest the presence of melanocyte precursors in the skin, such as the repigmentation of vitiligo patients' skin after phototherapy.

The bulge region of the hair follicles, whether in a mouse or a human, was the first known source of melanocyte stem cells. The bulge area, which points to the bottom of the permanent portion of hair follicles, is a portion of the outer root sheath that serves as the arrector pili muscle's insertion point. Melanocyte stem cells are activated and hair follicles regenerate with each hair loss. Pluripotent, morphologically undifferentiated cells found in the bulge region give rise to melanoblasts and keratinocyte progenitors, which are responsible for both the epidermis and hair. These cells migrate into the basal layer of the epidermis following stimulation, where they differentiate into mature melanocytes.

Nonetheless, there is mounting proof that melanocytes are also stored in the dermis. Little progress has been made in identifying the melanocyte-producing stem cells in human skin, and the majority of advancements in melanocyte development have been made in murine models. The answer to the question "Where are melanoblasts located in the dermis?" is insufficient. Melanocytes resulting from the migration of a multipotent precursor cell along nerve projections have been traced thanks to recent developmental studies that use model organisms and lineage tracing. It is highly likely that the cutaneous nerves contain stem cell-like cells, but even if they do, they remain in this stem cell state until the signal from the end of the cutaneous nerve encourages them to differentiate into melanocytes. However, some melanoblasts from the dorsal route of NCC migration have also been observed to remain in the dermis until the second trimester of pregnancy, following the conclusion of the epidermis inoculation. It is still unclear if they can endure in the adult human dermis.

The absence of a set of melanoblast markers makes it difficult to identify melanoblasts in adult skin. The melanocyte populations in the dermis and epidermis appear to be biologically distinct from one another (Aoki et al., 2009).

1.3.2. Merkel Cells

Merkel cells are slow-adapting, oval-shaped type I mechanoreceptors that are connected to basal keratinocytes through desmosomal junctions and found in areas with high tactile sensitivity. Merkel cells can be found in the outer root sheath of hair follicles, lips, digits, and oral cavity regions. They can also occasionally be assembled into specialized structures called tactile discs or touch domes. Merkel cells release a chemical signal that causes an action potential in the nearby afferent neuron, which then transmits the signal to the brain, in response to relatively minor deformations of neighboring keratinocytes. Higher tactile resolution and sensitivity are the result of smaller, more densely packed receptive fields, which are caused by the high concentration of Merkel cells in specific areas, such as the fingertips (Figure 1.4).

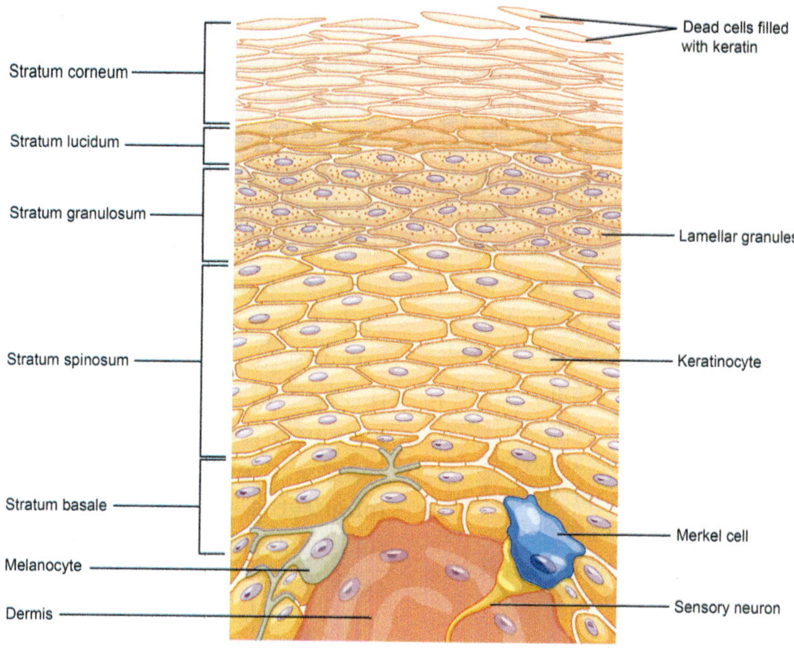

Figure 1.4. *Merkel cells.*

Source: By OpenStax College: J. Gordon Betts, Peter Desaix, Eddie Johnson. – Anatomy & Physiology, Connexions Web site. http://cnx.org/content/col11496/1.6/, Jun 19, 2013., CC BY 3.0, https://commons.wikimedia.org/w/index.php?curid=30131304.

1.3.2.1. Structure

All vertebrates have Merkel cells in their skin and in certain areas of their mucosa. These are transparent cells with a diameter of about 10 μm that are located in the stratum basale of the epidermis, at the base of sweat duct ridges in mammalian skin. These oval-shaped mechanoreceptors are present in vertebrate skin and are crucial for the perception of light touch. They form synaptic connections with somatosensory afferent nerve fibers and are widely distributed in extremely sensitive skin, such as the skin on human fingertips. Additionally, they can be found in rete ridges, which are epidermal invaginations of the plantar foot surface.

When referred to as Merkel nerve endings, they are most frequently connected to sensory nerve endings (also called a Merkel cell-neurite complex). They are connected to somatosensory nerve fibers that slowly adapt (SA1). They respond to deep static touches, such as edges and shapes, and low vibrations (5–15 Hz). They are highly concentrated in places like the fingertips because they have a small receptive field (very detailed information); because they are not covered (shelled), they can withstand pressure for extended periods of time.

1.3.2.2. Developmental

For more than 20 years, experts have been debating the origin of Merkel cells. Although studies on skin grafts in birds suggest that they originate from the neural crest, more recent research in mammals has shown that they have an epidermal origin.

1.3.2.3. Function

Merkel cells are sometimes known as touch cells, or Tastzellen, after the German anatomist Friedrich Sigmund Merkel. Because of the close physical relationship between Merkel cells and sensory nerve endings, this proposed function was debatable and difficult to verify until recently. On the other hand, recent research using mice and other model organisms shows that touch is intrinsically converted by Merkel cells into electrical signals that are sent to the nervous system. PIEZO2, a mechanosensitive ion channel that reacts to mechanical forces, is expressed by Merkel cells. Mice that have had Piezo2 specifically knocked out in skin cells—as opposed to sensory neurons—show reduced behavioral reactions to light touch.

Due to the presence of dense core granules, which suggests that they may also have a neuroendocrine function, Merkel cells are occasionally referred to as APUD cells (an older definition, more commonly classified as a part of a dispersed neuroendocrine system).

1.3.3. Langerhans Cell

A Langerhans cell (LC) was previously believed to be a resident dendritic cell in the skin but is now recognized as a tissue-resident macrophage. These cells contain organelles known as Birbeck granules and can be found in all layers of the epidermis, with a higher concentration in the stratum spinosum. Langerhans cells are also present in the papillary dermis, particularly near blood vessels, as well as in the mucosa of the mouth, foreskin, and vaginal epithelium. They may also be found in other tissues, such as lymph nodes, especially in cases of Langerhans cell histiocytosis (LCH).

1.3.3.1. Function

The local Langerhans cells in skin infections absorb and process microbial antigens to develop into fully functional antigen-presenting cells. Tissue-resident macrophages are generally engaged in the uptake of apoptotic bodies and immune homeostasis. But Langerhans cells can also adopt the phenotype of a dendritic cell and move into lymph nodes to engage in interactions with T-cells that are still naive. In the first trimester of pregnancy, primitive erythro-myeloid progenitors arise in the yolk sac outside the embryo. Under normal circumstances, Langerhans cells persist throughout life, replenishing themselves through local proliferation as needed. When an infection causes severe inflammation of the skin, blood monocytes are drawn to the affected area and undergo differentiation into replacement limbal cells.

Langerin is a protein found in Langerhans cells and dendritic cells. LCs are rich in cannabinoid receptor type 2 (CB2), which, when activated by agonists, reduces ear swelling and eosinophil recruitment in chronic contact dermatitis brought on by repeated challenges.

1.4. The Dermal-Epidermal Junction

A porous basement membrane zone forms the interface between the epidermis and dermis, allowing fluid and cell exchange while maintaining the integrity of the two layers. The most significant constituents of the dermal-epidermal junction structures are basal keratinocytes; dermal fibroblasts are also involved, albeit to a lesser degree.

The basal lamina, produced by basal cells of the epidermis, is primarily composed of type IV collagen, dermal microfibrils, and anchoring fibrils, forming the lamina densa and the electron-lucent lamina lucida. Hemidesmosomes, resembling rivets, attach basal cell plasma membranes to the basal lamina, transmitting tensile or shearing forces across the epithelium. The dermal-epidermal junction provides developmental signals, maintains epidermal integrity, determines cell polarity and growth direction, organizes the basal cell cytoskeleton, and functions as a semipermeable barrier between skin layers.

1.4.1. Role of the Dermal-Epidermal Junction

The dermal-epidermal junction has several functions:

- To bind tightly the epidermis to the dermis
- To determine the polarity of the basal keratinocytes, the spatial keratinocyte organization and the epidermal architecture; the epidermal stratification proceeds with the proliferating keratinocytes remaining attached to the basement membrane and the daughter cells migrating into the upper layers
- To serve as a selective barrier allowing the control of molecular and cellular exchanges between the two compartments
- It also has a fundamental role during the wound reepidermisation, by serving through its constitutive glycoproteins (mainly laminins) as a substrate for the adhesion and migration of keratinocytes.

1.4.2. Structure of the Dermal-Epidermal Junction

The dermal-epidermal junction may be divided into four morphological regions:

- The bottom portion of the basal epidermal cell membrane within the keratinocyte contains specialized junctional structures called hemidesmosomes. However, melanocytes, and Merkel cells do not possess hemidesmosomes. Melanocytes have focal adhesion systems, while Merkel cells have densifications of their plasma membrane in contact with the associated nerve end.
- Laminin 332 (= laminin-5) and 311 (= laminin-6) rich anchoring filaments traverse the 20–40 nm thick lamina lucida. These filaments interact with the extracellular domain of α6 β4 integrin at the keratinocyte cell surface to form an adhesion structure with the hemidesmodomes. Anchoring filaments are less common and have a different makeup between the hemidesmosomes; the integrin a3b1 is linked to the complex laminin 332-laminin 311 or 321.
- The lamina densa is made up primarily of type IV collagen and varies in thickness from 30 to 60 nm with age. It also contains nidogen, heparan sulfate proteoglycans, with perlecan being one of the major ones, and laminins 511 (previously laminin-10) and 322 (previously laminin 7). It serves as the intermediary anchorage zone for the anchoring fibrils that emerge from the dermal fibrillar zone and the anchoring filaments that come from the epidermis. The lamina densa merges with the surrounding lamina at the level of Merkel cells. Whereas the lamina lucida is similar in thickness in both sexes, the lamina densa is thicker in men than in women. Beneath the melanocytes, the lamina densa and lamina lucida are thinner.
- The anchoring fibrils, which are 20 to 60 nm thick, enlarge at their extremities and have bands with an irregular periodicity, either dense and thick or clear and thin, on their median part, are included in the fibrillar

zone. Type VII collagen makes up the anchoring fibrils. They either form intermingled loops that connect two distinct areas of the lamina densa or they establish the connection between the lamina densa and the papillary dermis anchoring plaques.

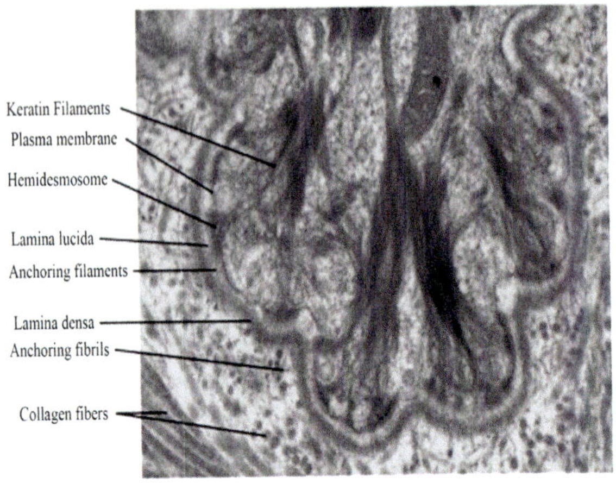

Figure 1.5. *Ultrastructural view of the dermal-epidermal junction in human skin.*

Source: https://biologiedelapeau.fr/spip.php?article18.

According to recent research, the arrangement of the dermal-epidermal junction may indicate contacts between its constituents that are closer than previously believed. As a result, there may be a direct interaction between the laminin-332 of the anchoring filaments and the type VII of anchoring fibrils.

1.4.3. Hemidesmosomes

The hemidesmosomes act as bridges between the keratin cytoskeleton and the basement membrane. They are composed of 3 dense plaques:

- An internal plaque with plectin and the bullous pemphigoid antigen, known as BP230, with a molecular weight of 230 KDa, is connected to the keratin intermediate filaments. The cytoplasmic domain of BP180 and the β4 integrin subunit are associated with the amino-terminal ends of plectin and BP 230, while their carboxy-terminal ends interact with keratin intermediate filaments (K5 and K14).
- An external plaque near the plasma membrane that includes the two hemidesmosomal transmembrane proteins, the cytoplasmic portions of BP180 and the β4 integrin subunit, as well as two less well-characterized proteins, P200 and IFAP 300.
- A sub-basal plaque in the lamina lucida, corresponding to the junction of the β4 integrin subunit with laminin-332 and the external parts of BP180. Starting from the sub-basal plaque, the anchoring filaments made of laminin 332 and the external portion of BP 180 cross the lamina lucida and engage with the anchoring fibrils located within the lamina densa.
- The keratin intermediate filaments (K5 and K14), the dense plaque (BPAG1 and plectin), the external plaque (integrins α6 β4, BP 180) and the sub-basal plaque (integrins α6 β4, BP 180, and laminin-332) of the hemidesmosome, the anchoring filaments (integrins α6 β4, BP 180, and laminin-332), the lamina densa (type IV collagen, nidogen, perlecan, laminin 511 and 322), the anchoring fibrils (type VII collagen), and the collagen fibers (type I and III collagens) of the papillary dermis are responsible for the adhesion of the epidermis to the dermis.

1.5. Epidermal Appendages

The skin adnexa is a collection of ectodermally derived appendages that start as downgrowths from the epidermis during development. These include ducts, pilosebaceous units, and eccrine and apocrine glands. All adnexal structures can reepithelialize following damage through the migration of keratinocytes from the adnexal epithelium to the epidermal surface. Reepithelialization happens more quickly following injury in areas with a higher concentration of pilosebaceous units, like the face and scalp, than in areas with a lower concentration of adnexal structures, like the back.

1.5.1. Eccrine Sweat Glands

The back has the least amount of eccrine sweat glands compared to the soles of the feet, which are involved in heat regulation. The epidermal ridge is the source of the sweat glands, which begin as a band of epithelial cells growing downward. The intraepidermal spiral duct, the straight dermal portion, and the coiled secretory duct are the three composite parts of the eccrine sweat unit that are created during development from this tubular, or ductal, structure. Dermal duct cells that have moved upward make up the spiral duct, which opens onto the skin's surface. Within the duct, cells go through a process called cornification, and the resulting corneocytes eventually join the cornified layer. The inner secretory section of the gland is connected to the superficial spiral duct by the straight dermal segment.

The glycogen-rich clear secretory cells, the dark mucoidal cells, and the myoepithelial cells with contractile specialized properties make up the secretory coil of the eccrine unit, which is located deep within the dermis or within the superficial panniculus. Clear cells create intercellular canaliculi where two clear cells next to each other and rest either on the basement membrane or on the myoepithelial cells. The canaliculi open straight into the gland's lumen. Sweating is triggered by heat and is initiated by large, glycogen-rich inner epithelial cells. The darker mucoidal cells in the dermal duct and secretory coil actively reabsorb sodium from sweat in the duct, starting with an isotonic solution and ending with an extremely hypotonic solution that is emitted onto the skin surface through the intraepidermal spiral duct. This reaction preserves sodium while encouraging cooling.

The sympathetic nervous system is the only one that innervates eccrine glands. Depending on the target structure, postganglionic sympathetic fibers innervating the cutaneous district can release either acetylcholine or noradrenaline as neurotransmitters. The primary source of discharge for the sympathetic cholinergic fibers that connect to the sweat glands is variations in the body's core temperature or deep tissue temperature. The glands on the palms and soles release a substance when under emotional stress in addition to reacting to temperature cues.

1.5.1.1. Secretion

The electrolyte solution secreted by eccrine glands is sterile and diluted, containing sodium chloride (NaCl), potassium, bicarbonate, and other minor components like glucose, pyruvate, lactate, immunoglobulins, cytokines, and antimicrobial peptides like dermcidin, among many others.

Sweat has substantially less Na+ ion concentration than plasma and extracellular fluid (~40 mM in sweat versus ~140 mM in plasma and extracellular fluid). Sweat initially contains a high concentration of Na^+ ions within the eccrine glands. The epithelial sodium channels (ENaCs), which are found on the apical membrane of the cells that make up the eccrine gland ducts, allow the Na+ ions to be reabsorbed into the tissue. This Na^+ ion reabsorption lessens the amount of Na+ lost through perspiration. Due to their inability to reabsorb salt from their perspiration, people with mutations in the ENaC subunit genes who have systemic pseudohypoaldosteronism syndrome have salty sweat. These Na^+ ion concentrations can occasionally rise significantly to 180 mmol/L.

The sweat glands, especially the exocrine glands, overreact to stimuli and are generally overactive in persons with hyperhidrosis, causing them to secrete more sweat than usual. Similarly, salty sweat is also produced by those who have cystic fibrosis. However, in these instances, the issue lies with the CFTR chloride transporter, which is likewise found on the apical membrane of the eccrine gland ducts.

1.5.2. Apocrine Sweat Glands

An apocrine sweat gland consists of a straight portion that inserts and secretes into the infundibular portion of the hair follicle and a coiled secretory portion that is situated at the intersection of the dermis and subcutaneous fat. Only a few areas of the human body—the axillae (armpits), the areola and nipples of the breast, the ear canal, the eyelids, the nostril wings, the perineal region, and certain sections of the external genitalia—have apocrine sweat glands. The ciliary glands (glands of Moll) in the eyelids, the ceruminous glands (which produce ear wax), and the mammary glands (which produce milk) are examples of modified apocrine glands. They are not to be confused with the body's eccrine sweat glands.

1.5.2.1. Structure

The excretory duct, which sometimes opens to the skin surface next to the hair, and a glomerulus of secretory tubules comprise the apocrine gland. The excretory duct also opens into a hair follicle. Large and spongy, the gland is situated deep within the dermis in the subcutaneous fat. Its lumen diameter is greater than that of the eccrine sweat gland. Apocrine gland secretory tubules are single-layered structures, but unlike eccrine secretory tubules, they only contain one kind of ductal epithelial cell, which can branch off into multiple ducts and vary in diameter depending on where it is located. Myoepithelial cells, which are more developed than those found in eccrine glands, encircle the tubules.

1.5.2.2. Sweating

Apocrine glands are found throughout the body in a five-month-old human fetus; however, within a few weeks, they are confined to specific regions, such as the armpits and external genitalia. They remain dormant until puberty-related hormonal fluctuations activate them.

1.5.2.3. Mechanism

Before microbial activity, the apocrine gland secretes an oily, odorless fluid containing proteins and lipids. In the same hair follicle where sebaceous glands open, it is visible on the skin's surface combined with sebum. The apocrine sweat glands secrete in irregular spurts, in contrast to the continuous secretion of eccrine sweat glands.

It was previously believed that apocrine sweat glands exclusively secreted apocrine substances, which are released when vesicles break off from the secretory cells and decompose in the secretory lumen. It has also been demonstrated by more recent studies that merocrine secretion occurs.

Around the secretory cells, myoepithelial cells form a smooth muscle lining. When the muscles contract, the secretory ducts are squeezed, forcing the accumulated fluid out of the hair follicle. At the hair follicle, sweat, and sebum combine to form the epidermal surface. The apocrine sweat has a pH of 6–7, is hazy, viscous, and is initially odorless. It is composed of NaCl, water, protein, and waste material from carbohydrates. Only after being broken down by bacteria, which releases volatile odor molecules, does sweat take on its distinctive smell. A stronger smell is caused by more bacteria, particularly corynebacteria. Because axillary hairs collect secretions, debris, keratin, and bacteria, they also contribute to the stench being stronger.

1.5.3. Apoeccrine Sweat Glands

During puberty, eccrine-like precursors give rise to the apocrine sweat gland (AEG), which opens directly to the skin. The adult axillae contain the AEG, which was found during the isolation of human axillary sweat from patients suffering from axillary hyperhidrosis, a condition marked by abnormally high rates of perspiration. The relative frequency of the AEG varies from person to person. The AEG opens directly to the skin's surface, just like eccrine glands do. Because the AEG secretes at a rate up to 10 times higher than the eccrine gland's, it is believed that the AEG plays a role in axillary hyperhidrosis.

1.5.4. Hair Follicles

In addition to providing protection from the weather and distributing sweat-gland products, hair serves many important biological purposes. Moreover, it plays a significant psychosocial role in society. Hair follicles all share the same basic structure, although they differ greatly in size and shape based on where they are located. No more hair follicles are added after birth; the quantity and distribution of hair follicles throughout the body, as well as the eventual phenotype of each hair, are determined during fetal development. Genes that are expressed very early in the follicle morphogenesis determine the specific spacing and allocation of the follicles. During embryogenesis, mesenchymal cells in the fetal dermis group together beneath the basal layer of the epidermis. These mesenchymal cell sites are covered by basophilic cells in the basal cell layer of the epidermis, which are stimulated to grow downward and into the dermis. The follicle keeps growing until it eventually broadens at the base and encircles the collection of mesenchymal cells that gives rise to the dermal papilla in the form of a bulb.

The hair cone is formed by differentiation at the base of the hair follicle, which also forms the hair, cuticle, and two inner root sheaths later on. Prior to the growing hair cone reaching the upper follicle, differentiation also takes place in the upper segments of the follicle that produce the hair canal in the upper dermis, through the epidermis, and opening to the surface (Figure 1.6).

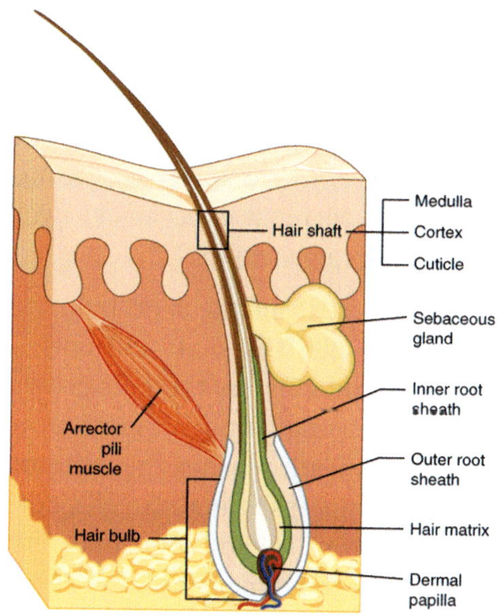

Figure 1.6. *Hair follicle.*

Source: Open Resources for Nursing (Open RN); Ernstmeyer K, Christman E, editors. Nursing Skills [Internet]. 2nd edition. Eau Claire (WI): Chippewa Valley Technical College; 2023. Chapter 14 Integumentary Assessment. Available from: https://www.ncbi.nlm.nih.gov/books/NBK596743/.

The fetal hair follicle produces a bud that develops into the sebaceous gland. Another bud forms into the attachment point for the arrector pili muscle below the sebaceous gland, on the same side of the follicle. A bundle of smooth muscles called the arrector pili (AP) is attached to the follicle's external root sheath. At the level of the papillary dermis, the distal end of the AP muscle exhibits several branches. The zone of follicular attachment of the AP muscle is known as the bulge, and it is believed to contain epithelial stem cells that play a vital role in the hair growth cycle by regenerating follicles. A third bud that forms above the sebaceous gland plane on the opposing side of the follicle gives rise to the apocrine gland. The isthmus is the area of the follicle between the AP attachment and the sebaceous duct, and the infundibular segment is the portion of the follicle above the sebaceous gland. The inferior portion, which lies beneath the isthmus, houses the hair bulb and the base of the follicle. While the infundibular and isthmus portions remain fixed throughout life, the inferior segment experiences cycles of involution and regeneration.

The matrix cells in the hair bulb rapidly divide to create the hair shaft and both inner and outer root sheaths. As the hair grows, the inner root sheath and hair shaft move upwards until the inner sheath reaches the isthmus and is shed. The compressed matrix cells entering the rigid inner root sheath determine the size of the hair, while the dimensions and curvature of the inner root sheath dictate the shape of the hair. For example, Caucasians have round scalp hairs, while pubic, facial, and eyelash hairs are oval. People of African descent have oval scalp hairs, resulting in curly hair.

Melanosome distribution within the hair shaft determines hair color. Melanocytes in the hair bulb produce melanosomes, which are then transferred to the keratinocytes in the bulb matrix. Melanosomes in African Americans are typically larger than those in Caucasians, whose melanosomes are smaller and aggregate into membrane-bound complexes. Melanosomes in red hair are spherical in shape. Graying hair is a result of melanocyte loss brought on by aging, which also reduces melanosome synthesis. The growth of hair happens in cycles, but every follicle is a separate entity. The three stages of the hair growth cell cycle are anagen, catagen, and telogen. On the scalp, anagen, or the active growth stage, normally lasts three to five years. During this time, hairs grow at a rate of 0 to 33 mm per day. The anagen phase's duration shortens with age and sharply shortens in alopecia patients.

Catagen, which results in the formation of club hair after numerous cells in the outer root sheath undergo apoptosis, typically lasts for two weeks. Hairs in the telogen phase, which is a resting phase on the scalp, eventually push out of the growing anagen hair shaft and last for three to five months. Most body hair is shorter and stays in one place longer at other parts of the body where telogen and anagen phases are longer, respectively.

The secreted molecules fibroblast growth factor and insulin-like growth factor 1 may play significant roles in the development and cycling of hair follicles. Both are made by the dermal papilla in mice and primarily have receptors in the matrix cells that cover them. Growth hormone, prolactin, retinoids, glucocorticoids, thyroid hormones, and estrogens are some of the hormonal factors that affect hair growth. The androgens, which function through androgen receptors in the dermal papilla, are the hormones that have the most remarkable effect. These include testosterone and its active metabolite, dihydrotestosterone. During adolescence, these hormones cause hair follicles in androgen-dependent areas, like the beard area, to enlarge. But later in life, they may cause the scalp's follicles to shrink, which can lead to androgen alopecia or male pattern baldness.

Hair loss and unwanted hair growth are regarded as reversible events because they reflect deviations in hair follicle cycling, except rare congenital hair defects brought on by mutations in keratins or other structural proteins and scarring alopecias. Numerous distinct physiologic factors can influence the hair cycle. For instance, a pregnancy frequently causes the telogen phase to last longer and the anagen phase to produce more scalp hairs. Telogen hairs are lost and anagen hairs are concurrently converted to telogen when estrogen levels stabilize after delivery; this significant loss of telogen hairs occurs in three to five months. Telogen effluvium, the synchronous termination of anagen or telogen, is frequently seen following trauma, including childbirth, surgery, weight loss, and extreme stress. It is also linked to medication use, endocrine disorders, anemia, and malnourishment. Unless there is a metabolic or nutritional deficit, regrowth usually ensues.

1.5.5. Sebaceous Gland

Mammals' hair and skin are lubricated by sebum, an oily or waxy substance secreted by microscopic exocrine glands in the skin called sebaceous glands or oil glands. Sebaceous glands are most abundant on the face and scalp in humans, but they are also present on every other area of the skin except for the palms and soles of the feet. Meibomian glands, also known as tarsal glands, are a type of sebaceous gland found in the eyelids that secrete a particular kind of sebum into tears. Areolar glands are specialized sebaceous glands that surround and lubricate the female nipple. Fordyce spots are benign sebaceous glands that are visible and typically located on the lips, gums, inner cheeks, and genitalia.

1.5.5.1. Structure

1.5.5.1.1. Location

All parts of the skin, except the palms and soles of the feet, are covered in sebaceous glands. Sebaceous glands come in two varieties: those that are attached to hair follicles and those that stand alone.

Sebaceous glands are attached to hair follicles and found in areas covered in hair. Each hair follicle may have one or more glands surrounding it. The arrector pili muscles encircle the glands, creating a unit known as the pilosebaceous system. The glands have an acinar structure, which resembles a berry with many lobes, where a central duct branches off of several glands. Sebum is secreted by the glands onto the hair shafts, where it is then carried to the skin's surface. The structure is an epidermal invagination known as a pilosebaceous unit, and it consists of hair follicles, arrector pili muscles, and sebaceous gland.

Sebaceous glands can be found in hairless areas such as the eyelids, nose, penis, labia minora, inner mucosal membrane of the cheek, and nipples. Some of these glands have specific names, such as Fordyce spots on the lip and mucosa of the cheek, Meibomian glands on the eyelids, and Montgomery's glands on the breasts.

1.5.5.1.2. Development

During the thirteenth to sixteenth week of fetal development, sebaceous glands first protrude as bulgings off hair follicles. The same tissue that gives rise to the skin's epidermis is where sebaceous glands develop. The presence of sebaceous glands is more likely when the signaling factors Wnt, Myc, and SHH are overexpressed. A substance known as vernix caseosa, a waxy, translucent white substance covering newborns' skin, is secreted by the sebaceous glands of human fetuses. Following birth, the glands' activity diminishes until it nearly stops between the ages of two and six, at which point it rises to a peak during puberty as a result of elevated androgen levels.

1.5.5.2. Function

Sebaceous glands are made up of enormous cells with numerous large vesicles that contain sebum, in contrast to the keratinocytes that make up the hair follicle. ENaC, CFTR, and the ion channels Na^+ and Cl^- are expressed by these cells.

Sebum, an oily, waxy material secreted by sebaceous glands, is composed of triglycerides, wax esters, squalene, and metabolites of fat-producing cells. In mammals, the hair and skin are lubricated by sebum. Together with apocrine glands, sebaceous secretions have a significant role in thermoregulation. When it's hot outside, the secretions emulsify the sweat that the eccrine sweat glands produce, creating a layer of sweat that doesn't evaporate quickly into droplets. This is crucial for postponing the loss of fluids. Sebum's lipidic nature becomes more pronounced in colder weather, effectively repelling rain from the skin and hair.

The production of sebum occurs through a holocrine process in which the sebaceous gland's cells burst and fragment while releasing sebum, and the remaining cells are secreted with the sebum. At the base of the duct, mitosis continuously replaces the cells.

1.5.5.2.1. Sebum

In humans, the sebaceous gland secretes sebum. Triglycerides make up approximately 41% of it, followed by wax esters (26%), squalene (12%), and free fatty acids (16%). Different species' sebum compositions differ. Sebum is the only place in the body where wax esters and squalene are produced as finished products. Acne is thought to be caused by sapenic acid, a sebum fatty acid that is specific to humans. Although sebum has no smell, bacteria can produce strong odors when they break it down. The rate at which sebum secretion occurs is known to be influenced by sex hormones; it has been demonstrated that estrogens inhibit and androgens, like testosterone, stimulate secretion. In hair follicles and the prostate, dihydrotestosterone functions as the main androgen.

1.5.5.2.2. Immune Function and Nutrition

The integumentary system of the body includes sebaceous glands, which act as a barrier against microbes. Acids that make up the acid mantle are secreted by sebaceous glands. This is a thin layer of skin that is slightly acidic and serves as a barrier to any microorganisms that might try to penetrate the skin. The skin's pH ranges from 4 to 6, which is acidic and helps offset the alkaline properties of impurities. Sebaceous lipids provide the skin with vitamin E and aid in preserving the integrity of the skin barrier.

1.5.5.2.3. Unique Sebaceous Glands

The fetus's sebaceous glands create vernix caseosa, a waxy white substance that covers the skin to shield it from amniotic fluid, during the final three months of the fetus's development.

The areolar glands are in the areola that surrounds the nipple in the female breast. These glands secrete an oily fluid that lubricates the nipple and also secrete volatile compounds that are thought to serve as an olfactory stimulus for the newborn. During pregnancy and lactation these glands, also called Montgomery's glands, become enlarged.

Tear evaporation is slowed down by meibum, a type of sebum secreted onto the eye by meibomian glands in the eyelids. Their lipid content also keeps the eyelids from adhering to one another, helping to form an airtight seal when the eyes are closed. They affix straight to the eyelash follicles, which are situated inside the tarsal plates of the eyelids in a vertical arrangement. On the genitalia and oral mucosa, there are ectopic sebaceous glands known as Fordyce spots or granules. They manifest as milk spots, or yellowish-white milia.

A portion of the sebum secreted by ear canal glands is what makes up earwax. These secretions offer good lubrication because they are thick and contain a lot of lipids.

1.5.6. Nails

In addition to improving feeling and shielding the fingertips, fingernails also make it possible to grasp small objects. The nail matrix that underlies the nail bed is made up of melanocytes, blood vessels, and nerves. It also features parallel rete ridges. Keratinocytes in a matrix form the nail plate.

The average daily growth of fingernails is 0.1 mm, which is two-three times faster than the growth of toenails. Toenails can reveal information about a disease or toxic exposure that occurred many months ago due to their slow growth rate. For instance, Mees lines—horizontal hypopigmentation that runs the length of all nail plates—may result from arsenic poisoning (Daniel and Scher, 1997).

1.6. The Dermis

The dermis is an integrated system of fibrous, filamentous, and amorphous connective tissue that allows fibroblasts, mast cells, neurons, and vascular networks to enter the skin in response to stimuli. In response to different stimuli, other blood-borne cells such as lymphocytes, plasma cells, and other leukocytes also penetrate the dermis. The majority of the skin is made up of the dermis, which also gives the skin its elasticity, pliability, and tensile strength. It has receptors for sensory stimuli, binds water, helps regulate body temperature, and shields the body from mechanical harm. To preserve the characteristics of both tissues, the dermis and epidermis interact. The two regions work together during development to form the epidermal appendages and dermal-epidermal junction. They also work together to repair and remodel the skin after wounds heal. The structure and organization of the connective tissue components are predictable in a depth-dependent manner, but the dermis does not go through an obvious sequence of differentiation that parallels epidermal differentiation. Collagen and elastic connective tissue are two examples of matrix components that vary depth-dependently and undergo turnover and remodeling in pathologic processes, normal skin, and response to external stimuli.

All of the components of the dermis are mesodermal, except nerves, which come from the neural crest along with melanocytes. The dermis is nothing more than a collection of dendritic-shaped cells containing acid-mucopolysaccharides, which are the building blocks of fibroblasts, up until the sixth week of fetal life. Fibroblasts begin actively synthesizing collagen, elastic fibers, and reticulum fibers by the twelfth week. By the 24th week, a vascular network has formed and fat cells have emerged beneath the dermis. The adult dermis has thicker collagen bundles than the infant dermis, which is made up of smaller collagen bundles. The dermis of an infant contains a large number of fibroblasts, but few remain in the adult form.

Collagen is the primary component of the dermis and is a fibrous family of proteins found in human skin. There are at least 15 genetically distinct types of collagen in the skin, making it a major structural protein for the entire body. Collagen is also found in tendons, ligaments, bones, and the dermis, making it a key stress-resistant material for the skin. Elastic fibers, on the other hand, help maintain elasticity but do not resist deformation and tearing as effectively as collagen. Collagen fibers are constantly being degraded by proteolytic enzymes known as collagenases and replaced by new fibers. Collagen makes up 70% of the skin's dry weight.

The procollagen molecule, a particular helical polypeptide chain, is integrated by fibroblasts. The fibroblasts are then secreted by the cell and coalesce into collagen fibrils. Collagen is greatly enhanced by the amino acids hydroxyproline, hydroxylysine, and glycine. The majority of the group, and the most prevalent proteins in the body, are the fibrillar collagens found in the skin. Type I collagen is the main component of the dermis. The reticular dermis has dense collagen bundles, while the adventitial and papillary dermis contain loosely positioned collagen fibers. Collagen type VII, which is mostly produced by keratinocytes, is the main structural element of anchoring fibrils. Type IV collagen is found in the basement membrane zone.

Elastic fiber is made up of two parts: an amorphous protein called elastin and protein filaments. It is structurally and chemically distinct from collagen. Elastic fiber is fused to the glycosaminoglycan-rich extracellular matrix of the dermis by the fibroblast. In the reticular dermis, the fibers are coarse, and in the papillary dermis, they are fine. The main mucopolysaccharide that builds up in pathologic conditions is hyaluronic acid, which makes up a small portion of the dermis in a healthy state.

1.6.1. Vasculature

The two intercommunicating plexuses that make up the dermal vasculature are the lower plexus at the dermal-subcutaneous interface and the subpapillary or superficial plexus, which is made up of postcapillary venules located at the intersection of the papillary and reticular dermis. The superficial plexus's venules, end arterioles, and capillaries supply the dermal papillae. Larger blood vessels supply the deeper plexus, which has more intricate adnexal structures.

The preoptic-anterior hypothalamus regulates blood flow in the human skin, causing significant variations in response to heat stress. Sweating, vasodilation, and increased skin blood flow are all essential for dissipating heat when exercising in the heat. Vasoconstriction in the skin reduces heat loss from the body when exposed to cold, helping to avert hypothermia. The ability to regulate skin blood flow can be severely compromised when it comes to maintaining a normal body temperature. For instance, during times of high outside temperatures, patients with type II diabetes may be more susceptible to heat exhaustion and heat stroke due to deficiencies in cutaneous vascular control. In a similar vein, hot flashes are caused by menopausal hormones.

1.6.2. Muscles

The areolas surrounding the nipples, AP, and tunica dartos of the external genitalia are examples of the involuntary or smooth muscle of the skin. Smooth muscle differs from striated muscle due to the nucleus's placement in the middle of the muscle cell and the lack of striations. The muscle fibers of the arrectores pilorum are connected to the hair follicle beneath the sebaceous glands and are found in the upper dermal connective tissue. They are positioned so that, when the hair follicle contracts, the angle at which they are situated causes the hair follicle to be drawn vertically, deforming the skin and resulting in "gooseflesh." Small bundles of smooth muscle of the muscularis of veins and arteries have various configurations. Glomus bodies are specialized smooth muscle aggregates that are present on the digits and lateral aspects of the palms and soles, situated between the venules and arterioles. They shunt blood and control body temperature. Striated or voluntary muscle is present as the platysma in the skin of the neck and as the expression muscle in the skin of the face. The complex network of muscle, fascia, and aponeuroses that connects muscles to the parts they move is known as the superficial muscular aponeurotic system.

1.6.3. Nerves

Neurovascular bundles of the dermis contain a large number of nerve bundles, arterioles, and venules. Meissner corpuscles, which are mostly located on the ventral sides of the hands and feet and are part of the dermal papillae, aid in mediating touch. Meissner corpuscles are more prevalent on the hands, with the fingertips having the highest concentration. Large nerve-end organs called Vater-Pacini corpuscles are found in the deeper layer of the dermis of weight-bearing surfaces and genitalia. They produce a sensation of pressure. They are also frequently observed in the anogenital and nipple areas. The pain, temperature, and itchy sensation are sensed by unmyelinated nerve fibers that terminate at the papillary dermis and hair follicles.

The autonomic nervous system's postganglionic adrenergic fibers control vasoconstriction. This system controls the contraction of the AP muscles in hair follicles as well as the secretions of apocrine glands. Cholinergic fibers, on the other hand, mediate eccrine sweat secretions.

1.6.4. Mast Cells

Specialized secretory cells called mast cells are found in the body's connective tissues and are derived from bone marrow. They are found in the subcutaneous fat as well, despite being more prevalent in the papillary dermis. Mast cells have an oval to spindle-shaped appearance in the normal dermis, with a round to-oval nucleus positioned in the middle. There are a lot of mast cells surrounding blood vessels, particularly postcapillary venules. Mast cells exhibit multiple long, large villi around their periphery when magnified. Mast cell granules are membrane-bound, spherical, oval, or angular structures that include serine proteinases, heparin, histamine, and some cytokines. The cell's surface contains hundreds of thousands of glycoprotein receptor sites for immunoglobulin E. Type I or connective tissue mast cells are located in the dermis and submucosa. Type II or mucosal mast cells are located in the respiratory tract mucosa and in the bowel.

Because of aberrant migration, proliferation, and apoptosis failure during mastocytosis, mast cells build up in the skin. Although these cells have historically been linked to the allergic response, more recent research indicates that they may also be able to control innate immunity, host defense, and inflammation. Antigens or allergens acting through the high-affinity receptor for immunoglobulin E, superoxides, complement proteins, neuropeptides, and lipoproteins can activate mast cells. Histamine, leukotrienes, prostanoids, proteases, and numerous cytokines and chemokines are all expressed by mast cells following activation. Some mediators might play a key role in the development of an inflammatory response. Mast cells are believed to be actively involved in a variety of illnesses, including allergies, parasite infections, atherosclerosis, cancer, asthma, pulmonary fibrosis, and arthritis, due to their location and mediator expression.

1.6.4.1. Structure

Mast cells and basophil granulocytes, a subset of white blood cells, are similar in that they are both granulated cells that have anticoagulant heparin and histamine. The mast cell nucleus is round, but the basophil nucleus is lobulated. This is how their nuclei differ from one another. IgE's paratopes attach to an antigen, causing mast cells and basophils to release histamine and other inflammatory mediators. This is how the Fc region of IgE binds to these cells. Many have hypothesized that mast cells are basophils that have settled on tissues as a result of these similarities. Additionally, they have a common precursor that expresses the CD34 molecule in bone marrow. While mast cells circulate in an immature form and only mature once in a tissue site, basophils exit the bone marrow already mature. An immature mast cell's specific properties are most likely determined by the location in which it settles. A pure population of mouse mast cells was successfully differentiated and grown *in vitro* for the first time using a conditioned medium made from splenocytes stimulated with concanavalin A. Subsequent research revealed that the element in the conditioned media necessary for mast cell differentiation and growth was T cell-derived interleukin 3.

Mucosal mast cells and connective tissue-type mast cells are the two subtypes of mast cells that are traditionally distinguished in rodents. T-cells are necessary for the latter's functions.

Mast cells are found in most tissues that are typical of surrounding lymphatic, pulmonary, and digestive tract mucosa as well as blood vessels. They are particularly noticeable in areas that mark the boundaries between the internal and external environments, such as the skin, digestive tract mucosa, lungs, mouth, and nose.

1.6.4.2. Function

A crucial part of the inflammatory process is played by mast cells. When a mast cell is activated, it can release mediators, or substances that cause inflammation, from storage granules into the local microenvironment either slowly (known as piecemeal degranulation) or quickly (known as anaphylactic degranulation). Mast cells can be activated to degranulate by a variety of means, including allergens via immunoglobulin E receptors (e.g., FcεRI), physical injury via damage-associated molecular patterns (DAMPs), microbial pathogens via pathogen-associated molecular patterns (PAMPs) and various compounds via ligand-gated ion channels or G-protein coupled receptors (e.g., morphine via opioid receptors). Additionally, complement proteins can activate mast cell membrane receptors for a variety of purposes.

The least abundant part of the antibodies, the Fc region of IgE, has a high-affinity receptor (FcεRI) expressed by mast cells. Because of this receptor's extreme affinity, binding of IgE molecules to it is essentially irreversible. IgE, which is produced by plasma cells—the immune system's cells that produce antibodies—thus coats mast cells. Usually, IgE antibodies are restricted to a single antigen.

Mast cells in allergic reactions do not become active until an allergen attaches to the IgE that has already been coated on the cell. Additional membrane activation events have the potential to either work in concert with FcεRI signal transduction or prime mast cells for their subsequent degranulation. Allergens are typically polysaccharides or proteins. The variable regions of the IgE molecules bound to the mast cell surface are where the allergen binds to the antigen-binding sites. It seems that to activate the mast cell, two or more IgE molecules must bind together, a process known as cross-linking. The complex series of events within the mast cell that result in its activation are caused by the clustering of the intracellular domains of the cell-bound Fc receptors, which are linked to the cross-linked IgE molecules. It seems that this reaction has developed as a defense mechanism against bacteria and parasites, even though it is best understood in the context of allergies (Herskovitz et al., 2015).

A Closer Look

The Habitat of the Skin

The distinct populations of microorganisms that are adapted to their particular niche are chosen by the physical and chemical characteristics of the skin. The skin is generally cold, acidic, and desiccated, but the thickness, folds, and density of hair follicles and glands within the skin define specific habitats. The epidermis is a strong physical barrier that keeps moisture and nutrients inside the body while preventing the entry of germs and possible toxins. Squames, or terminally differentiated, enucleated keratinocytes, make up the stratum corneum, the top layer of the epidermis. The "bricks and mortar" of the epidermis are made up of keratin fibrils and crosslinked, cornified envelopes encased in lipid bilayers. Since the skin is a constantly self-renewing organ, squames, which started their migration from the basal layer about four weeks earlier, constantly shed from the skin's surface as the last stage of terminal differentiation.

Invaginations and appendages

The skin has various invaginations and appendages, such as sweat glands (eccrine and apocrine), sebaceous glands, and hair follicles, each likely hosting its own unique microbiota. Eccrine glands, more abundant than apocrine glands, are present on all skin surfaces and release a secretion primarily composed of water and salt, aiding in thermoregulation by dissipating heat through evaporation. They also play a role in excreting water and electrolytes and maintaining skin acidity to prevent microbial colonization. Apocrine glands, located in specific areas like the armpits, nipples, and genitoanal regions, produce milky, viscous secretions in response to adrenaline. These secretions may contain pheromones that influence certain behaviors in others. The characteristic odor associated with sweat comes from bacteria processing apocrine secretions. Sebaceous glands secrete sebum, a lipid-rich substance, and are linked to hair follicles to form the pilosebaceous unit. Sebum is a hydrophobic layer that lubricates, shields, and protects skin and hair from germs. Propionibacterium acnes, a common skin commensal bacterium, and other facultative anaerobes can grow in sebaceous glands because they are relatively anoxic. Propionibacterium acnes's whole genome sequencing has identified several genes that encode lipases, which break down sebum-containing lipids in the skin. *Propionibacterium acnes* releases free fatty acids onto the skin by hydrolyzing the triglycerides found in sebum. The bacteria can then stick to these free fatty acids, which might help the sebaceous gland colonize. The skin's surface has an acidic pH of approximately five due to the presence of free fatty acids. An acidic pH inhibits the growth of many common pathogens, including *Streptococcus pyogenes* and *Staphylococcus aureus*. This promotes the growth of corynebacteria and coagulase-negative staphylococci. On the other hand, skin occlusion causes an elevated pH, which promotes the growth of *S. aureus* and *S. pyogenes*. *Propionibacterium acnes* is more common on human skin than it is on the skin of other mammals due to the fact that humans produce significantly more triglyceride-containing sebum than other mammals.

Topography

Due to regional variations in skin anatomy, the skin surface varies topographically. Based on studies using culture-based methods, these regions are known to harbor different kinds of microorganisms. Certain areas of the skin, like the toe web, axillary vault, and groin, are partially occluded. The higher temperatures and humidity in these areas promote the growth of microorganisms that prefer moist environments, such as *Staphylococcus aureus*, coryneforms, and Gram-negative bacilli. Another variable that affects the skin microbiota depending on the area is the density of sebaceous glands. The face, chest, and back are regions with a high density of sebaceous glands, which promote the growth of lipophilic microorganisms (*Propionibacterium* spp. alongside *Malassezia* spp.). The skin on the arms and legs is more dried out and has more temperature variations on its surface than other skin sites. These regions were found to contain quantitatively fewer organisms than moist areas of the skin surface using culture-based methods.

Host factors

Factors such as age, location, and sex of the host play a significant role in the diversity of microbial flora found on the skin. The microenvironment of the skin is greatly influenced by age, with colonization of microbiota starting immediately after birth. Research is needed to understand how microbial communities on the skin develop and stabilize during the early years of life. Puberty brings about changes in sebum production, affecting the levels of lipophilic bacteria on the skin. Differences in sweat, sebum, and hormone production between males and females contribute to the microbial variations observed between genders on the skin.

Environmental factors

Individual-specific environmental factors, like clothing choices, occupation, and antibiotic use, can influence how the skin microbiota colonizes an area. Molecular techniques have been used to study the impact of antibiotic treatment on the gut microbiota; however, to our knowledge, no comparable evaluation of the skin microbiota in healthy individuals has been done. Skin microbiota variation may also be influenced by moisturizers, soaps, cosmetics, and hygiene products. These products change the skin barrier's conditions, but it's still unknown how they will affect the skin microbiota. When compared to high-temperature low-humidity conditions, quantitative culture showed that high-temperature and high-humidity conditions are linked to increased quantities of bacteria on the feet, axillary vaults, and back. In the same study, there was a correlation between a higher frequency of Gram-negative bacteria on the back and feet and high humidity and low temperature. One can imagine that geographical variability in skin microbiota correlates with the longitudinal and/or latitudinal variation in UV exposure. Ultraviolet (UV) light is a well-documented bactericidal treatment.

Summary

- The skin is the largest organ of the body, accounting for about 15% of the total adult body weight. It performs many vital functions, including protection against external physical, chemical, and biological assailants, as well as prevention of excess water loss from the body and a role in thermoregulation.
- The epidermis is a stratified, squamous epithelium layer that is composed primarily of two types of cells: keratinocytes and dendritic cells.
- Keratinocytes are the primary type of cell found in the epidermis, the outermost layer of the skin. In humans, they constitute 90% of epidermal skin cells.
- The basal layer, also known as the stratum basale, contains column-shaped keratinocytes that attach to the basement membrane zone with their long axis perpendicular to the dermis.
- Intercellular spaces between spinous cells are bridged by abundant desmosomes that promote mechanical coupling between cells of the epidermis and provide resistance to physical stresses.
- Horny cells (corneocytes) of the cornified layer provide mechanical protection to the underlying epidermis and a barrier to prevent water loss and invasion by foreign substances.
- Melanocytes molecularly are recognizable by the identification of melanocyte-specific proteins as tyrosinase (TYR), tyrosinase-related proteins 1 and 2 (TYRP1, TYRP2/DCT), melanosomal matrix proteins (Pmel17, MART-1), microphthalmia transcription factor (MITF).
- Melanogenesis is a biochemical pathway responsible for melanin synthesis. It takes place in melanocytes, in separate cytoplasmic organelles called melanosomes.
- Merkel cells are oval-shaped, slow-adapting, type I mechanoreceptors located in sites of high tactile sensitivity that are attached to basal keratinocytes by desmosomal junctions.
- A Langerhans cell (LC) is a tissue-resident macrophage of the skin once thought to be a resident dendritic cell. These cells contain organelles called Birbeck granules.
- The interface between the epidermis and dermis is formed by a porous basement membrane zone that allows the exchange of cells and fluid and holds the two layers together.
- The skin adnexa are a grouping of ectodermal derived appendages, including eccrine and apocrine glands, ducts, and pilosebaceous units that originate as downgrowths from the epidermis during development.
- The dermis is an integrated system of fibrous, filamentous, and amorphous connective tissue that accommodates stimulus-induced entry by nerve and vascular networks, epidermally derived appendages, fibroblasts, macrophages, and mast cells.

References

1. Andersson, T., Ertürk Bergdahl, G., Saleh, K., Magnúsdóttir, H., Stødkilde, K., Andersen, C. B. F., Lundqvist, K., Jensen, A., Brüggemann, H., & Lood, R. (2019). Common skin bacteria protect their host from oxidative stress through secreted antioxidant RoxP. *Scientific Reports, 9*(1), 3596.

2. Aoki, H., Yamada, Y., Hara, A., et al. (2009). Two distinct types of mouse melanocyte: Differential signaling requirement for the maintenance of non-cutaneous and dermal versus epidermal melanocytes. *Development, 136*(15), 2511–2521.
3. Chu, D. H. (2008). Overview of biology, development, and structure of skin. In K. Wolff, L. A. Goldsmith, S. I. Katz, B. A. Gilchrest, A. S. Paller, & D. J. Leffell (Eds.), *Fitzpatrick's Dermatology in General Medicine* (7th ed., pp. 57–73). New York, NY: McGraw-Hill.
4. Daniel, R. C., & Scher, R. K. (1997). Nail changes secondary to systemic drugs and ingestants. In R. K. Scher & R. C. Daniel (Eds.), *Nails: Therapy, Diagnosis, Surgery* (2nd ed., pp. 251–258).
5. Herskovitz, I., Macquhae, F., Fox, J. D., & Kirsner, R. S. (2016). Skin movement, wound repair and development of engineered skin. *Experimental Dermatology, 25*(2), 99–100.
6. Kanitakis, J. (2002). Anatomy, histology and immunohistochemistry of normal human skin. *European Journal of Dermatology, 12*(4), 390–401.
7. Kerr, J. F., Wyllie, A. H., & Currie, A. R. (1972). Apoptosis: A basic biological phenomenon with wide-ranging implication in tissue kinetics. *British Journal of Cancer, 26*(4), 239–257.
8. Ravara, B., Hofer, C., Kern, H., Guidolin, D., Porzionato, A., De Caro, R., & Albertin, G. (2018). Dermal papillae flattening of thigh skin in Conus Cauda Syndrome. *European Journal of Translational Myology, 28*(4), 7914.
9. Slominski, A. T., Manna, P. R., & Tuckey, R. C. (2015). On the role of skin in the regulation of local and systemic steroidogenic activities. *Steroids, 103*, 72–88.
10. Tenea, D., Dinkel, J., Becker, J. C., & van der Walt, E. (2019). Merkel cell carcinoma of the head in a young African albino woman with HIV/HTLV-1 coinfection associated with multiple squamous cell carcinomas. *Case Reports in Dermatology, 11*(1), 113–122.
11. Vern-Gross, T. Z., & Kowal-Vern, A. (2014). Erythema multiforme, Stevens-Johnson syndrome, and toxic epidermal necrolysis syndrome in patients undergoing radiation therapy: A literature review. *American Journal of Clinical Oncology, 37*(5), 506–513.
12. Wagner, T., Beer, L., Gschwandtner, M., Eckhart, L., Kalinina, P., Laggner, M., Ellinger, A., Gruber, R., Kuchler, U., Golabi, B., Tschachler, E., & Mildner, M. (2019). The differentiation-associated keratinocyte protein cornifelin contributes to cell-cell adhesion of epidermal and mucosal keratinocytes. *Journal of Investigative Dermatology, 139*(11), 2292–2301.

Chapter

INFLAMMATORY SKIN DISEASES

2

Contents

Introduction

The body uses inflammation as a vital defense mechanism to identify and react to pathogens, irritants, damaged cells, and other threats. Inflammation is also required for the healing process to start. On the other hand, excessive inflammation can harm our tissues. Inflammatory skin conditions have a significant patient burden and are consistently one of the most difficult medical conditions to treat. It can be difficult to diagnose and treat skin inflammation and rashes, which can result in redness, pain, itching, and dryness. Poison oak and poison ivy, dermatitis, and drug rashes are common inflammatory skin conditions.

Orientation and Directional Terms

Term	Definition	Illustration
Psoriasis	Psoriasis is a chronic (long-lasting) disease in which the immune system becomes overactive, causing skin cells to multiply too quickly. Patches of skin become scaly and inflamed, most often on the scalp, elbows, or knees, but other parts of the body can be affected as well	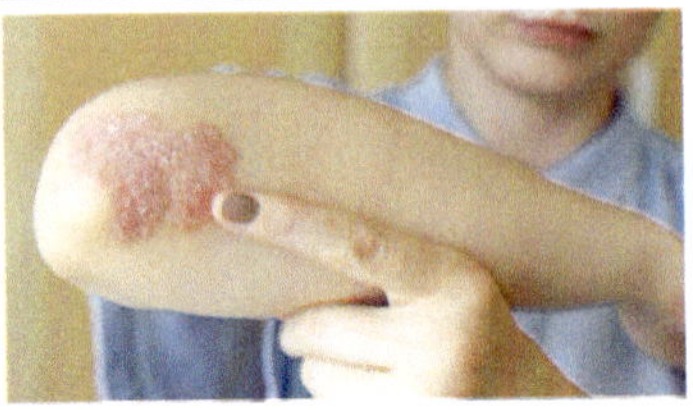
Eczema	Eczema is a common skin condition that causes itchiness, rashes, dry patches, and infection. It's a type of dermatitis, which is a group of conditions that can inflame or irritate your skin.	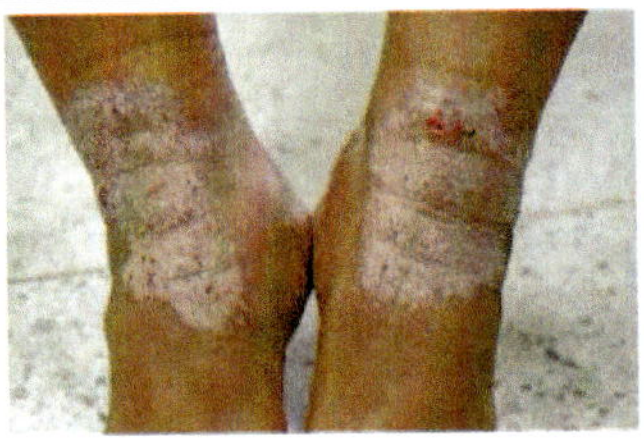
Skin biopsy	A skin biopsy is a procedure that involves removing a small sample of skin for examination under a microscope. It's a common diagnostic procedure used to identify skin conditions like skin cancer, infections, psoriasis, or rashes.	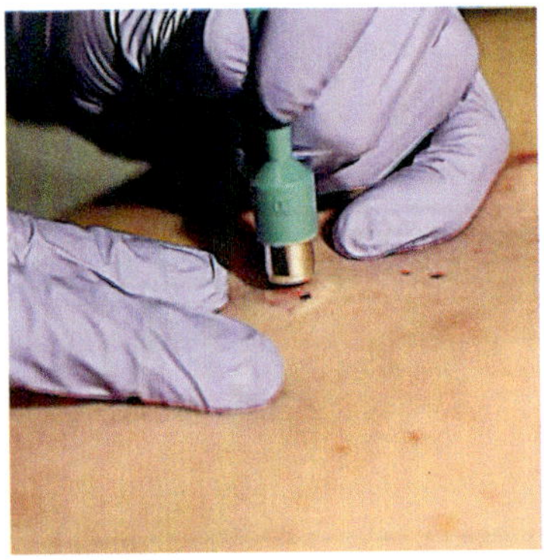
Lichen planus	Lichen planus is a chronic inflammatory disease that affects the skin, nails, hair, and mucous membranes. It's characterized by itchy, violet papules and plaques that can appear on the skin, inside the mouth, or on the nails.	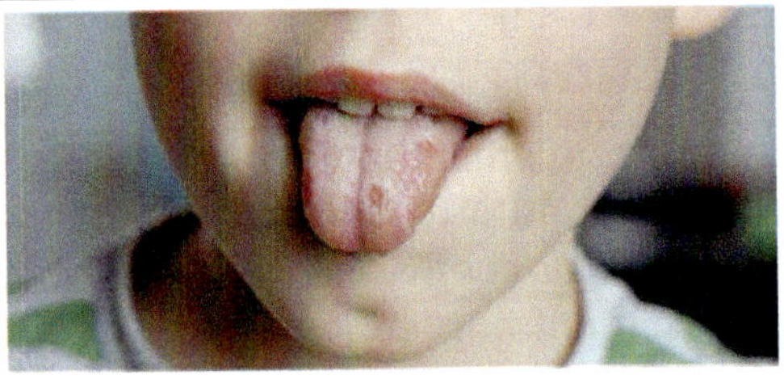

2.1. Psoriasis

Psoriasis is a chronic inflammatory skin condition with a high immune-mediated genetic susceptibility and autoimmune pathogenic features. In pathophysiological pathways, acquired, and cellular immunity interact in complex ways. The population is impacted by the disease's complex multifactorial etiology. The condition is most often caused by a combination of environmental and hereditary factors. There is a correlation between the disorder's severity and prevalence. Psoriasis is known medically as psoriasis vulgaris. Still, another name for it is plaque-type psoriasis. The extremities have a patchy appearance throughout. Roughly 90% of patients have the chronic plaque form of psoriasis. Traditional clinical manifestations consist of erythematous, pruritic, and distinct-bordered patches covered in silvery scaling.

There are five primary forms of psoriasis: erythrodermic, guttate, inverse, pustular, and plaque. About 90% of cases are plaque psoriasis, commonly referred to as psoriasis vulgaris. Usually, it appears as red areas with white scaling on top. The backs of the forearms, shins, navel region, and scalp are the body parts most frequently impacted. Lesions in guttate psoriasis are shaped like drops. Small, pus-filled blisters that are not contagious are the hallmarks of pustular psoriasis. Red patches in skin folds are caused by inverse psoriasis. Any of the other types of psoriasis can progress to erythrodermic psoriasis, which happens when the rash gets extremely widespread. Most psoriasis sufferers at some point experience problems with their fingernails and toenails. This could include variations in nail color or pits in the nails.

Most people believe that psoriasis is a genetic condition brought on by environmental factors. If two twins are identical, the other twin has a three times higher chance of developing psoriasis than if they are not. This implies that psoriasis is predisposed to genetic factors. Wintertime and certain medications, like NSAIDs or beta blockers, can exacerbate symptoms. Psychological strain and infections may also be factors. The immune system responding to skin cells is the underlying mechanism. Signs and symptoms are usually used to make the diagnosis (Elman et al., 2018).

Psoriasis has no known cure, although there are treatments that can help manage the symptoms. Steroid creams, vitamin D3 creams, UV light, immunosuppressive medications like methotrexate, and biologic therapies that target particular immunologic pathways are some of these treatments. With creams alone, about 75% of skin involvement improves. Two to 4% of people are afflicted by the illness. Equal numbers of men and women experience this problem. Although it can strike at any age, the disease usually first manifests in adults. An increased risk of lymphomas, depression, Crohn's disease, cardiovascular disease, and psoriatic arthritis is linked to psoriasis. Of those with psoriasis, up to 30% develop psoriatic arthritis.

2.1.1. Signs and Symptoms

2.1.1.1. Plaque Psoriasis

Psoriasis vulgaris, which accounts for 85–90% of cases of psoriasis, is the most common type. It is also referred to as chronic stationary psoriasis or plaque-like psoriasis. The classic presentation of plaque psoriasis is elevated, inflammatory skin patches covered in silvery-white, scaly skin. These regions, known as plaques, are most frequently seen on the back, scalp, elbows, and knees.

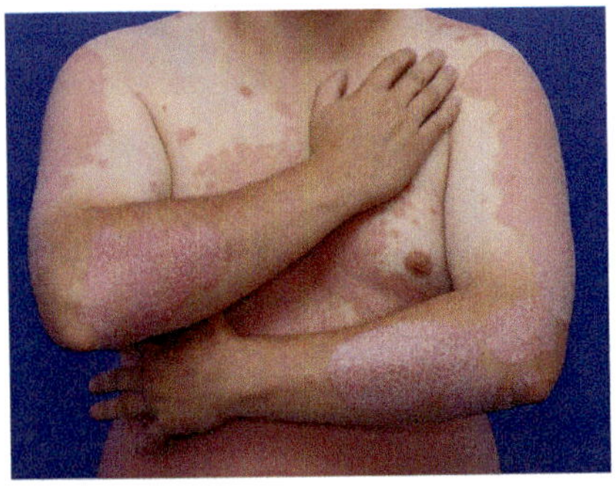

Figure 2.1. *Plaque psoriasis.*

Source: https://www.ncbi.nlm.nih.gov/books/NBK430879/figure/article-27295.image.f1/?report=objectonly.

2.1.1.2. Other Forms

Roughly 10% of cases are of other types of psoriasis. They include forms that resemble seborrheic dermatitis, pustular, inverse, napkin, guttate, and oral.

1. **Pustular Psoriasis:** Pustular psoriasis presents as raised bumps full of noninfectious pus, surrounded by red and tender skin. It can manifest as either localized or widespread on the body. Two types of localized pustular psoriasis, pustulosa palmoplantaris and acrodermatitis continua of Hallopeau, specifically affect the hands and feet (Figure 2.2).

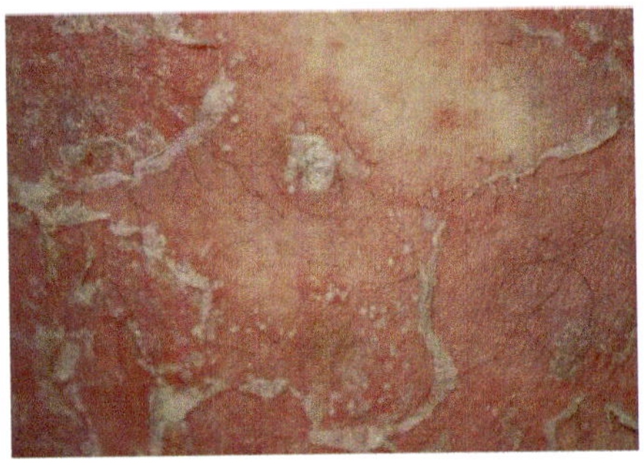

Figure 2.2. *Pustular psoriasis.*

Source: https://www.ncbi.nlm.nih.gov/books/NBK493189/figure/article-36078.image.f1/?report=objectonly.

2. **Inverse Psoriasis:** Smooth, irritated patches of skin are the hallmark of flexural psoriasis, another name for inverse psoriasis. Skin folds are commonly affected by the patches, especially those around the genitals (between the thigh and groin), the armpits, the panniculus, the intergluteal cleft, the skin folds under the breasts, and between the buttocks. This unusual type of psoriasis is believed to be caused by heat, trauma, and infection.
3. **Napkin Psoriasis:** Napkin psoriasis is a type of psoriasis that is frequently seen in infants under two years old. It is identified by red bumps covered in silver scales in the diaper area, and these can sometimes spread to the torso or limbs. Napkin psoriasis is often mistaken for diaper rash. As children grow older, this condition usually improves but may reappear later in life as plaque psoriasis or inverse psoriasis.
4. **Guttate Psoriasis:** An inflammatory disease called guttate psoriasis is typified by a large number of tiny, scaly, red or pink, droplet-like lesions (papules). Large portions of the body, mostly the trunk, limbs, and scalp, are covered in these numerous papules; however, the palms and soles are usually spared. The onset of guttate psoriasis usually happens 1–3 weeks after a streptococcal infection, either oropharyngeal or perianal. The diagnosis of guttate psoriasis is usually based on the history and results of a clinical examination, and it is most common in children and young adults. It is also possible to perform a skin biopsy, which usually reveals a psoriasiform reaction pattern with rete ridge elongation and epidermal hyperplasia (Figure 2.3).

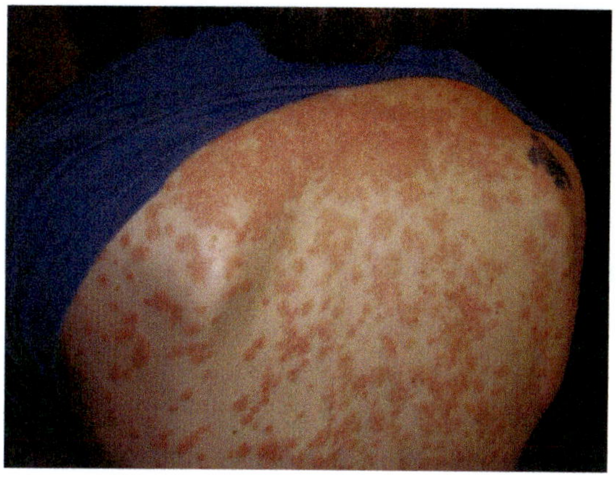

Figure 2.3. *The late stages of Guttate Psoriasis where the droplets spread all over body parts.*

Source: https://www.researchgate.net/figure/It-shows-the-late-stages-of-Guttate-Psoriasis-where-the-droplets-spread-all-over-body_fig2_331859346.

Although there isn't enough data to determine the optimal course of treatment for guttate psoriasis, topical corticosteroids are usually the first line of treatment for mild cases. For moderate to severe cases of guttate psoriasis, phototherapy is an option. The use of biological therapies to treat guttate psoriasis has not been thoroughly researched.

Guttate psoriasis generally has a more favorable outcome compared to plaque psoriasis, usually clearing up within 1–3 weeks. However, around 40% of patients with guttate psoriasis may develop plaque psoriasis over time.

5. **Erythrodermic Psoriasis:** *Psoriatic erythroderma*, or *Erythrodermic psoriasis*, is marked by widespread skin inflammation and exfoliation, often covering more than 90% of the body's surface. This condition may cause severe dryness, itching, swelling, and pain, and can develop from any form of psoriasis. It commonly occurs when unstable plaque psoriasis exacerbates, especially following sudden withdrawal from systemic glucocorticoids. Due to the extensive inflammation and exfoliation, the body's ability to regulate temperature and maintain barrier functions is impaired, making this form of psoriasis potentially life-threatening.
6. **Mouth:** Unlike lichen planus, another common papulosquamous disorder that frequently affects both the skin and the mouth, oral psoriasis is extremely uncommon. Psoriasis that affects the oral mucosa, or the lining of the mouth, can cause white or grey-yellow plaques to form. It can also be asymptomatic. The most prevalent symptom of oral psoriasis is fissured tongue, which affects 6.5–20% of those with psoriasis affecting the skin, according to reports. Psoriasis and the microscopic appearance of oral mucosa affected by geographic tongue (migratory stomatitis) are strikingly similar. Geographic tongue may be a predictor of psoriasis, according to a recent study that discovered a correlation between the two disorders.
7. **Seborrheic-Like Psoriasis:** Commonly occurring psoriasis with clinical features similar to both psoriasis and seborrheic dermatitis, seborrheic-like psoriasis can be challenging to differentiate from the latter. In regions where sebum production is higher, such as the scalp, forehead, skin folds next to the nose, the skin around the mouth, the skin on the chest above the sternum, and in skin folds, this type of psoriasis usually appears as red plaques with greasy scales.

2.1.1.3. Psoriatic Arthritis

A type of chronic inflammatory arthritis known as psoriatic arthritis usually coexists with skin and nail psoriasis and presents with a highly variable clinical presentation. It can occur in any joint, but most commonly affects the joints in the fingers and toes. Usually, it involves excruciating inflammation of the joints and surrounding connective tissue. Dactylitis, a swelling of the fingers and toes resembling a sausage, may ensue from this. In addition, psoriatic arthritis can cause spondylitis, hip, knee, and sacroiliac joint pain (sacroiliitis). About 30% of people who have psoriasis will also get psoriatic arthritis. In roughly 75% of cases, the skin symptoms of psoriasis appear before the arthritic ones.

2.1.1.4. Nail Changes

Psoriasis can cause a range of changes in the appearance of fingers and toenails, including damage to the nails. In 40–45% of cases of skin psoriasis, nail psoriasis manifests itself, and in 80–90% of cases of psoriatic arthritis over the course of a lifetime. These changes include yellow-reddish discoloration of the nails known as the oil drop or salmon spots, whitening of the nail, small areas of bleeding from capillaries under the nail, dryness, thickening of the skin under the nail (subungual hyperkeratosis), loosening, and separation of the nail (onycholysis), and crumbling of the nail. 70% of patients with nail psoriasis have pitting of the nails.

2.1.1.5. Medical Signs

Medical professionals may use specific medical signs in addition to the rash's appearance and distribution to aid in diagnosis. These could include the Koebner phenomenon (psoriatic skin lesions brought on by trauma to the skin), Auspitz's sign (pinpoint bleeding when scale is removed), and pain and itching that is restricted to papules and plaques.

2.1.2. Causes

Psoriasis's etiology is not entirely understood. Different types of psoriasis have been linked to genetics, seasonal variations, climate change, skin damage, immunocompromised states, certain infections, and the use of certain medications.

2.1.2.1. Genetics

Approximately one-third of individuals with psoriasis have a family history of the disease, and scientists have pinpointed genetic markers linked to the condition. Studies on identical twins indicate a 70% likelihood of one twin developing psoriasis if the other twin has it, while the risk decreases to around 20% for fraternal twins. These results indicate a combination of genetic predisposition and environmental factors contributing to the development of psoriasis.

There is a strong genetic component to psoriasis, and numerous genes are linked to the condition, although it is unknown how these genes interact. The majority of the genes that have been found are associated with the immune system, specifically T cells and the major histocompatibility complex (MHC). Because genetic studies can identify molecular mechanisms and pathways for additional research as well as possible targets for medications, they are valuable.

Using traditional genome-wide linkage analysis, nine loci on various chromosomes have been linked to psoriasis. They are referred to as PSORS1 through PSORS9, or psoriasis susceptibility 1 through 9. Genes related to inflammatory pathways are located within those loci. In psoriasis, specific variants (mutations) of those genes are frequently observed. Thanks to genome-wide association searches, additional genes that are changed to psoriasis-specific variations have been found. Certain genes are responsible for the expression of inflammatory signal proteins, which impact immune system cells linked to psoriasis. Other autoimmune diseases are associated with some of these genes. PSORS1 is the main factor, likely responsible for 35–50% of the heritability of psoriasis. It regulates genes that impact immune function or encode skin proteins overexpressed in psoriasis. PSORS1 regulates critical immune functions and is found on chromosome 6 of the MHC. Psoriasis vulgaris is strongly correlated with three genes in the PSORS1 locus: CDSN, variant allele 5, which encodes corneodesmosin, a protein expressed in the granular and cornified layers of the epidermis and upregulated in psoriasis; HLA-C variant HLA-Cw6, which encodes an MHC class I protein; and CCHCR1, variant WWC, which encodes a coiled-coil protein overexpressed in psoriatic epidermis.

Interleukin-12 subunit beta (IL12B) on chromosome 5q, which expresses interleukin-12B, and IL23R on chromosome 1p, which expresses the interleukin-23 receptor and is involved in T cell differentiation, are two important immune system genes that are currently being studied. Psoriasis has been closely associated with both the interleukin-23 receptor and IL12B. The inflammatory process that results in psoriasis involves T cells. These genes are on the pathway that upregulates two inflammatory genes, nuclear factor κB and tumor necrosis factor-α. The PSORS2 locus's CARD14 gene was found to be the first gene specifically connected to psoriasis. For plaque psoriasis, which is the most common type of psoriasis, a rare mutation in the gene encoding for the CARD14-regulated protein along with an environmental trigger was sufficient.

2.1.2.2. Lifestyle

Seasonal and climatic changes, chronic infections, and stress have all been linked to the disease's worsening. Hot water, scratching psoriasis skin lesions, dry skin, excessive alcohol consumption, cigarette smoking, and obesity are additional factors that may exacerbate the condition. As of 2019, research on the effects of quitting alcohol abuse or smoking cigarettes has not been completed.

2.1.2.3. HIV

Psoriasis rates among people living with HIV/AIDS are similar to those among HIV-negative people, although psoriasis tends to be more severe in HIV-positive individuals. HIV-positive people with psoriasis have a far higher incidence of psoriatic arthritis than people without the virus. Cellular signals from the T_h2 subset of CD4+ helper T cells are generally indicative of an immune response in HIV-positive individuals, while a pattern of cellular signals characteristic of the T_h1 subset of CD4+ helper T cells and T_h17 helper T cells is indicative of an immune response in psoriasis vulgaris patients. It is believed that the overactivation of CD8+-T cells, which exacerbates psoriasis in HIV-positive individuals, is brought on by a decreased presence of CD4+-T cells. In people living with HIV/AIDS, psoriasis is frequently severe and may not respond to standard treatment. A recent HIV infection can cause a severe flare-up of psoriasis and/or psoriatic arthritis in people with long-term, well-controlled psoriasis.

2.1.2.4. Microbes

It has been reported that psoriasis develops after strep throat and can be exacerbated by *Staphylococcus aureus* or Malassezia species colonization of the skin or gut. along with *Candida albicans*. Children and teenagers are frequently affected by guttate psoriasis, which can be brought on by a recent group A streptococcal infection (tonsillitis or pharyngitis).

2.1.2.5. Medications

Beta-blockers, lithium, antimalarial drugs, nonsteroidal anti-inflammatory drugs, terbinafine, calcium channel blockers, captopril, glyburide, granulocyte colony-stimulating factor, interleukins, interferons, lipid-lowering drugs, and, ironically, TNF inhibitors like infliximab or adalimumab can all cause drug-induced psoriasis. Because of the rebound effect, stopping corticosteroids (topical steroid cream) can make psoriasis worse.

2.1.3. Pathophysiology

The skin's epidermal layer grows abnormally quickly and excessively in psoriasis patients. The pathological events that cause psoriasis lead to both an excess of skin cells and abnormal skin cell production, particularly during wound repair. Psoriasis is thought to have two phases of pathological events: an initiation phase, during which an immune system activation event (such as skin trauma, infection, or medication) occurs, and a maintenance phase, during which the disease progresses chronically. In psoriasis, skin cells replace every 3–5 days instead of the typical 28–30 days. These alterations are thought to be the result of keratinocytes maturing too soon, which is caused by an inflammatory cascade in the dermis that includes T cells, macrophages, and dendritic cells—three different subtypes of white blood cells. These immune cells migrate from the dermis to the epidermis and secrete cytokines, which are chemical signals that cause inflammation. Examples of these cytokines include interleukin-36γ, interleukin-1β, interleukin-6, and interleukin-22. It is thought that these released inflammatory cues encourage the growth of keratinocytes. One theory is that psoriasis is caused by a malfunction in the regulatory cytokine interleukin-10 and regulatory T cells. Similar to psoriatic skin lesions, inflammatory cytokines are also detected in psoriatic nails and joints (in the case of psoriatic arthritis), indicating a shared inflammatory mechanism.

Gene mutations of proteins implicated in the barrier function of the skin have been recognized as indicators of psoriasis susceptibility.

DNA released from dying cells stimulates certain dendritic cells' receptors, causing them to release the cytokine interferon-α, which in turn acts as an inflammatory stimulus in psoriasis. Keratinocytes also secrete cytokines like interleukin-1, interleukin-6, and tumor necrosis factor-α in response to these chemical signals from dendritic cells and T cells. These signals alert downstream inflammatory cells to arrive and cause more inflammation.

The innate and adaptive immune systems are connected by dendritic cells. They stimulate the growth of T cells and type 1 helper T cells (Th1) and are more prevalent in psoriatic lesions. Psoralen and ultraviolet A (PUVA) therapy, along with targeted immunotherapy, can decrease the number of dendritic cells and promote the secretion of TH2 cell cytokines rather than Th1/Th17 cell cytokines. Psoriatic T cells secrete interleukin-17 and interferon-γ as they migrate from the dermis into the epidermis. It is known that interleukin-23 stimulates the synthesis of interleukin-17 and interleukin-22. When combined with interleukin-17, interleukin-22 causes keratinocytes to release cytokines that draw neutrophils.

2.1.4. Diagnosis

The appearance of the skin is typically used to diagnose psoriasis. Psoriasis is characterized by scaly, erythematous plaques, papules, or skin patches that can itch and cause pain. Usually, the diagnosis can be made without the need for any specialized blood tests or diagnostic procedures.

Dermatological conditions with similar appearances to psoriasis include discoid eczema, seborrheic eczema, pityriasis rosea (which can be mistaken for guttate psoriasis), nail fungus (which can be mistaken for nail psoriasis), and cutaneous T cell lymphoma (which is initially misdiagnosed in 50% of cases). Psoriasis should not be mistaken for dermatological signs of systemic diseases, such as the rash associated with secondary syphilis (Perez-Chada et al., 2018).

A skin biopsy or scraping may be done to confirm the diagnosis and rule out other conditions if the clinical diagnosis is unclear. Under microscopy, clubbed epidermal projections from a biopsy skin sample interdigitate with the dermis. Another typical histologic finding of psoriasis lesions is epidermal thickening. In psoriatic lesions, the stratum granulosum layer of the epidermis is frequently absent or markedly reduced; additionally, the skin cells from the skin's most superficial layer are aberrant since they never fully mature. These epithelial cells maintain their nuclei, in contrast to their mature counterparts. On microscopy, inflammatory infiltrates are usually visible when looking at psoriasis-affected skin or joint tissue. While the inflammatory infiltrates of the dermal layer of skin and the joints are primarily composed of CD4+ T cells, epidermal skin tissue affected by psoriatic inflammation frequently contains a high concentration of CD8+ T cells.

2.1.4.1. Classification

2.1.4.1.1. Morphological

As a papulosquamous disorder, psoriasis is typically classified into several categories according to histological features. Plaque, pustular, guttate, and flexural psoriasis are some of the variations. Every form has its own unique ICD-10 code. There are two more types of psoriasis: nonpustular and pustular.

2.1.4.1.2. Pathogenetic

Gene and demographic factors are taken into account in another classification scheme. Type 1 is linked to the human leukocyte antigen HLA-Cw6, begins before the age of 40, and has a positive family history. On the other hand, type 2 is not linked to HLA-Cw6, does not exhibit a family history, and manifests after the age of 40. Roughly 75% of psoriasis sufferers are type 1 carriers.

There is a great deal of controversy surrounding the designation of psoriasis as an autoimmune condition. Psoriasis and psoriatic arthritis have been described differently by researchers; some have categorized them as autoimmune diseases, while others have distinguished them from autoimmune diseases and called them immune-mediated inflammatory diseases.

2.1.4.1.3. Severity

There is disagreement over the best way to categorize psoriasis severity. A percentage of body surface area (BSA) of at least 10, a Psoriasis Area and Severity Index (PASI) score of at least 10, and a Dermatology Life Quality Index (DLQI) score of at least 10 are considered indicators of mild psoriasis. According to the same group, BSA >10, PASI >10, and DLQI >10 were considered to be indicators of moderate to severe psoriasis.

The DLQI is a 10-item assessment tool designed to gauge how various dermatological conditions affect day-to-day functioning. Higher scores indicate greater social or occupational impairment. The DLQI score is calculated using a range of 0 (minimum impairment) to 30 (maximum impairment), with each answer receiving a point value of 0–3.

The most popular method for measuring psoriasis is the PASI. It generates a single score ranging from 0 (no disease) to 72 (maximal disease) by evaluating the extent of lesions and the impacted area. However, there have been attempts to make the PASI more user-friendly for clinical use because it can be too complicated to use outside of research settings.

2.1.5. Comorbidities

Psoriasis extends beyond its skin condition. Sometimes the effects of psoriasis symptoms extend beyond the skin and negatively affect the lives of those who have it. Furthermore, co-morbidities raise the cost and treatment burden of psoriasis and should be taken into account when managing this illness.

2.1.5.1. Cardiovascular Complications

People who have psoriasis are at a 2:2 increased risk of developing cardiovascular problems. In addition, psoriasis increases a person's risk of stroke and myocardial infarction, or heart attacks. There is conjecture that psoriasis is associated with systemic inflammation, which is thought to be the cause of the "psoriatic march" and other inflammatory consequences, such as cardiovascular issues. A study measuring aortic vascular inflammation in psoriasis patients with fluorodeoxyglucose F-18 positron emission tomography computed tomography (FDG PET/CT) discovered elevated coronary artery disease indices in psoriasis patients, including total plaque burden, luminal stenosis, and high-risk plaques. Similarly, when the PASI score is reduced by 75%, it was discovered that there is an 11% decrease in aortic vascular inflammation.

2.1.5.2. Depression

28–55% of psoriasis sufferers have depression or depressive symptoms. Because psoriasis causes visible skin disfigurement, people with the condition are frequently stigmatized. Although social stigmatization is a risk factor for depression, there may be other immune system factors contributing to the higher incidence of depression seen in psoriasis patients. There is evidence that those who suffer from chronic inflammatory diseases, such as psoriasis, may also be more susceptible to depression due to elevated inflammatory signals in the body.

2.1.5.3. Type 2 Diabetes

Individuals with psoriasis have a higher likelihood of developing type 2 diabetes, with a roughly 1.5 odds ratio. A genetic study utilizing genome-wide analysis identified four shared genetic loci between psoriasis and type 2 diabetes – ACTR2, ERLIN1, TRMT112, and BECN1. These loci are linked through the inflammatory NF-κB pathway.

2.1.6. Management

Psoriasis cannot be cured, however there are numerous treatment options. For mild disease, topical medications are usually used, phototherapy for moderate disease, and systemic medications for severe disease. For acute guttate psoriasis or an acute guttate flare-up of chronic psoriasis, there is no evidence to support the efficacy of biological therapy, phototherapy, or conventional topical and systemic medications.

2.1.6.1. Topical Agents

When applied consistently for eight weeks, topical corticosteroid preparations prove to be the most efficacious agents; coal tar and retinoids were found to have minimal benefit and may even be no better than a placebo. In certain situations, very strong topical corticosteroids might be beneficial; however, they should only be used for a maximum of four weeks at a time, and only in conjunction with less strong topical treatments, if none of the other options are working.

Paricalcitol and other vitamin D analogs are better than placebos. For chronic plaque psoriasis, vitamin D is better than coal tar, and combination therapy involving both corticosteroids and vitamin D is preferable to either treatment alone.

A 2016 review discovered that corticosteroid monotherapy or dual therapy (vitamin D analogs and topical corticosteroids) was safer and more effective than topical vitamin D analogs alone for treating scalp psoriasis. Corticosteroid monotherapy seems to be a suitable course of treatment for short-term use because of its comparable safety profiles and the negligible advantage of dual therapy over monotherapy.

It has been discovered that emollients and moisturizers like mineral oil, petroleum jelly, calcipotriol, and decubal—an oil-in-water emollient—increase the removal of psoriatic plaques. When paired with phototherapy, several emollients have been demonstrated to be even more successful in removing psoriatic plaques. Some emollients, however, have no effect on the clearance of psoriasis plaque or even lessen the clearance that is achieved with phototherapy. For example, salicylic acid, an emollient, shares structural similarities with para-aminobenzoic acid, which is frequently found in sunscreen and is known to interfere with phototherapy for psoriasis. It has been discovered that using coconut oil as an emollient in psoriasis reduces the amount of plaque that is cleared by phototherapy. When applied topically to psoriatic plaques, medicated creams and ointments can help lower skin turnover, eliminate accumulated scale, lessen inflammation, and remove plaques from the affected skin. Coal tar, dithranol, corticosteroids (like desoximetasone), fluocinonide, vitamin D3 analogs (like calcipotriol), and retinoids are commonly found in ointments and creams.

When combined with steroids, vitamin D analogs may be beneficial as side effects from steroids alone are more common. Analogs of vitamin D might make it possible to use fewer steroids.

One type of topical treatment for psoriasis is balneotherapy, which entails taking daily baths in the Dead Sea. The benefit of sun exposure, particularly UVB light, is generally attributed to this four-week regimen. This has been promoted as a successful non-medication method of treating psoriasis and is also reasonably priced. It is common to see reductions in PASI scores of more than 75% as well as remission lasting several months. Mild side effects include sunburn, itchiness, folliculitis, and poikiloderma. There may also be a theoretical risk of melanoma or nonmelanoma cancer. According to certain studies, there is no long-term elevated risk of melanoma. The evidence supports the theory that the treatment is linked to a higher risk of benign forms of sun-induced skin damage, such as liver spots or actinic elastosis, but is inconclusive regarding the risk of nonmelanoma skin cancer. Psoriatic arthritis can also be effectively treated with Dead Sea balneotherapy. Balneophototherapy, which combines salt baths with ultraviolet B-light (UVB), may be more effective than UVB alone in treating chronic plaque psoriasis, according to preliminary research. Another successful treatment for psoriasis is glycerin.

2.1.6.2. UV Phototherapy

Phototherapy using sunlight has been a longstanding treatment for psoriasis, with UVB wavelengths of 311–313 nanometers being the most commonly used. Special lamps have been created for this purpose to regulate exposure time and prevent skin damage. These lamps typically come equipped with timers to ensure safe usage. The dosage of UVB light is gradually increased during treatment to acclimate the skin. While there is a slight increase in the risk of cancer with this therapy, studies have shown that narrowband UVB therapy is just as effective as PUVA therapy for psoriasis treatment. In fact, a 2013 meta-analysis concluded that there is no significant difference in efficacy between the two treatments, with narrowband UVB therapy being more convenient for patients.

One issue with clinical phototherapy is the challenge many individuals face in accessing a facility. Indoor tanning services are now widely available and could serve as an alternative option for those unable to access dermatologist-administered phototherapy. Many people already use indoor tanning as a treatment for psoriasis, with some facilities reporting that a significant percentage of their clientele seek treatment for psoriasis. However, there is a concern that tanning beds primarily emitting UVA may not be as effective in treating psoriasis, as compared to those emitting UVB. Research suggests that plaque psoriasis can respond to erythemogenic doses of both UVA and UVB, with exposure to either type leading to the reduction of psoriatic plaques. It may require more energy, however, to reach these effective doses with UVA light.

Tanning beds are not an exception to the rule that UV light therapies carry risks; the World Health Organization has classified them as carcinogens. It is well known that exposure to UV light raises the risk of melanoma as well as squamous cell and basal cell carcinomas. Younger individuals with psoriasis, especially those under 35, are more vulnerable to melanoma from UV light treatment. According to a review of studies, patients who are at risk for skin cancer should use UV light therapy with caution.

Pyrimidine dimer induction of DNA damage is one of the main mechanisms of NB-UVB. Since these dimers' formation disrupts and ends the cell cycle, phototherapy of this kind is effective in treating psoriasis. The NB-UVB-induced disruption of the cell cycle is antagonistic to the psoriasis-specific fast skin cell division. NB-UVB phototherapy treatments also effectively suppress the activity of various immune cell types present in the skin. Redness of the skin is the most frequent short-term side effect of this type of phototherapy; less frequently occurring side effects of NB-UVB phototherapy include skin that itches and blisters, eye irritation in the form of corneal or conjunctival inflammation, or cold sores brought on by the herpes simplex virus reactivating in the skin around the lips. Typically, eye protection is provided during phototherapy sessions.

Psoralen applied topically or orally combined with ultraviolet A (UVA) light exposure is known as photodynamic therapy (PUVA). Although PUVA's exact mode of action is unknown, it most likely involves UVA light activating psoralen, which prevents the abnormally fast cell formation seen in psoriatic skin. PUVA has a variety of modes of action, some of which include immune system effects on the skin. PUVA is linked to symptoms such as headache, nausea, exhaustion, burning, and itching. Squamous cell carcinoma and long-term treatment go hand in hand (but not with melanoma). Although PUVA plus acitretin was a beneficial combination therapy for moderate to severe psoriasis, acitretin use has been linked to liver damage and birth defects.

2.1.6.3. Systemic Agents

Oral medication or injectable therapies are examples of systemic therapies for psoriasis that is resistant to topical and phototherapy treatments. Regular blood and liver function tests are necessary for patients receiving systemic treatment to screen for drug toxicities. For the majority of these treatments, pregnancy must be avoided. The majority of patients who stop receiving systemic treatment for their psoriasis eventually develop new outbreaks.

Common non-biologic systemic treatments for psoriasis include methotrexate, ciclosporin, hydroxycarbamide, fumarates like dimethyl fumarate, and retinoids. Methotrexate and ciclosporin are immunosuppressive medications, while retinoids are synthetic versions of vitamin A. These treatments are often considered the first choice for psoriatic erythroderma. However, oral corticosteroids should be avoided as they can worsen psoriasis when discontinued.

Manufactured proteins known as biologics block the immune system's role in psoriasis. Biologics, as opposed to generalized immunosuppressive medications like methotrexate, target particular immune system components that are linked to psoriasis. Biologics are safe for long-term use in patients with moderate to severe plaque psoriasis based on limited long-term outcome data, and these drugs are typically well-tolerated. Nevertheless, biologics have been linked to a slight increase in the risk of infection because of their immunosuppressive effects.

According to guidelines, biologics are the third line of treatment for plaque psoriasis when topical medication, phototherapy, and non-biologic systemic treatments have not produced the desired results. Pregnancy and biologics: safety has not been evaluated. According to European guidelines, women who intend to become pregnant should refrain from taking biologics, and people who are HIV-positive or chronic carriers of the hepatitis B virus should not use anti-TNF therapies like infliximab.

A number of monoclonal antibodies target cytokines, which are messenger molecules used by cells to communicate inflammation. One of the primary inflammatory cytokines that is executed is TNF-α. To inhibit TNF-α signaling, four monoclonal antibodies (MAbs) have been developed: infliximab, adalimumab, golimumab, and certolizumab pegol. Additionally, one recombinant TNF-α decoy receptor, etanercept, has been developed. Apart from anti-TNF-α antibodies, other monoclonal antibodies have been developed against pro-inflammatory cytokines, such as ixekizumab, which inhibits the inflammatory pathway at a different point. The FDA-approved drug ustekinumab targets the same domain, p40, that is shared by IL-12 and IL-23. The US FDA approved guselkumab in 2017 to treat plaque psoriasis. Studies on the effectiveness of anti-TNF drugs for childhood psoriasis are scarce. According to one randomized control study, children's psoriasis was less severe after 12 weeks of etanercept treatment, and there were no long-term side effects.

Two drugs called alefacept and efalizumab target T cells. A monoclonal antibody called efalizumab selectively targets the LFA-1 CD11a subunit. Additionally, it inhibits the adhesion molecules on blood vessels lining endothelial cells, which draw T cells. In February 2009, efalizumab was voluntarily removed from the European and American markets. S. market by the manufacturer in June 2009 as a result of the drug's correlation with cases of progressive multifocal leukoencephalopathy. Alefacept also inhibits the molecules that T cells and dendritic cells use to communicate, and it even triggers the death of T cells by natural killer cells, which helps to reduce inflammation. Premilast can be applied as well.

Psoriasis sufferers may acquire antibodies that neutralize monoclonal antibodies. In a laboratory test, neutralization happens when an antidrug antibody stops a monoclonal antibody, like infliximab, from binding antigen. Neutralization specifically happens when the anti-drug antibody attaches to the antigen-binding site of infliximab rather than TNF-α. Infliximab stops reducing inflammation and potentially exacerbates psoriasis when it can no longer bind to tumor necrosis factor-alpha. There have been no reports of neutralizing antibodies directed against the biological drug etanercept, which is a fusion protein consisting of two TNF-α receptors. The development of immune tolerance and the innate presence of the TNF-α receptor are likely the main causes of the lack of neutralizing antibodies against etanercept. The best biologics for treating moderate to severe cases of psoriasis are infliximab, metekizumab, ixekizumab, and ranibizumab, according to compelling data. Additionally, there is some evidence in favor of the use of certolizumab, ustekinumab, guselkumab, brodalumab, and secukinumab. Anti-IL17, anti-IL12/23, anti-IL23, and anti-TNF alpha biologics have all been demonstrated to outperform conventional systemic therapies in general. Psoriasis's immune pathways include IL-22, Th9, Th17, and Th1 lymphocytes. The biologic agents mentioned earlier obstruct various aspects of these pathways.

2.1.7. Prognosis

The majority of psoriasis sufferers only have minor skin lesions that are effectively treated with topical medications. People's quality of life may be negatively impacted by severe physical discomfort and some disability, contingent on the severity and location of outbreaks. Itching and pain can make it difficult to take care of oneself or sleep. Activities such as playing sports, working in certain jobs, and taking care of family members may become challenging for people who have plaques on their hands or feet. Because flaky plaque in the hair can be mistaken for dandruff, plaque on the scalp can be especially embarrassing.

People who have psoriasis may have negative self-images and feel self-conscious about their appearance due to psychosexual worries and a fear of being rejected by others. Depression is more common in people with psoriasis, and the condition has been linked to low self-esteem. The false belief that psoriasis is contagious is a common cause of prejudice towards people who have the condition. Significant depression and social isolation can result from psychological distress; psoriasis has been linked to a high rate of suicidal thoughts. The quality of life of patients with psoriasis and other dermatological conditions can be measured using a variety of instruments. According to clinical research, people frequently have a lower quality of life. Youngsters who have psoriasis may face bullying.

Obesity, cardiovascular disease, and metabolic disorders are among the conditions linked to psoriasis. These are more common in the elderly. When it comes to concurrent conditions, nearly half of psoriasis sufferers over 65 have at least three, and two-thirds have at least two.

2.1.7.1. Cardiovascular Disease

Obesity and a variety of cardiovascular and metabolic issues have been linked to psoriasis. Individuals with psoriasis have a 27% higher chance of developing diabetes compared to those without the condition. Severe psoriasis may pose an even greater risk for diabetes compared to milder cases, especially in younger individuals. People with psoriasis or psoriatic arthritis also have a slightly elevated risk of heart disease and heart attacks. The severity and duration of psoriasis seem to be connected to the risk of cardiovascular disease. However, there is no clear evidence to suggest that psoriasis increases the risk of death from heart-related issues. Methotrexate treatment may offer some protection for heart health in individuals with psoriasis.

The odds of having hypertension are 1.58 times (i.e., 58%) higher in people with psoriasis than those without the condition; these odds are even higher with severe cases of psoriasis. A similar association was noted in people who have psoriatic arthritis—the odds of having hypertension were found to be 2.07 times (i.e., 107%) greater when compared to the odds of the general population. The link between psoriasis and hypertension is not currently understood. Mechanisms hypothesized to be involved in this relationship include the following: dysregulation of the renin–angiotensin system, elevated levels of endothelin 1 in the blood, and increased oxidative stress. The number of new cases of heart rhythm abnormality atrial fibrillation is 1.31 times (i.e., 31%) higher in people with mild psoriasis and 1.63 times (i.e., 63%) higher in people with severe psoriasis. There may be a slightly increased risk of stroke associated with psoriasis, especially in severe cases. Treating high levels of cholesterol with statins has been associated with decreased psoriasis severity, as measured by PASI score, and has also been associated with improvements in other cardiovascular disease risk factors such as markers of inflammation. These cardioprotective effects are attributed to the ability of statins to improve blood lipid profile and because of their anti-inflammatory effects. Statin use in those with psoriasis and hyperlipidemia was associated with decreased levels of high-sensitivity C-reactive protein and TNFα as well as decreased activity of the immune protein LFA-1. Compared to individuals without psoriasis, those affected by psoriasis are more likely to satisfy the criteria for metabolic syndrome.

2.1.7.2. Other Diseases

When compared to the general population, the rates of Crohn's disease and ulcerative colitis are higher by a factor of 3.8 and 7.5, respectively. Psoriasis sufferers are also more likely to develop celiac disease. The relationship between psoriasis and multiple sclerosis has been questioned and has not been thoroughly studied. Systemic therapy, especially methotrexate, is thought to be the cause of the 16% overall relative risk increase for non-skin cancer that has been linked to psoriasis. Individuals receiving long-term systemic therapy for psoriasis are 54% more likely to develop lung and bronchus cancers, 205% more likely to develop upper gastrointestinal tract cancers, 31% more likely to develop urinary tract cancers, 90% more likely to develop liver cancer, and 46% more likely to develop pancreatic cancers. Additionally, there is a higher chance of developing skin cancers other than melanoma. The risk of squamous cell carcinoma of the skin is increased by 431% and the risk of basal cell carcinoma is increased by 100% in individuals with psoriasis. Psoriasis is not linked to a higher risk of melanoma. Cancer risk is higher in those who have psoriasis.

2.2. Atopic Dermatitis

Atopic dermatitis (AD), sometimes referred to as atopic eczema, is a chronic form of skin inflammation (dermatitis). Skin that is red, swollen, cracked, and itchy is the result. The affected areas may release a clear fluid that thickens with time. Eczema, a term that generally refers to a larger group of skin conditions, is another name for AD.

20% of people will at some point in their lives experience atopic dermatitis. It affects younger children more frequently. Compared to men, women are marginally more impacted. Many people with the condition outgrow it.

Although the illness can strike anyone at any age, it usually first manifests in childhood and gets worse with time. The face, limbs, and a large portion of the body may be impacted in infants under a year old. The most commonly affected areas in children as they age are the folds of the elbows, the insides of the knees, and the neck region. The hands and feet are typically impacted in adults. Scratching the eczema-affected areas makes it worse and raises the possibility of skin infections. Atopic dermatitis patients frequently experience asthma attacks or hay fever (Johansson et al., 2004) (Figure 2.4).

Although the exact cause is unknown, it is thought to be related to genetics, immune system issues, environmental exposures, and problems with skin permeability. The other identical twin has an 85% chance of having the same condition if one of them is impacted. People who reside in arid climates and cities are more likely to be impacted. The symptoms worsen with exposure to specific chemicals or frequent hand washing. Although it might exacerbate the symptoms, emotional stress is not the root cause. The illness cannot be spread. Usually, a diagnosis is made in light of the symptoms, signs, and family history.

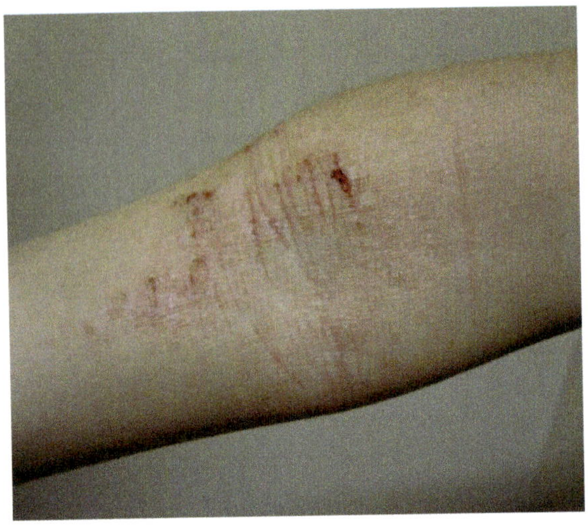

Figure 2.4. *Atopic dermatitis of the inside crease of the elbow.*

Source: By James Heilman, MD – Own work, CC BY-SA 3.0, https://commons.wikimedia.org/w/index.php?curid=10429479.

The three main components of treatment are treating the underlying skin inflammation, improving the skin barrier with skin care, and avoiding things that exacerbate the condition. Creams with added moisture help to hydrate the skin and stop AD flare-ups. Creams containing anti-inflammatory corticosteroids are applied to manage flare-ups. If other methods fail to control flare-ups, creams based on calcineurin inhibitors (tacrolimus or pimecrolimus) may be utilized. Some antihistamine medications may provide relief from itching. Seasonal variations, stress, and house dust mites are common things that aggravate it. For certain people, phototherapy might be helpful. In most cases, antibiotics—whether taken orally or topically—are ineffective unless the patient is ill or has a secondary bacterial infection. Dietary exclusion is only necessary if food allergies are suspected, and it is not beneficial for the majority of people. Systemic medications like cyclosporin, methotrexate, dupilumab, or baricitinib may be necessary in more severe cases of AD.

2.2.1. Signs and Symptoms

Signs describe the outward changes brought on by AD, while symptoms are the feelings that people with the disease experience.

The primary sign of AD is itching, which can get very bad. Some people feel pain, soreness, or burning.

Individuals with AD frequently experience dry skin, which can appear gray to those with darker skin tones. The inflammatory areas associated with AD are usually poorly defined, appearing red in individuals with light skin tones or purple or dark brown in those with darker skin tones.

Surface changes include:

- scaling cracking (fissures).
- swelling (edema).
- scratch marks (excoriation).
- bumpiness (papulation).
- oozing of clear fluid.
- thickening of the skin (lichenification) where the AD has been present for a long time.

When a child is a newborn, eczema usually begins on the cheeks, outer limbs, and body. As the child grows, eczema often settles in skin folds such as behind the knees, elbow folds, around the neck, wrists, and under the buttock folds. AD can impact any area of the body.

AD frequently affects the eyelids, where skin swelling can cause Dennie-Morgan infraorbital folds—an extra-prominent crease that forms beneath the eyelid. Infra-auricular fissures, which can cause pain, can develop beneath the ears.

Postinflammatory pigmentation, which can be either lighter or darker than normal skin, is a common result of AD inflammation. If the underlying AD is adequately treated, these marks eventually return to normal over a few months. They are not scars.

People with AD frequently have extremely itchy red, splotchy, raised lesions that form in the creases of their arms, legs, face, and neck. They also frequently have dry, scaly skin that covers their entire body, with the possible exception of the diaper area.

2.2.2. Causes

Though there is evidence pointing to immunologic, environmental, and possibly genetic factors, the exact cause of AD is unknown.

2.2.2.1. Pollution

In the US and the UK, the prevalence of atopic dermatitis has increased three to six times since 1970. Even now, the risk of developing atopic dermatitis increases dramatically for people who migrate to industrialized nations before the age of four. This risk increases even further for those who live in urbanized areas of the industrialized nation. These and other data, which strongly imply that early life industrial exposures may cause atopic dermatitis, have been clarified by recent work. Chemicals like xylene and (di)isocyanates stop skin bacteria from making lipids that belong to the ceramide-sphingolipid family. Lack of these lipids in the early years of life predicts which children will develop atopic dermatitis. Additionally, these substances directly stimulate the TRPA1 itching receptor in the skin. Beginning in 1970, there was a significant increase in the industrial production and use of xylene and diisocyanates, which increased the average exposure to these chemicals. For instance, these substances are present in some exposures that have been shown to either raise the risk of developing atopic dermatitis or exacerbate symptoms, such as car exhaust, paints, wallpaper adhesives, non-latex foam furniture, wildfires, and fabrics like spandex, polyester, and nylon.

2.2.2.2. Climate

Patients with atopic dermatitis are more likely to experience flare-ups and to have low humidity and low temperature.

2.2.2.3. Genetics

Atopy has been a family or personal history for many people with AD. Atopy is a term used to characterize people with high IgE production. These people are more likely to experience allergic rhinitis, eczema, hay fever, asthma, and urticaria. IgE levels specific to allergens or total are elevated in up to 80% of patients with atopic dermatitis.

Atopic dermatitis patients who have mutations in the gene that produces filaggrin (FLG) about 30% of the time have an increased risk of developing asthma and atopic dermatitis at an early age. Nevertheless, there is no predictive value for atopic dermatitis risk based on the expression of the filaggrin protein or breakdown products.

2.2.2.4. Hygiene Hypothesis

The hygiene hypothesis states that by aiding in the immune system's development, early exposure to specific microorganisms (such as gut flora and helminth parasites) protects against allergic diseases. In a modern, hygienic setting, this exposure is restricted, and the immune system's improper development makes it more likely for innocuous substances to cause allergies.

There is some evidence to support this theory in relation to AD. Atopic dermatitis is less common in people who were raised around dogs. Furthermore, epidemiological research backs up helminths' ability to prevent AD. Similarly, kids who drink unpasteurized milk and have poor hygiene are less likely to develop AD.

2.2.2.5. Allergens

Atopic dermatitis (AD) can occasionally be brought on by sensitization to certain foods, like milk. However, it is generally accepted that skin barrier dysfunction resulting from AD is more likely to cause skin problems than food allergies. Atopic dermatitis can occasionally be linked to both non-coeliac gluten sensitivity and celiac disease. In these cases, gluten appears to be the cause of AD because a gluten-free diet (GFD) improves symptoms. Fruit-rich diets appear to offer protection against AD, while diets high in processed foods appear to have the opposite effect.

Allergen exposure, whether from food or the surroundings, can make atopic dermatitis worse. For example, it is thought that dust mite exposure increases the chance of developing AD.

2.2.2.6. Role of Staphylococcus aureus

In people with atopic dermatitis, the bacteria *S. aureus* frequently colonizes the skin. *S. aureus* takes advantage of abnormalities in the skin barrier of people with AD to cause cytokine expression, which exacerbates the illness. However, since atopic dermatitis is not contagious, it cannot be directly brought on by a pathogenic organism. Additionally, there is not enough data to support the efficacy of anti-staphylococcal therapies in treating *S. aureus* in eczema, whether it is infected or not.

2.2.2.7. Hard Water

The presence of atopic dermatitis in children may be associated with the calcium carbonate content, or "hardness" of household drinking water. Residing in regions with hard water may contribute to the onset of AD during childhood. Nevertheless, once AD has been diagnosed, utilizing water softeners at home does not alleviate the severity of the symptoms.

2.2.3. Pathophysiology

Excessive type 2 inflammation underlies the pathophysiology of atopic dermatitis.

One important theory regarding the pathophysiology of AD is that disruption of the epidermal barrier is a major factor. Allergens can enter the skin's deeper layers through the epidermis when the epidermal barrier is disrupted. This causes innate lymphoid and epidermal inflammatory dendritic cells to become activated, which in turn draws Th2 CD4+ helper T cells to the skin. The eczematous lesions are assumed to be the result of this dysregulated Th2 inflammatory response. As a result of Th2 helper T cell activation, inflammatory cytokines such as IL-4, IL-13, and IL-31 are released, activating downstream Janus kinase (Jak) pathways. Inflammation is caused by activated Jak pathways, which also activate B cells and plasma cells. These cells then release IgE that is specific to particular antigens, which exacerbates the inflammation. The Th1, Th17, and Th22 pathways are additional CD4+ helper T-cell pathways that are hypothesized to be involved in the inflammatory process of atopic dermatitis. The phenotypic presentation of atopic dermatitis varies amongst populations, which may be explained by the fact that some CD4+ helper T-cell inflammatory pathways are more frequently activated in particular ethnic groups with AD (for instance, the Th-2 and Th-17 pathways are commonly activated in Asian people). The skin barrier is also compromised by mutations in the FLG gene, filaggrin, which adds to the pathophysiology of AD. The horny layer of the epidermis contains keratinocytes, which are epidermal skin cells that produce filaggrin. Filaggrin induces the release of lipid matrix material and moisturizing factors from skin cells, which promote keratinocyte adhesion and strengthen the skin barrier. This lipid matrix and external moisturizing factors are lost due to a loss-of-function mutation in filaggrin, which ultimately disrupts the skin barrier. The compromised skin barrier causes antigen and allergen penetration of the epidermal layer as well as transdermal water loss, which results in xerosis, or dry skin, that is frequently observed in AD. Filaggrin mutations are also linked to a reduction in the skin's naturally occurring antimicrobial peptides, which can disrupt the skin's flora and cause bacterial overgrowth, most commonly *Staphylococcus aureus* overgrowth or colonization.

The skin's release of pruritogens—molecules that cause pruritus or itching—is also linked to atopic dermatitis. Pruritogens are released into the skin by keratinocytes, mast cells, eosinophils, and T cells. This activation of Aδ and Group C nerve fibers in the epidermis and dermis results in pain and pruritus sensations. The Th2 cytokines IL-4, IL-13, IL-31, histamine, and different neuropeptides are among the pruritogens. In addition to mechanical stimulation, scratching lesions can also cause the release of pruritogens, which feeds the cycle of pruritus or itching that follows scratching. Prolonged scratching of lesions can result in prurigo nodularis, which is a condition in which the skin becomes thicker or lichenified (generalized nodules that are severely itchy).

2.2.4. Treatments

Although there is no known cure for AD, some treatments can lessen the intensity and frequency of flare-ups. Topical corticosteroids are the most often used topical treatments for AD; they help control flare-ups, while moisturizers, or emollients, help maintain control. Clinical trials frequently use a severity scale, like the SCORAD index or the Eczema Area and Severity Index, to assess the effectiveness of treatments.

2.2.4.1. Moisturisers

The goal of daily basic care is to maintain the skin's barrier function and lessen its susceptibility to allergen penetration and irritation. Those who are affected frequently state that when skin hydration improves, AD symptoms also improve. Emollients, also known as moisturizers, can lessen illness flare-ups and increase skin comfort. They can be applied topically, as bath additives, or as an alternative to soap. Although there are many different products available, lotions, creams, gels, and ointments make up the majority of leave-on treatments (from least to most greasy). Since all of the various kinds of moisturizers work just as well, consumers should select one or more products based on factors such as age, the body part being moisturized, season, climate, and personal preference. It's also possible that over-the-counter moisturizers are just as effective as non-medicated prescription moisturizers.

There is no proof that using emollient bath additives more frequently is advantageous.

2.2.4.2. Medication

2.2.4.2.1. Topical

Atopic dermatitis has been successfully treated with topical corticosteroids, which are applied directly to the skin. Modern corticosteroids, like mometasone furoate and fluticasone propionate, are safer and more effective than their predecessors. More potent corticosteroids have a greater effect than less potent ones. Additionally, they are usually safe when taken in short bursts to treat AD flare-ups. One daily application has the same effect as two or more daily applications. As first-line treatments for atopic dermatitis, topical calcineurin inhibitors like tacrolimus or pimecrolimus are also advised in addition to topical corticosteroids. In AD, using tacrolimus or pimecrolimus is both safe and effective. For mild-to-moderate AD, crisaborole, an inhibitor of PDE-4, is a safe and effective topical treatment option. The safety and effectiveness of the Janus kinase inhibitor rufolitinib are unknown.

2.2.4.2.2. Systemic

Systemic immunosuppressants like ciclosporin, methotrexate, interferon gamma-1b, mycophenolate mofetil, and azathioprine are among the oral drugs used to treat AD. Naltrexone and antidepressants can be used to manage pruritus (itchiness).

Research has not yet confirmed the effectiveness of leukotriene receptor antagonists like montelukast for treating AD, although they may hold some promise.

Some monoclonal antibodies (mAb) have a slight increase in conjunctivitis risk but are very effective in treating atopic dermatitis. The US and EU have approved the use of monoclonal antibodies dupilumab (Dupixent) and tralokinumab (Adtralza, Adbry) to treat moderate-to-severe eczema. For the treatment of moderate-to-severe AC, lebrikizumab (Ebglyss) is also approved in the EU; however, due to manufacturing issues, its approval was denied in the US.

As of January 2022, certain JAK inhibitors, including upadacitinib, also known as Rinvoq, and abrocitinib, also known as Cibinqo, have been licensed for the treatment of moderate-to-severe eczema in the US. Although these treatments have uncertain serious harms, they are among the most effective systemic treatments.

The symptoms of AD may be effectively treated with allergen immunotherapy, but there is a higher chance of unfavorable side effects. A series of injections or drops of an allergen-containing solution under the tongue make up this treatment.

Antibiotics are often used orally or topically to combat excessive *S. aureus* in the skin of individuals with AD. However, there is not enough evidence to support the effectiveness of anti-staphylococcal treatments in treating *S. aureus* in eczema, whether infected or uninfected.

2.2.4.3. Diet

Although the exact function of vitamin D in atopic dermatitis is unknown, taking supplements of the vitamin may help with symptoms. Omega 3 long-chain polyunsaturated fatty acids (LCPUFA) have no discernible advantages for expectant mothers in terms of preventing the onset of AD in their offspring. Several probiotics seem to have a positive effect, with a roughly 20% reduction in the rate of AD.

Probiotics containing multiple strains of bacteria seem to work the best. A gluten-free diet helps people with celiac disease and non-celiac gluten sensitivity manage their symptoms and stops new outbreaks.

The effectiveness of using blood-specific IgE or skin prick tests to determine dietary exclusions to improve disease severity or control is a topic of debate. Clinicians differ in their utilization of these tests for such purposes, and there is minimal evidence supporting any benefits.

2.2.4.4. Lifestyle

Medical professionals frequently advise individuals with AD to moisturize their skin by taking regular, lukewarm baths, particularly in salt water. Only patients with *Staphylococcus aureus* should benefit from diluted bleach baths, which may be beneficial for those with moderate to severe eczema.

It is often advised for individuals with AD to steer clear of woolen or scratchy fabrics, as they have the potential to incite a flare-up.

2.2.4.5. Light

During phototherapy, ultraviolet (UV) light in the broad or narrow band is exposed to the patient. It has been discovered that exposure to UV radiation has a localized immunomodulatory effect on impacted tissues; this effect may be utilized to lessen the intensity and frequency of flare-ups. Of all the phototherapies available, only narrowband (NB) ultraviolet B (UVB) exposure may be able to reduce AD symptoms and reduce itching. However, UV therapy is not risk-free because UV radiation has also been linked to some skin cancers. Due to the risk of skin cancer from prolonged use or exposure, UV phototherapy is not recommended for young adults or children.

2.2.4.6. Alternative Medicine

Although many Chinese herbal remedies are designed to treat atopic eczema, there is insufficient proof to suggest that using these remedies topically or orally will lessen the severity of eczema in either adults or children.

2.3. Acne

Acne vulgaris, another name for acne, is a chronic skin condition that develops when oil and dead skin cells block hair follicles. Pimples, oily skin, blackheads or whiteheads, and potential scarring are typical symptoms of the condition. It mostly affects the skin on the face, upper chest, and back that have a comparatively high number of oil glands. The appearance that results can cause low self-esteem, anxiety, lack of confidence, and, in severe situations, suicidal thoughts or depression (Barnes, et al., 2012).

In 80% of cases, acne susceptibility is primarily genetic. It's unclear how diet and cigarette smoking contribute to the illness, and it doesn't seem like cleanliness or sun exposure do either. Androgen hormones appear to play a role in the underlying mechanism in both sexes by inducing an increase in sebum production. Excessive growth of the skin-resident bacteria *Cutibacterium acnes* is another common factor (Figure 2.5).

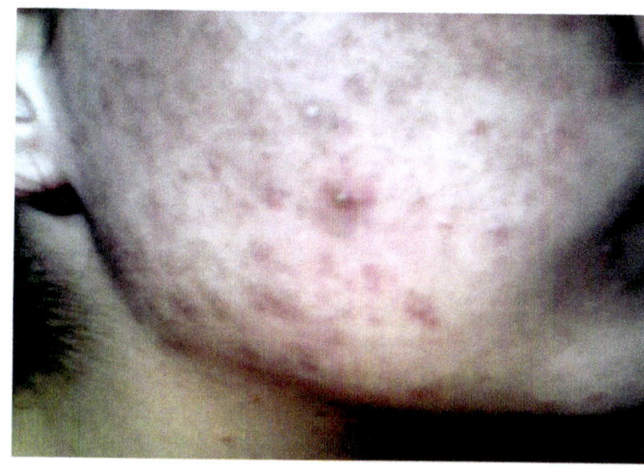

Figure 2.5. *Presentation of acne on the face of the patient.*

Source: By Diariodaj – Personal file, Public Domain, https://commons.wikimedia.org/w/index.php?curid=8106273.

There are various ways to treat acne, such as dietary adjustments, pharmaceuticals, and medical procedures. Reducing the consumption of simple carbohydrates, like sugar, may lessen the symptoms. Benzoyl peroxide, salicylic acid, and azelaic acid are common topical treatments for inflammatory skin conditions.

For the treatment of acne, formulations containing retinoids and antibiotics that are applied topically and taken orally are available. Antibiotic therapy, however, may lead to the development of antibiotic resistance. Many forms of birth control tablets shield women from acne. Because isotretinoin pills have a higher potential for side effects, doctors usually save them for cases of severe acne. Some in the medical community believe that treating acne aggressively and early on will lessen its overall long-term effects on patients.

2.3.1. Signs and Symptoms

Acne is commonly characterized by increased oily sebum production by the skin, microcomedones, comedones, papules, nodules (large papules), pustules, and frequently leaves scars. Acne manifests differently in different skin tones. Social and psychological issues could arise from it.

2.3.1.1. Scars

Inflammation in the dermis causes acne scars, affecting a large majority of individuals with acne vulgaris. The scars result from abnormal healing processes and dermal inflammation, more commonly seen in severe cases of acne but can occur with any form of acne vulgaris. The classification of acne scars is based on whether the healing response after dermal inflammation leads to an excess of collagen deposition or loss at the acne lesion site.

Atrophic acne scars, which make up about 75% of all acne scars, are the most prevalent type of acne scars due to the loss of collagen during the healing response. Atrophic acne scars can have various subtypes, such as rolling, boxcar, and ice-pick scars. Boxcar scars range in size from 1.5 to 4 mm across and are round or ovoid indented scars with sharp borders. Ice-pick scars are deep, narrow scars that penetrate the dermis and measure less than 2 mm in diameter. Rolling scars have a wave-like pattern of depth in the skin and are wider (4–5 mm across) than ice-pick and boxcar scars.

Scars that are hypertrophic are rare and are distinguished by a higher level of collagen following an aberrant healing reaction. Firm and elevated from the skin, that is how they are described. While keloid scars can form scar tissue outside of the original wound borders, hypertrophic scars stay inside the wound's original borders. Acne scars that are keloidal in nature typically affect the trunk of the body and are more common in men and people with darker skin tones.

2.3.1.2. Pigmentation

Postinflammatory hyperpigmentation (PIH) is the term for the common darkening of the skin in the vicinity of an inflamed nodular acne lesion after it resolves. The skin appears darker as a result of inflammation stimulating melanocytes, which are specialized skin cells that produce melanin pigment. PIH is more common in those with darker skin tones. The term "pigmented scar," which is often used to describe PIH, is misleading because it implies that the color change is irreversible. When the nodule is kept from getting worse, PIH is frequently preventable and eventually goes away. Untreated photoaging can, however, persist for several months, years, or even permanently if it affects deeper skin layers. Sunlight exposure, even at low levels, can cause hyperpigmentation of the skin. Using sunscreen with an SPF of 15 or higher every day helps reduce this risk. Azelaic acid, arbutin, or other whitening agents can be used to improve hyperpigmentation.

2.3.2. Causes

Apart from heredity, no clear-cut risk factors have been found for the development of acne. Stress, food, infections, and hormones are a few possible secondary contributors. Research on how smoking affects acne severity and frequency has yielded conflicting results. Acne is not linked to cleanliness or sunlight.

2.3.2.1. Genes

It seems that acne is highly heritable; 81% of population variation can be attributed to genetics. Acne is strongly inherited, as evidenced by studies done on affected twins and first-degree relatives. Given that the disease does not follow a traditional (Mendelian) inheritance pattern, acne susceptibility is most likely the result of multiple genes influencing one another. These candidate genes include variants in the IL-1 alpha, CYP1A1, and tumor necrosis factor-alpha (TNF-alpha) genes, among others. An elevated risk of acne is linked to the 308 G/A single nucleotide polymorphism variation in the TNF gene. Rare genetic conditions like Apert's syndrome can manifest as acne. XYY syndrome may be linked to severe acne.

2.3.2.2. Hormones

Hormonal activity, which happens during puberty and menstruation cycles, maybe a factor in acne development. The sex hormones known as androgens increase during puberty, causing the skin follicle glands to enlarge and produce more oily sebum. Acne is associated with the androgen hormones testosterone, dihydrotestosterone (DHT), and dehydroepiandrosterone (DHEA). Severe acne is also linked to high levels of insulin-like growth factor 1 (IGF-1) and growth hormone (GH). Acne does not develop in people with complete androgen insensitivity syndrome (CAIS) or Laron syndrome (insensitivity to GH, resulting in very low IGF-1 levels), suggesting that both androgens and IGF-1 are necessary for acne to occur.

Acne can occur in patients with medical conditions that frequently result in a high-androgen state, such as congenital adrenal hyperplasia, polycystic ovary syndrome, and tumors that secrete androgen. On the other hand, acne is rare in those who do not produce androgenic hormones or who are not sensitive to the effects of androgens. Germination can raise androgen levels, which in turn can raise the production of oily sebum. The use of anabolic steroids or testosterone replacement therapy may have a side effect of acne. Supplements for bodybuilding and nutrition sold over-the-counter frequently have anabolic steroids added to them illegally.

2.3.2.3. Infections

The role of the anaerobic bacterial species *Cutibacterium acnes* in the development of acne is not fully understood. Different strains of *C. acnes* are associated with varying levels of acne severity, with some strains found in normal skin and others in inflammatory acne. It is uncertain whether these harmful strains develop on the skin or are acquired from external sources. These strains can perpetuate the cycle of inflammation, excess oil production, and inadequate shedding of dead skin cells in acne pores. Additionally, the presence of the parasitic mite Demodex has been linked to acne development, although it is unclear if eradicating the mite improves acne symptoms.

2.3.2.4. Diet

Research has shown that high-glycemic-load diets can affect acne severity to varying degrees. Both randomized controlled trials and nonrandomized studies have indicated that adopting a lower-glycemic-load diet can help reduce acne. Some weak observational evidence suggests a link between consuming dairy milk and a higher frequency and severity of acne. This may be due to the presence of whey protein and hormones such as bovine IGF-1 and dihydrotestosterone precursors in milk, which have been found to promote the effects of insulin and IGF-1, leading to increased production of androgen hormones, sebum, and comedones. Studies have not found a significant association between consuming chocolate or salt and acne severity. Limited research has been conducted on the relationship between obesity and acne. Excessive intake of Vitamin B12 may trigger acne-like skin outbreaks or worsen existing acne.

2.3.2.5. Stress

There is limited evidence from high-quality studies to definitively prove that stress directly causes or exacerbates acne. However, some research suggests a potential link between higher stress levels and increased severity of acne in specific situations, such as hormonal fluctuations during premenstrual syndrome. Although this connection remains a topic of debate, further investigation is needed to fully understand the relationship between stress and acne.

2.3.2.6. Other

A few people notice a significant worsening of their acne when they are in hot, muggy weather; this is because certain bacteria and fungi like warm, moist conditions. We refer to this exacerbation of acne caused by climate change as tropical acne. Acne that already exists can worsen if skin follicles are mechanically blocked by helmets or chinstraps. On the other hand, technically speaking, acne that results from a mechanical obstruction is not classified as acne vulgaris; rather, it is referred to as acne mechanica, another type of acneiform eruption. Pre-existing acne, also known as acne medicamentosa, can exacerbate with some medications. Lithium, hydantoin, isoniazid, glucocorticoids, iodides, bromides, and testosterone are a few examples of such drugs. You can refer to acne medicamentosa as “steroid acne” if it is specifically brought on by anabolic-androgenic steroids.

People who are genetically predisposed to acne may experience polymorphous light eruption, which is brought on by exposure to artificial and natural UV light. *Acne aestivalis* is the name of this type of acne that is specifically brought on by prolonged exposure to UVA rays. Seasonal acne outbreaks on the upper arms, shoulder girdle, back, and chest are common in affected individuals. Usually, the breakouts happen one to three days following intense UVA radiation exposure. In contrast to other types of acne, this one does not affect the face; this could be due to the pathophysiology of polymorphous light eruption, which affects the skin in areas that have recently been exposed to high UV radiation. Throughout life, faces are usually kept uncovered, so there’s very little chance that an eruption will occur there. Research indicates that the application of a broad-spectrum sunscreen in conjunction with topical antioxidants can prevent both the breakout response of *Acne aestivalis* and polymorphous light eruption outbreaks.

2.3.3. Pathophysiology

Blockages in the skin’s hair follicles cause acne vulgaris, a chronic skin disease of the pilosebaceous unit. Acne vulgaris, which is typically associated with adolescence, can affect adults, including women who have gone through menopause. Adult female acne (AFA), characterized as a chronic inflammatory disease of the pilosebaceous unit, is the manifestation of acne vulgaris in adult females. AFA is characterized by a hormonal shift that can cause acne due to a relative increase in androgen levels during the menopausal transition, which happens when estrogen levels start to decline. Although most AFA women have normal androgen levels and few acne lesions, baseline investigations, such as an androgen testing panel, can help rule out associated comorbidities like polycystic ovarian syndrome, congenital adrenal hyperplasia, or tumors.

Four abnormal processes lead to the blockages in the skin’s hair follicles that cause acne vulgaris manifestations: increased production of oily sebum (influenced by androgens); excessive keratin deposition resulting in the formation of comedones; colonization of the follicle by the bacteria *Cutibacterium acnes*; and local release of pro-inflammatory chemicals in the skin.

The development of a plug, or microcomedone, is the first pathologic alteration. It is mainly caused by the overgrowth, multiplication, and accumulation of skin cells in the hair follicle. Dead skin cells in healthy skin rise to the surface and leave the hair follicle through its pores. The higher production of oily sebum in acne sufferers leads to the accumulation of dead skin cells. The microcomedone is created when a buildup of oily sebum and dead skin cell debris clogs the hair follicle's pore. This process is made worse by the *C. acnes* biofilm inside the hair follicle. The skin pigment melanin is exposed to air if the microcomedone is superficial within the hair follicle, which causes it to oxidize and take on a dark appearance (also referred to as an open comedo or blackhead). On the other hand, a closed comedo, or whitehead, is formed if the microcomedone is located deep within the hair follicle.

Dihydrotestosterone is the primary hormone that stimulates the production of oily sebum in the skin. Another hormone called DHEA-S also plays a role in increasing sebaceous gland activity. During adrenarche, a stage of puberty, the adrenal glands release higher levels of DHEA-S, leading to an increase in sebum production. This creates an environment rich in sebum, allowing the skin bacterium *C. acnes* to thrive and potentially cause inflammation in and around the hair follicle by activating the immune system. *C. acnes* contributes to acne by promoting the production of inflammatory chemicals like IL-1α, IL-8, TNF-α, and LTB4, with IL-1α being crucial for comedo formation.

The primary mechanism of acne-related skin inflammation is the ability of *C. acnes* to bind to and activate toll-like receptors (TLRs), a class of immune system receptors that includes TLR2 and TLR4. TLR2 and TLR4 activation caused by C. Increased secretion of TNF-α, IL-8, and IL-1α is a result of acne. Th1 cells, neutrophils, and macrophages are among the immune cells drawn to the hair follicle by the release of these inflammatory signals. Comedo development is fueled by increased skin cell activity and reproduction, which is stimulated by IL-1α. Additionally, when TLR2 and TLR4 bind, sebaceous gland cells release more antimicrobial peptides like HBD1 and HBD2. *C. acnes* contributes to skin inflammation by changing the fatty composition of oily sebum. The oxidation of squalene by *C. acnes* is a key factor in this process, as it activates NF-κB and raises IL-1α levels. Additionally, squalene oxidation boosts 5-lipoxygenase activity, which converts arachidonic acid to leukotriene B4 and promotes skin inflammation through interaction with PPARα. This leads to the activation of AP-1 and NF-κB, attracting inflammatory T cells. The conversion of sebum triglycerides to pro-inflammatory free fatty acids by *C. acnes* through lipase secretion further reinforces its inflammatory effects, as these acids stimulate the production of cathelicidin, HBD1, and HBD2, leading to more inflammation. The activation of AP-1 in the inflammatory cascade can result in the development of inflammatory acne lesions such as papules, pustules, and nodules. In severe cases, the follicle may rupture into the deeper skin layers, leading to the formation of deep nodules. This process also triggers matrix metalloproteinases that contribute to tissue damage and scarring.

In addition to *C. acnes*, the bacterium *Staphylococcus epidermidis* (*S. epidermidis*) also plays a role in the development of acne vulgaris. The coexistence of S. epidermidis and *C. acnes* leads to the formation of biofilms, which obstruct the hair follicles and pores, leading to an anaerobic environment beneath the skin. This promotes the growth of both *C. acnes* and *S. epidermidis*. The overgrowth of *C. acnes* results in the formation of biofilms and a matrix that makes acne treatment even more challenging.

2.3.4. Diagnosis

The clinical judgment of a medical professional is used to diagnose acne vulgaris. When diagnosing someone with suspected acne, a thorough medical history regarding any family history of acne, a review of prescribed medications, and any indications of excessive androgen hormone, cortisol, or growth hormone production should all be taken into consideration. To diagnose acne, comedones (blackheads and whiteheads) must be visible. If they were absent, a different skin condition might be suggested by an appearance similar to acne. Under a microscope, microcomedones—the precursors to blackheads and whiteheads—can be seen that are invisible to the unaided eye when examining the skin. Numerous characteristics could suggest that a person's acne vulgaris is hormonally sensitive. The onset of acne between the ages of 20 and 30, its worsening the week before a woman's period, the prevalence of acne lesions over the jawline and chin, and the presence of inflammatory or nodular acne lesions are historical and physical indicators that may point to hormone-sensitive acne. There are several scales available to assess the severity of acne vulgaris, but there is still debate regarding the best one to use for diagnosis. Using photos, Cook's acne grading scale assigns a number between 0 and 8, with higher numbers denoting more severe acne. This scale was the first to evaluate the severity of acne using a standardized photographic protocol; it has undergone multiple revisions since it was first developed in 1979. By counting and classifying acne lesions on the face, back, and chest, the Leeds acne grading technique determines whether the lesions are inflammatory or not. Leeds scores go from 0 (least severe) to 10 (most severe), with a maximum score of 12 on modified scales. The Pillsbury acne grading system ranges from grade 1 (the least severe) to grade 4 (the most severe), depending on the severity of the acne.

2.3.4.1. Differential Diagnosis

Acneiform eruptions are a group of skin conditions that can resemble acne vulgaris. These ailments include, among others, rosacea, folliculitis, keratosis pilaris, milia, perioral dermatitis, angiofibromas, and epidermal cysts. One element that might aid in differentiating between these disorders is age. Skin conditions like keratosis pilaris and perioral dermatitis can resemble acne in appearance but are more common in children. Rosacea typically affects older adults more frequently. Additionally, facial redness that is brought on by heat, alcohol, or spicy food is more indicative of rosacea. Medical professionals can distinguish acne from other skin disorders that share similarities in appearance when comedones are present. Acne vulgaris can resemble chloracne and occupational acne caused by exposure to specific chemicals and industrial compounds.

2.3.5. Management

There are numerous approaches to treating acne. These consist of alpha hydroxy acid, antibiotics, antiseborrheic drugs, nicotinamide, retinoids, azelaic acid, benzoyl peroxide, hormonal therapies, keratolytic soaps, and salicylic acid. Treatments for acne operate in at least four different ways, such as decreasing inflammation, influencing hormones, and eliminating *C. acnes*, and restoring normal skin cell turnover and pore-level sebum production to avoid clogging. Topical therapies like benzoyl peroxide, retinoids, and antibiotics are common treatments. Systemic therapies include hormonal agents, antibiotics, and oral retinoids.

Benzoyl peroxide, topical or oral antibiotics, and topical retinoids are suggested treatments for acne vulgaris in the first instance. Due to their high cost and paucity of evidence, procedures like light therapy and laser therapy are not recommended as first-line treatments; instead, they are usually used as adjuncts.

The benefits of blue light therapy are unclear. The early phases of comedo formation are the focus of acne medications, which are typically ineffective for visible skin lesions. Acne usually clears up eight to 12 weeks after the start of treatment.

Acne is frequently thought of as a temporary condition, and some people even expect it to go away after puberty. This misconception may result in issues with long-term treatment adherence or a dependence on self-management. People can have a better understanding of what to expect from treatments if the long-term nature of the condition is communicated and they have better access to trustworthy information about acne.

2.3.5.1. Skin Care

People with acne are generally advised not to wash their affected skin more than twice a day. Applying a moisturizer devoid of fragrances to skin that is sensitive and prone to acne can potentially alleviate irritation. When using acne medications, skin irritation usually peaks two weeks after starting and then gradually gets better. Dermatologists advise using cosmetics that are marked as non-comedogenic, oil-free, and non-pore-clogging.

Patients with acne vulgaris, including those with oily skin, should prioritize moisturizing to help maintain the skin's moisture barrier. Skin barrier dysfunction can worsen acne symptoms, making it important to use moisturizers, especially those containing ceramides. These moisturizers can help alleviate dry skin and irritation often caused by acne treatments. Research indicates that ceramide-containing moisturizers play a vital role in skin care, improving adherence to acne therapy and enhancing the effectiveness of existing treatments. In a study with acne patients, the vast majority of patients had no cutaneous adverse events over the course of the study when they applied a micronized 0.05% tretinoin gel in the evening after using a 1.2% clindamycin phosphate/2.5% benzoyl peroxide gel in the morning. The results showed that the use of ceramide cleanser and ceramide moisturizing cream improved adherence to the regimen, produced favorable tolerability, and did not interfere with the effectiveness of the treatment. The scientific community generally agrees that protecting the acidic mantle and its barrier functions is crucial. For the skin surface to remain in its ideal, healthy state, a pH between 4.5 and 5.5 is thus necessary to maintain.

2.3.5.2. Diet

Rarely are diet/nutrition and dermatological conditions shown to be causally related. Rather, correlations between diet and outcomes, such as the severity of a patient's disease and the number of conditions they experience, have been discovered, some of which are compelling. There is growing evidence that medical nutrition therapy can help lessen the severity and occurrence of skin conditions like acne. Acne and diets with a high glycemic index have been linked by researchers. To treat acne, dermatologists also advise against eating a diet high in simple sugars. As of 2014, there is not enough data to support the use of milk restriction in this way.

2.3.5.3. Medications

2.3.5.3.1. Benzoyl Peroxide

Because of its efficiency and low risk of side effects, benzoyl peroxide (BPO) is the first choice for treating mild to moderate acne. (mainly skin irritation). Benzoyl peroxide oxidizes the proteins of *C. acnes* in the skin follicle by producing benzoic acid and oxygen-free radicals. These free radicals most likely disrupt the bacterium's capacity to metabolize and produce proteins. Benzoyl peroxide also inhibits inflammation and breaks down comedones with a mild effectiveness. Benzoyl peroxide is combined with a topical antibiotic or retinoid in combination products, such as benzoyl peroxide/clindamycin and benzoyl peroxide/adapalene. Benzoyl peroxide applied topically works well to treat acne.

Increased skin photosensitivity, dryness, redness, and sporadic peeling are among the side effects. Using sunscreen is frequently suggested while receiving treatment to avoid sunburn. While benzoyl peroxide comes with fewer side effects, lower concentrations work just as well to treat acne as higher concentrations. Benzoyl peroxide does not seem to cause bacterial antibiotic resistance, in contrast to antibiotics.

2.3.5.3.2. Retinoids

Retinoids are anti-inflammatory drugs that also balance out the life cycle of follicle cells and lower sebum production. They and vitamin A share structural similarities. Research indicates that primary care physicians and dermatologists underprescribe them for acne. It seems that the retinoid affects the follicle lining cells' life cycle. This lessens the possibility of a blockage caused by the buildup of skin cells inside the hair follicle. They are a first-line treatment for acne, particularly for those with darker skin tones. It is well known that retinoid treatment causes postinflammatory hyperpigmentation to improve more quickly.

Adapalene, retinol, retinaldehyde, isotretinoin, tazarotene, trifarotene, and tretinoin are examples of topical retinoids. They can seriously irritate the skin and frequently trigger the first bout of acne and facial flushing. Retinoids are generally advised for use at night because they make the skin more sensitive to sunlight. Of all the topical retinoids, tretinoin is the least costly and causes the most skin irritation; adapalene, on the other hand, causes the least irritation but is much more expensive. Benzoyl peroxide and tretinoin are not compatible in most formulations. Although it costs more and is the most effective topical retinoid, tazarotene is typically not as well tolerated. The FDA approved a tazarotene lotion formulation in 2019 that was marketed as a less irritating option. A similar but milder form of vitamin A is retinol, which is found in many over-the-counter moisturizers and other topical products.

For moderate acne that is resistant to other treatments, as well as for severe nodular acne, isotretinoin is an oral retinoid that works wonders. Usually, one to two months of use is sufficient to observe results. After a course of oral isotretinoin for four to six months, acne usually goes away completely or gets much better. Approximately 80% of patients report improvement after just one round of treatment, and over 50% report total remission. A second course is needed for about 20% of patients, but 80% of those patients report improvement, meaning the cumulative efficacy rate is 96%.

Isotretinoin side effects, such as depression, suicidality, and anemia, are a source of concern. Some of these claims are not well-supported by the available data. Certain studies have found that isotretinoin is more effective at reducing acne lesions than either antibiotics or placebos. A 2018 review, however, comparing inflammatory lesions following isotretinoin or antibiotic treatment, found no differences. When using isotretinoin, the frequency of adverse events was roughly twice as high; however, the majority of these events were connected to dryness. Incontrovertibly, no elevated risk of depression or suicide was discovered.

Due to its known negative effects during pregnancy, isotretinoin use in women of childbearing age is strictly regulated by medical authorities. Such a woman must use an effective method of birth control and have a confirmed negative pregnancy test to be eligible for isotretinoin. The iPLEDGE program was launched in the US in 2008 to discourage the use of isotretinoin while pregnant. The woman who signs the iPledge pledge must take two negative pregnancy tests and use two different forms of birth control for at least one month before the start of isotretinoin therapy and one month thereafter. The ongoing non-adherence to contraception raises questions about the efficacy of the iPledge program.

2.3.5.3.3. Antibiotics

Antibiotics can be taken orally or applied topically to treat acne. They function by eliminating *C.acnes* as well as lessening inflammation. Many recommendations urge medical professionals to lower the amount of oral antibiotic prescriptions they write, but many do not abide by these recommendations. For acne, oral antibiotics are still the most often recommended systemic treatment. Antibiotic-resistant *C.acnes* has become more common as a result of the widespread overuse of broad-spectrum antibiotics for acne. *C. acnes* strains found throughout the world, particularly the widely used macrolide and tetracycline antibiotics (like doxycycline) (e.g., topical erythromycin). Antibiotics are therefore preferred by dermatologists to be used in combination therapy rather than on their own.

Often used antibiotics include clindamycin, erythromycin, metronidazole, sulfacetamide, and tetracyclines (e.g., doxycycline or minocycline), which can be applied topically or taken orally. A low-dose of 40 milligrams of doxycycline taken daily seems to be just as effective as 100 milligrams but with fewer adverse effects on the gastrointestinal tract. Nevertheless, the FDA has not approved the use of low-dose doxycycline to treat acne. For mild to moderately severe acne, topical antibiotics are usually used. Oral antibiotics cause inflammatory acne lesions to resolve more quickly than topical treatments and are typically more effective than topical antibiotics. The Global Alliance to Improve Outcomes in Acne advises against using oral and topical antibiotics concurrently.

Oral antibiotic courses should not be used for longer than three months as they are linked to the emergence of antibiotic resistance and offer no discernible advantages over shorter courses. To reduce the chance of *C. acnes* developing antibiotic resistance, it is advised to use benzoyl peroxide or a retinoid concurrently with long-term oral antibiotics that last longer than three months.

When applied topically, the antibiotic dapsone effectively treats inflammatory acne. Because of its higher price and unclear superiority over other antibiotics, it is typically not the first choice. For women or those with sensitive skin or darker skin tones, topical dapsone therapy may be the recommended course of action. Because of the possibility of resulting in yellow-orange skin discoloration when combined with benzoyl peroxide, it is not advised to use this combination. Although minocycline works well to treat acne, it is not recommended as a first-line antibiotic because there is insufficient proof that it is superior to other therapies and because there are questions regarding its safety about other tetracyclines.

The FDA has approved the use of seromycin, the most recent oral antibiotic created especially for the treatment of acne, in patients nine years of age and older for the management of moderate to severe inflammatory acne. It is a narrow-spectrum tetracycline antibiotic with a low propensity to cause antibiotic resistance and the required antibacterial activity against pathogens associated with acne vulgaris.

Sarecycline showed clinical efficacy in reducing inflammatory acne lesions as early as three weeks and truncal acne, or acne on the back and chest, in clinical trials.

2.4. Hidradenitis suppurativa

Inflammatory and swollen lumps are a common feature of the long-term dermatological condition hidradenitis suppurativa (HS) (Figure 2.6). These usually hurt and burst, releasing pus or liquid. The groin, buttocks, perineum, underarms, and under breasts are the regions most frequently impacted. Even after healing, scar tissue persists. Many daily activities, such as walking, hugging, moving, and sitting down, may be severely restricted by HS. Patients with lesions in the sacral, gluteal, perineal, femoral, groin, or genital regions may have difficulty sitting, and prolonged sitting can exacerbate their skin conditions.

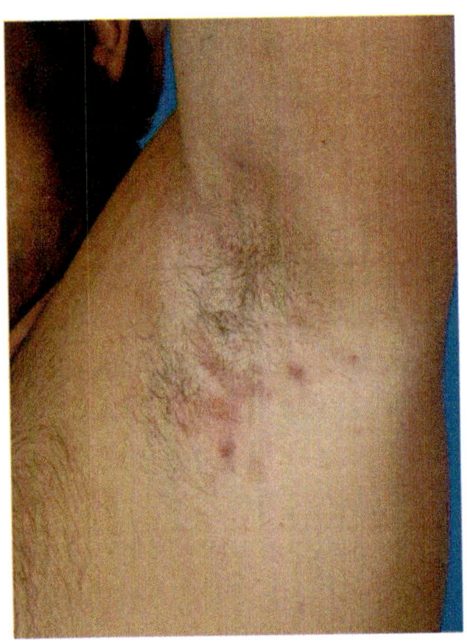

Figure 2.6. *Hidradenitis suppurativa (HS).*

Source: By Ziyad Alharbi†Email author, Jens Kauczok† and Norbert Pallua – https://bmcdermatol.biomedcentral.com/articles/10.1186/1471-5945-12-9, CC BY 2.5, https://commons.wikimedia.org/w/index.php?curid=51362653.

Although the precise cause is frequently unknown, a mix of environmental and genetic factors are thought to be involved. A family member with the illness affects about one-third of those who have it. The risk factors for obesity and smoking are also present. Neither bad personal hygiene nor deodorant use nor infections are the cause of the condition. Rather, it is thought to be brought on by an obstruction of the hair follicles, with the nearby apocrine sweat glands being heavily involved in this obstruction. There's a chance that the sweat glands themselves are inflamed. The symptoms are used to make a diagnosis (Yang et al, 2018).

2.4.1. History and Physical

The diagnosis of hidradenitis suppurativa is frequently delayed by seven years on average because of its similarities to other conditions. Identification of distinctive morphological characteristics (nodules, tunnels, and scars), location (intertriginous areas), and chronicity are all necessary for a clinical diagnosis. Prodromal symptoms, which can occur 12 to 48 hours before the lesion appearance, include burning, stinging, pain, pruritus, warmth, and hyperhidrosis in half of the patients. Menstruation, weight gain, stress, hormonal shifts, extreme heat, and sweating are examples of triggers. Unless there is an advanced illness or a secondary infection, patients are typically well-looking and afebrile when they are presented.

Primary hidradenitis suppurativa lesions are characterized by deep-seated nodules that last for days to months. These lesions are usually 0.5–2 cm in size. The lesions may have serosanguinous discharge, which can turn purulent and malodorous, and is frequently misdiagnosed as furuncles or boils. In contrast to furuncles, these nodules can form intercommunicating tunnels and tracts that have the potential to ulcerate or drain. They are also deep, recurrent, and rupture-prone. These tracts can be seen with an ultrasound examination or an injection of lidocaine. In advanced stages, there may be open comedones called tombstone comedones and thick, fibrotic scars and plaques that distort architecture.

The most typical site of hidradenitis suppurativa lesions is the axilla. Inguinal, inner thigh, perianal, perineal, inframammary, gluteal, pubic, scrotal, vulvar, and trunk regions are among the other frequently affected areas. Less commonly affected areas include the scalp and retroauricular areas. Pertinent history includes recurrent lesions and intermittent improvement, usually starting during puberty and continuing into young adulthood. Confirmation of the diagnosis is aided by a family history of a related condition.

Once the history and physical exam are complete, the Hurley staging system may be used to classify the disease. This system categorizes lesions as follows:

- Hurley Stage I: Abscesses lack tunnels and scars.
- Hurley Stage II: Recurrent abscesses have tunnels and scars, and the lesions may be single or multiple but widely separated.
- Hurley Stage III: Lesions diffusely involve the skin, i.e., multiple interconnected sinus tracts are present, and abscesses occupy large areas, leaving little to no uninvolved skin.

The follicular occlusion tetrad includes pilonidal sinus, acne conglobata, and dissecting scalp cellulitis in addition to hidradenitis suppurativa. When hidradenitis suppurativa is diagnosed, it is important to look for potential co-occurring conditions. During assessment, clinicians should also take into account associations with spondyloarthropathy, hypertension, diabetes mellitus, dyslipidemia, metabolic syndrome, and inflammatory bowel disease (especially Crohn's disease). Particular attention should also be paid to syndromes such as pyogenic arthritis, pyoderma gangrenosum, acne, suppurative hidradenitis (PAPASH) and pyoderma gangrenosum, acne suppurative hidradenitis (PASH), which may be linked to a mutation in the PSTPIP1 gene.

2.4.2. Causes

In recent times, there has been significant disagreement among experts regarding the exact cause of hidradenitis suppurativa. On the other hand, the illness most likely has a combination of environmental and genetic roots. In particular, an immune-mediated pathology has been postulated, while the possibility of environmental influences still exists.

Lesions will occur in any areas with hair follicles, and/or sweat glands, although areas such as the axilla, groin, and perineal region are more commonly involved. This theory includes most of these potential indicators:

- Post-pubescent individuals.
- Blocked hair follicles or blocked apocrine sweat glands.
- Excessive sweating.
- Androgen dysfunction.
- Genetic disorders that alter cell structure.

According to the disease's historical understanding, inflammation, pain, and an enlarged lesion are caused by malfunctioning apocrine glands or dysfunctional hair follicles that may be caused by a blocked gland.

2.4.2.1. Triggering Factors

Several triggering factors should be taken into consideration:

- Obesity is an exacerbating rather than a triggering factor, through mechanical irritation, occlusion, and skin maceration.
- Tight clothing, and clothing made of heavy, nonbreathable materials
- Deodorants, depilation products, and shaving of the affected area – their association with HS is still an ongoing debate among researchers.
- Drugs, in particular oral contraceptive pills, cigarette smoking, and lithium.
- Hot and especially humid climates.
- Stress

2.4.2.2. Predisposing Factors

- Genetic factors: an autosomal dominant inheritance pattern has been proposed.
- Endocrine factors: sex hormones, especially an excess of androgens, are thought to be involved, although the apocrine glands are not sensitive to these hormones. Women often have outbreaks before their menstrual period and after pregnancy; HS severity usually decreases during pregnancy and after menopause.

2.4.3. Treatment/Management

Relief of lesion-related symptoms (such as pain), a decrease in the frequency of recurrences and the formation of new lesions, and the prevention of disease and comorbidity progression are the main objectives of treatment for hidradenitis suppurativa. The majority of treatment approaches are determined by consensus and expert opinion because there have been few comparative studies.

Monitoring the frequency, severity, extent, and morphology of lesions is part of the assessment of treatment response. Validated instruments are also used to assess changes in quality of life and the assessment of the progression to associated comorbidities. The severity of the condition and its response to treatment are assessed using a variety of scales and scoring systems, such as the Sartorius score, the International Hidradenitis Suppurativa Severity Scoring System, the Hidradenitis Suppurativa Physician Global Assessment, and the Hidradenitis Suppurativa Core Outcome Set International Collaboration.

Regardless of the stage of the disease, comorbidities that are causing or exacerbating hidradenitis suppurativa should be addressed in the course of treatment. Given that obesity and smoking are linked to more severe disease progression, counseling, and support for weight loss and quitting are essential. It's also critical to minimize skin trauma, which can be done by staying away from adhesive dressings, harsh cleaning agents, and tight clothing. Draining lesions can be kept from becoming more irritated by using nonocclusive dressings or soft dressings with clear petroleum jelly.

Patients suffering from hidradenitis suppurativa should receive comprehensive education regarding the nature of their condition, wound care, and pain management. Plans for individualized pain management need to take inpatient admissions into consideration. Both inflammatory and noninflammatory sources, such as scarring (which causes tensile pain), keloids, abscesses, open ulcerations, sinus tracts, frictional pain, lymphedema, anal fissures, and arthritis, can cause pain associated with hidradenitis suppurativa. Depending on the severity of the condition and the type of pain, treatments may involve topical medications like lidocaine, systemic nonsteroidal anti-inflammatory drugs, acetaminophen, atypical anticonvulsants like gabapentin or pregabalin, and serotonin-norepinephrine reuptake inhibitors. Those who have co-occurring depression may benefit most from duloxetine.

The psychosocial component of treatment for hidradenitis suppurativa is a vital but frequently disregarded component. Patients' quality of life is negatively impacted by pain, drainage, odor, and involvement of sensitive areas. People who have this illness may become socially isolated, struggle to find work because they miss work during flare-ups, and have increased dysfunction in relationships or in their sexual lives. Reassurance that this illness is not spread by others or the consequence of bad hygiene may be beneficial. Support groups and counseling are frequently helpful supplements to treatment plans. Acute symptomatic lesions may be treated with topical resorcinol, punch debridement, and intralesional corticosteroid injection (usually triamcinolone). It is not advised to make an incision and drain.

The first line of treatment for early, uncomplicated disease is topical antibiotics. The most successful form of treatment has been shown to be topical clindamycin, which can be used as an appropriate oral therapy adjunct. Metformin, antiandrogens, such as spironolactone, and oral tetracycline antibiotics, such as doxycycline, can be used to treat Hurley stage I disease in the absence of skin tunneling or scarring. If the patient responds well to the treatment after two to three months, tetracyclines should be stopped and other medications should be continued. In the event that there is improvement but it is not sufficient, another tetracycline trial ought to be started. If, after two to three months on the same regimen or a second tetracycline trial, the clinical response is still not satisfactory, switching to a combination of oral clindamycin and rifampin, dapsone, or acitretin may be considered.

Hurley stages II and III are initially treated similarly to Hurley stage I disease. While planning a therapeutic intervention, potential side effects must be taken into account. Before beginning a regimen of these medications, patients should be informed of their side effects. If the patient does not improve after two to three months of initial therapy, does not improve after two to three months of a second therapeutic trial, or if the Hurley stage I case is not responding to treatment, surgery or biologic therapy should be considered.

Adalimumab is the recommended biologic agent for hidradenitis suppurativa because of its strong research support. As substitutes, consider acitretin, infliximab, or secukinumab. Treating this condition with etanercept has not proven to be effective. If, after three to four months of biologic therapy, the patient shows progressive improvement, the treatment has to be continued. Metformin and oral antiandrogens may be added as adjuvants.

If the response is not satisfactory, it is recommended to switch to a different class of biologics and then reevaluate in three to four months for further treatment or to explore other options. For severe, refractory hidradenitis suppurativa, surgical management and adjunctive therapies such as intravenous ertapenem may be considered. As an alternative to stop the inflammatory process, pulsed light therapy and localized laser therapy might be available.

To eliminate areas of active disease and reduce complications, surgical management can be pursued at any stage; however, it must be used in conjunction with medical therapy. Antibiotics, corticosteroids (such as prednisone or glucocorticoids), and anti-inflammatory drugs (such as biologics or cyclosporine) should all be part of preoperative care. Wide excision, deroofing, and punch debridement are examples of local procedures. A 5- to 7-mm circular punch biopsy tool is used in punch debridement to remove an inflamed lesion. After achieving hemostasis, the lesion is allowed to heal secondary intentionally with a petrolatum dressing. Deroofing is the process of entering skin tunnels and using a carbon dioxide laser or scissors to gradually remove the roofs.

To debride a lesion until only the subcutaneous fat is left, a wide excision with reconstruction may be carried out. The repair strategy may involve primary closure or a larger flap, contingent on the anatomic location. Grafting is an additional option that entails debriding the afflicted subepidermal skin and using the epidermis to recycle as a skin graft. Additionally, negative pressure wound therapy has been applied. Postoperatively, it is advised to use petroleum-based nonadherent dressings to prevent friction. When using these dressings, patients should be informed about the possibility of bleeding, infection, or developing a new illness.

Neodymium-doped yttrium aluminum garnet (Nd:YAG) laser therapy, bimekizumab, anakinra, ustekinumab, cyclosporine, tacrolimus, apremilast, zinc, photodynamic therapy, golimumab, risankizumab, liraglutide, microwave ablation (not currently recommended), cryoinsufflation, injections of botulinum toxin, and ionizing radiation are some other treatments that may be taken into consideration.

2.4.4. Prognosis

Fistulae left unnoticed, undiagnosed, or untreated in stage III disease, according to Hurley's staging system, rarely result in the development of squamous cell carcinoma in the anus or other affected areas. Amyloidosis, arthropathy, anemia, and multilocalized infections are possible additional stage III chronic sequelae. Sepsis has been known to result from Stage III complications, although clinical data are still ambiguous.

2.4.4.1. Potential Complications

- Contractures and reduced mobility of the lower limbs and axillae due to fibrosis and scarring occur. Severe lymphedema may develop in the lower limbs.
- Local and systemic infections (meningitis, bronchitis, pneumonia, etc.), are seen, which may even progress to sepsis.
- higher risk for diabetes mellitus.
- Interstitial keratitis.
- Anal, rectal, or urethral fistulae.
- Normochromic or hypochromic anemia.
- People with HS may be at increased risk for autoimmune disorders including ankylosing spondylitis, rheumatoid arthritis, and psoriatic arthritis.
- Squamous cell carcinoma has been found on rare occasions in chronic hidradenitis suppurativa of the anogenital region. The mean time to the onset of this type of lesion is 10 years or more and the tumors are usually highly aggressive.
- Tumors of the lung and oral cavity, and liver cancer.
- Hypoproteinemia and amyloidosis, which can lead to kidney failure and death.
- Seronegative and usually asymmetric arthropathy: periarticular arthritis, polyarthritis/polyarthralgia syndrome.

2.4.4.2. Impact on Mental Health

In addition to being a painful and socially isolating illness, HS has a detrimental effect on mental health. 12% of HS patients have anxiety, and 21% have depression. Additionally, there is a higher chance of suicide attempts in those with HS (Barnes et al., 2012).

A Closer Look

Novel Insights into the Role of S100A8/A9 in Skin Biology

The non-ubiquitous cytoplasmic Ca^{2+}-binding proteins S100A8 (calgranulin A, also known as migration inhibitory factor-related protein 8; MRP-8) and S100A9 (calgranulin B, also known as MRP-14) are members of a multigenic family. Their designation as damage associated molecular pattern molecules (DAMPs), their differential expression in chronic inflammatory diseases, and their link to cancer have all sparked significant interest in them during the past few years. Patients with (auto)immune diseases such as type 1 diabetes, cystic fibrosis, chronic bronchitis, rheumatoid arthritis, multiple sclerosis, sepsis, autoimmune colitis, and psoriasis have elevated plasma levels of S100A8 and S100A9, which are expressed and specifically released from activated phagocytes.

Although S100A8 and S100A9 preferentially form heteromeric protein complexes known as S100A8/A9 or calprotectin, each S100 protein has also been shown to have a different function. Unlike other related cells like lymphocytes, basophils, and eosinophils, constitutive expression of S100A8/A9 is primarily limited to myeloid cells like neutrophils, monocytes, macrophages, and certain other myeloid cells. About 30–60% of all cytosolic proteins in neutrophils and 1–2% of all cytosolic proteins in monocytes are composed of S100A8/A9. Tight regulation of S100A8/A9 expression occurs during myeloid differentiation. It was recently shown that the production of S100A8/A9 was necessary for the induction of autoreactive $CD8^+$ T cells and the development of systemic autoimmunity in a mouse autoimmune model. In contrast, Cd40lg× $S100A9^{-/-}$ mice displayed a delayed onset and significantly reduced severity of dermatitis, while Cd40lg-transgenic mice developed autoimmune dermatitis and overt disease. S100A8/A9 expression was shown to be necessary for the functional development of autoreactive $CD8^+$ T cells in adoptive cell transfer experiments.

Because S100A8/A9 performs both intracellular and extracellular roles, its actions are complex. Its function in the spread of inflammation and the upregulation of proinflammatory cytokines has been demonstrated earlier. Toll-like receptor 4 (TLR4) or the receptor for advanced glycation end-products (RAGE) mediates some of the extracellular functions. Other research, though, also reveals anti-inflammatory properties.

Additionally, tumors of epithelial origin and non-myeloid cells like skin cells can be made to express S100A8 and S100A9. Taken together, these findings suggest that S100A8 and S100A9 have a part in the pathophysiology of some skin conditions.

S100A8/A9 play important roles in non-myeloid cells

While the current focus of attention is on the function of S100A8/A9 in inflammatory cells, there is mounting evidence that these S100 proteins play a significant role in non-myeloid cells as well. It has previously been shown that in apolipoprotein E-deficient ($ApoE^{-/-}$) mice, whole-body S100a9 deficiency reduces atherosclerosis by reducing arterial macrophage accumulation. The effects of whole-body S100A9 deficiency were thought to be mediated by myeloid-derived S100A8/A9 due to the abundance of this protein in myeloid cells relative to non-myeloid cells. To investigate this theory, bone marrow from S100a9$^{-/-}$ mice or wild-type littermate controls was transplanted into low-density lipoprotein receptor-deficient (Ldlr$^{-/-}$) mice, who were subsequently given a high-fat diet for 20 weeks. On the other hand, atherosclerotic lesions, artery macrophage or neutrophil accumulation, were not lessened by bone marrow S100A9 deficiency. These findings may be explained by S100A8/A9 playing a bigger role in non-myeloid cells than previously thought. Consequently, S100A8/A9 are thought to have pro-atherosclerotic effects in endothelial and vascular smooth muscle cells, where they are expressed. The relative contributions of distinct cell types at particular stages of the disease progression may determine how S100A8/A9-deficiency affects different pathologies and diseases. These new results call into question the function of S100A8/A9, which is expressed in epithelial cells, in the healing of wounds and other skin conditions.

S100A8 and S100A9 expression in psoriasis

Several studies have shown the important role of S100A8/A9 in psoriasis. Both proteins were found in the skin lesions of psoriasis patients, with low expression in healthy skin from the same individuals. Elevated levels of S100A8/A9 in the blood of psoriatic patients are associated with disease activity, indicating a possible role for these proteins in the condition. The PSORS4 locus on chromosome 1q21, near the S100 gene cluster which includes S100a8 and S100a9 genes, has been linked to psoriasis susceptibility. This region also contains genes for epidermal differentiation markers such as profilaggrin and involucrin.

Two transgenic mouse models of psoriasis demonstrated that the expression of the S100a8 and S100a9 genes is an early molecular event in the development of psoriasis. The induction of S100a8/a9 gene expression occurs before any histological alterations or cytokine deregulation is observed. These models suggest that Jun proteins (JunB and c-Jun) or STAT3 may play a role in controlling S100A8/A9 expression during skin inflammation.

Another possible explanation for the elevated expression of S100A8/A9 in psoriatic skin is high concentrations of either IL-22 or epithelium-derived growth factor. Furthermore, psoriatic skin contains oncostatin M (OM), which induces S100A8/A9 but suppresses the expression of the "classical" epidermal differentiation markers. Strong evidence that OM induces S100A9 through the STAT3-signaling cascade was found in the S100a9 promoter analysis. However, direct STAT3 binding to the promoter was not seen, indicating that STAT3 may regulate S100A9 induction indirectly. To clarify the precise mechanism of the upregulation and, more importantly, to determine whether S100A8/A9 are causal in nature for psoriasis, more investigation is required.

Is S100A8/A9 involved in the keratinocyte response to injury?

The process of wound healing is the result of numerous interconnected biological events that are arranged chronologically in reaction to an injury and its surrounding conditions. The inflammatory, proliferative, and remodeling phases of wound healing are clearly defined as the three stages in which resident cells (fibroblasts and keratinocytes) and infiltrating leukocytes participate differently. Gene expression patterns in terms of both space and time are another characteristic of these interconnected biological events.

All phases of tissue repair involve the important roles played by neutrophils and monocytes. These cells are quickly drawn to the wound to carry out several host-defense tasks. In addition, macrophages secrete a wide range of cytokines, growth factors, and angiogenic factors that are thought to be crucial for controlling angiogenesis and bro-proliferation. Nevertheless, evidence from many mouse knockdown and knockout experiments shows that inflammatory cells are not necessary for effective wound healing. S100A9-deficient mice consistently show faster wound closure but about a 4-fold decrease in infiltrating granulocytes in 5-day wounds.

S100A8/A9 are found in differentiating suprabasal wound keratinocytes, especially in the first 12 to 24 hours after injury, with a gradual return to baseline expression over a 2-week period. Thus, during wound healing, there is a rapid increase of S100A8/A9 immunoreactivity that maps infiltration of recruited leukocytes (primarily neutrophils) followed by a sustained S100A8/A9 expression in wound keratinocytes that represent *de novo* synthesis of S100A8/A9. An interesting study on wild-type versus *Pu.1*$^{-/-}$ mice demonstrates that both keratinocytes and leukocytes express S100A9 (and S100A8) in wounds of wild-type mice, whereas S100A9 expression is limited to keratinocytes in wounds of *Pu.1*$^{-/-}$ mice. The macrophage-restricted transcription factor Pu.1 is required for normal adult myelopoiesis. *Pu.1* gene disruption affects the maturation of progenitors of the neutrophil or monocytic lineage and, therefore, the induction of *S100a9* gene expression during hematopoietic development. In wounds of wild-type mice, the S100A8/A9 proteins were expressed as early as 3 hours after injury, with expression peaking at 12 hours post-wounding, whereas in wounds from *Pu.1*$^{-/-}$ mice, expression was not observed until 12 hours post-wounding and S100A8/A9 levels were much reduced compared with that of wild-types. *In situ* hybridization clearly showed S100A8 and S100A9 to be expressed, in addition to keratinocytes, in the region of the wound populated by inflammatory cells in wild-type mice only. Interestingly, wounds in neonatal *Pu.1*$^{-/-}$ mice, which are essentially missing both neutrophils and macrophages, show both speedier repair and reduced scarring, consistent with the results from S100A9-deficient mice. Furthermore, S100A9 is increased in nonhealing as compared with healing wounds. In the healing wound, S100A9 staining is primarily observed in suprabasal keratinocytes at the hyperproliferative wound edge. In nonhealing wounds, on the other hand, S100A9 is observed in the papillary dermis, suprabasal layers of the hyperproliferative wound edge, and to some extent in CD11b positive myeloid cells.

All of these findings point to the possibility that S100A8/A9 expression in epithelial and inflammatory cells is crucial for wound healing. Studies on bone marrow transplants utilizing donors that are S100A9-deficient mice could provide insight into the relative roles played by inflammatory and epithelial cells expressing S100A8/A9 in wound healing.

What biological functions can be attributed to epithelial S100A8/A9?

Studies on over-expression have shown that intracellular S100A8/A9 stimulates epithelial NADPH oxidases, which in turn triggers NF-κB activation. This supports the theory that NF-κB is a transcription factor that is sensitive to redox. Significant roles in the control of keratinocyte growth, survival, and differentiation are played by the NF-κB pathway. NFκB activation causes epithelial cells to grow arrest, in contrast to immune cells. Overexpression of S100A8/A9 consistently reduces cell survival, proliferation, and differentiation. In fact, the level of differentiation is correlated with the expression of S100A9 in keratinocytes. In response to S100A8/A9, keratinocytes show increased differentiation and decreased proliferation. This could be significant for cellular processes that induce transient expression of S100A8/A9, such as wound healing, viral infection, and ultraviolet (UV) irradiation.

Overexpression of S100A8/A9 partially prevents UV-induced skin carcinogenesis. Apoptosis and growth arrest are also components of the innate immune response against viruses. Under these circumstances, the S100A8/A9-suppressed cell growth may serve as an extra checkpoint for cells deciding whether to begin self-healing or to undergo apoptosis. Following a skin injury, keratinocyte migration and proliferation are necessary for wound healing and re-epithelialization. Keratinocytes near the wound's edge recapitulate a portion of the epithelial-mesenchymal transition (EMT) process as the wound heals. Instead of migrating as individual cells, they seem to take on an intermediate phenotype called the "metastable" state, which permits them to move while retaining loose connections. Numerous findings point to S100A8 and S100A9's stimulatory function in epithelial migration. First, keratinocytes from wounds express S100A8/A9. Second, it has been proposed that the expression of the genes encoding the S100 family may be coordinated because they are located in a cluster on human chromosome 1q21 near the human epidermal differentiation complex. Third, MMP-9 induction and the transition to a migratory keratinocyte phenotype are correlated, and S100A8/A9-over expressing HaCaT keratinocytes exhibit significantly higher MMP-9 gene expression. Fourth, the expression of S100A8/A9 guards against anoikis. Fifth, there is evidence linking S100A8/A9 to the epidermal cytoskeleton in inflammatory dermatoses. They bind to keratin filaments.

Correlation of epithelial S100A8/A9 expression and skin diseases

While psoriasis keratinocytes exhibit hyperproliferation and abnormal differentiation, S100A8/A9 overexpression studies *in vitro* have demonstrated that S100A8/A9 mediates keratinocyte differentiation and inhibits the proliferation. The increased expression of S100A8/A9 in psoriasis keratinocytes may provide a negative feedback on the hyperproliferative state of these cells, which would explain these seemingly contradictory findings. It's also possible that the effects of S100A8 and S100A9 *in vivo* in psoriatic skin are not accurately modeled by the cell culture overexpression studies. A third theory is that intracellular S100A8/A9 mediates growth inhibition and promotes differentiation, while S100A8/A9 secreted from keratinocytes exhibits mitogenic activity in these cells. Furthermore, it is widely recognized that proinflammatory cytokines, which are released by immune cells and activated keratinocytes, promote keratinocyte proliferation and intensify the hyperproliferative reaction to barrier disruption.

S100A8/A9 expression in atopic dermatitis (AD) is below detection thresholds. A calcineurin inhibitor called piperculolimus has been effectively used to treat AD patients and prevent their condition from returning. Recent research has demonstrated that this medication causes the up-regulation of genes critical to the healthy function of the skin's barrier, including S100A8/A9. It will take more research to determine whether S100A8/A9 mediates the positive effect of pimecrolimus.

Summary

- Inflammation is an essential defense mechanism in the body, where our immune systems recognize and respond to damaged cells, irritants, pathogens, etc.
- A chronic inflammatory skin condition known as psoriasis has autoimmune pathogenic characteristics and a high immune-mediated genetic susceptibility.
- The five main types of psoriasis are plaque, guttate, inverse, pustular, and erythrodermic. Plaque psoriasis, also known as psoriasis vulgaris, makes up about 90% of cases. It typically presents as red patches with white scales on top.
- Psoriasis in the mouth is very rare, in contrast to lichen planus, another common papulosquamous disorder that commonly involves both the skin and mouth.
- Psoriatic arthritis is a form of chronic inflammatory arthritis that has a highly variable clinical presentation and frequently occurs in association with skin and nail psoriasis.
- Atopic dermatitis (AD), also known as atopic eczema, is a long-term type of inflammation of the skin (dermatitis). It results in itchy, red, swollen, and cracked skin.
- Acne, also known as acne vulgaris, is a long-term skin condition that occurs when dead skin cells and oil from the skin clog hair follicles. Typical features of the condition include blackheads or whiteheads, pimples, oily skin, and possible scarring.
- Acne vulgaris is a chronic skin disease of the pilosebaceous unit and develops due to blockages in the skin's hair follicles.
- Benzoyl peroxide (BPO) is a first-line treatment for mild and moderate acne due to its effectiveness and mild side effects (mainly skin irritation).
- *Hidradenitis suppurativa* (HS) is a long-term dermatological condition characterized by the occurrence of inflamed and swollen lumps. These are typically painful and break open, releasing fluid or pus.

References

1. Barnes, L. E., Levender, M. M., Fleischer, A. B., & Feldman, S. R. (2012). Quality of life measures for acne patients. *Dermatologic Clinics, 30*(2), 293–300.
2. Cunliffe, W. J., Holland, K. T., Bojar, R., et al. (2002). A randomized, double-blind comparison of a clindamycin phosphate/benzoyl peroxide gel formulation and a matching clindamycin gel with respect to microbiologic activity and clinical efficacy in the topical treatment of acne vulgaris. *Clinical Therapeutics, 24*, 1117–1133.
3. Elman, S. A., Weinblatt, M., & Merola, J. F. (2018). Targeted therapies for psoriatic arthritis: An update for the dermatologist. *Seminars in Cutaneous Medicine and Surgery, 37*(3), 173–181.
4. Gamret, A. C., Price, A., Fertig, R. M., Lev-Tov, H., & Nichols, A. J. (2018). Complementary and alternative medicine therapies for psoriasis: A systematic review. *JAMA Dermatology, 154*(11), 1330–1337.
5. Gasslitter, I., Häfner, H. M., & Kofler, K. (2022). Postoperative wound care with custom-made wound dressings for hidradenitis suppurativa: Wound care after radical excision with secondary wound closure. *Dermatologie (Heidelberg), 74*(12), 994–996.

6. Johansson, S. G., Bieber, T., Dahl, R., Friedmann, P. S., Lanier, B. Q., Lockey, R. F., et al. (2004). Revised nomenclature for allergy for global use: Report of the Nomenclature Review Committee of the World Allergy Organization, October 2003. *The Journal of Allergy and Clinical Immunology, 113*(5), 832–836.

7. Larsabal, M., Ly, S., Sbidian, E., Moyal-Barracco, M., Dauendorffer, J. N., Dupin, N., Richard, M. A., Chosidow, O., & Beylot-Barry, M. (2019). GENIPSO: A French prospective study assessing instantaneous prevalence, clinical features and impact on quality of life of genital psoriasis among patients consulting for psoriasis. *British Journal of Dermatology, 180*(3), 647–656.

8. Magin, P., Adams, J., Heading, G., et al. (2006). Psychological sequelae of acne vulgaris: Results of a qualitative study. *Canadian Family Physician, 52*, 978–979.

9. Nguyen, C. T., Bloch, Y., Składanowska, K., Savvides, S. N., & Adamopoulos, I. E. (2019). Pathophysiology and inhibition of IL-23 signaling in psoriatic arthritis: A molecular insight. *Clinical Immunology, 206*, 15–22.

10. Perez-Chada, L. M., Cohen, J. M., Gottlieb, A. B., Duffin, K. C., Garg, A., Latella, J., et al. (2018). Achieving international consensus on the assessment of psoriatic arthritis in psoriasis clinical trials: An International Dermatology Outcome Measures (IDEOM) initiative. *Archives of Dermatological Research, 310*, 701–710.

11. Shamim, H., Riemer, C., Weenig, R., Sokumbi, O., Sciallis, G., McEvoy, M., Mischke, D., & Comfere, N. (2021). Acneiform presentations of folliculotropic mycosis fungoides. *American Journal of Dermatopathology, 43*(2), 85–92.

12. Vinnicombe, Z., Singh, G. V., Spiers, J., Pouncey, A. L., McEvoy, H., & Lancaster, K. (2024). Comparison of negative pressure wound therapy with or without a split-thickness skin graft in the surgical management of axillary hidradenitis suppurativa: A retrospective cohort study. *Plastic Surgery (Oakville, Ont.), 32*(2), 314–320.

13. Yang, E. J., Beck, K. M., Sanchez, I. M., Koo, J., & Liao, W. (2018). The impact of genital psoriasis on quality of life: A systematic review. *Psoriasis (Auckland, N.Z.), 8*, 41–47.

14. Yiu, Z. Z., & Warren, R. B. (2018). Ustekinumab for the treatment of psoriasis: An evidence update. *Seminars in Cutaneous Medicine and Surgery, 37*(3), 143–147.

15. Zouboulis, C. C., Derumeaux, L., Decroix, J., et al. (2000). A multicenter, single-blind, randomized comparison of a fixed clindamycin phosphate/tretinoin gel formulation (Velac) applied once daily and a clindamycin lotion formulation (Dalacin T) applied twice daily in the topical treatment of acne vulgaris. *British Journal of Dermatology, 143*, 498–505.

Chapter

3

INFECTIOUS SKIN DISEASES

Contents

Introduction

Skin infections can be brought on by a variety of pathogens, including bacteria, viruses, fungi, and parasites. The cause will determine the symptoms, course of treatment, and prognosis. A mild infection can progress to a serious one. The majority of skin infections are very curable. On the other hand, if an infection penetrates deeper into the skin or covers a large portion of the body, it may worsen.

People with a weakened immune system have a higher risk of skin infections and complications from skin infections. This could be due to:

- a health condition, such as HIV, diabetes, poor circulation, or malnutrition.
- a side effect of medication, such as chemotherapy or biologic drug use.
- being older or very young.
- have skin folds due to obesity.

Orientation and Directional Terms

Term	Definition	Illustration
Skin infection	A skin infection is an infection of the skin in humans and other animals, that can also affect the associated soft tissues such as loose connective tissue and mucous membranes.	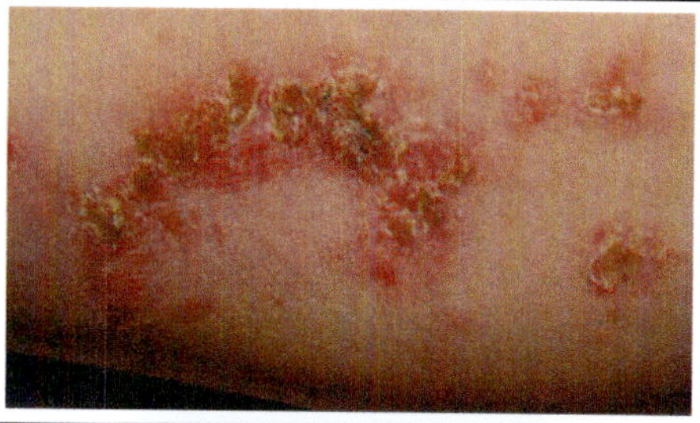
Staphylococcus	Staphylococcus is a genus of Gram-positive bacteria in the family Staphylococcaceae from the order Bacillales. Under the microscope, they appear spherical, and form in grape-like clusters. Staphylococcus species are facultative anaerobic organisms.	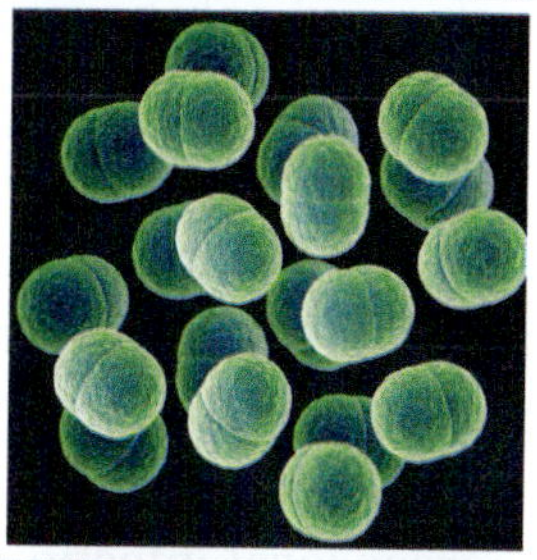
Bullous impetigo	Bullous impetigo is a bacterial skin infection caused by Staphylococcus aureus that results in the formation of large blisters called bullae, usually in areas with skin folds like the armpit, groin, between the fingers or toes, beneath the breast, and between the buttocks. It accounts for 30% of cases of impetigo, the other 70% being non-bullous impetigo.	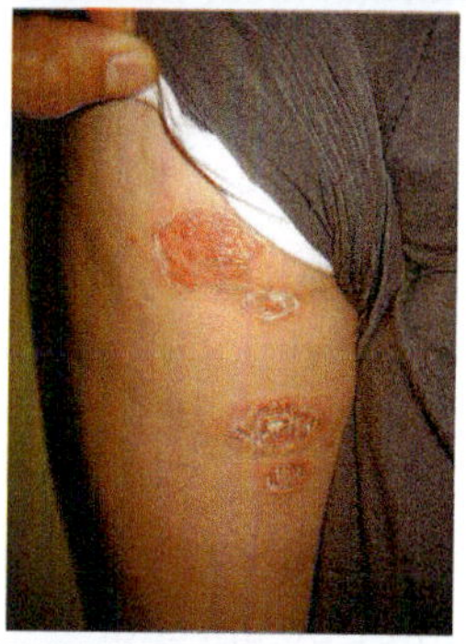
Ecthyma	Ecthyma is most often caused by the streptococcus bacteria. Sometimes, staphylococcus bacteria cause this skin infection on its own or in combination with streptococcus.	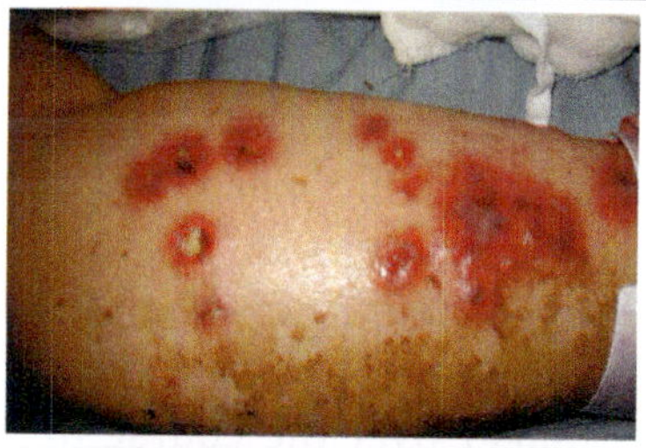
Herpes zoster	Herpes zoster is an infection that results when varicella-zoster virus reactivates from the dorsal root ganglia.	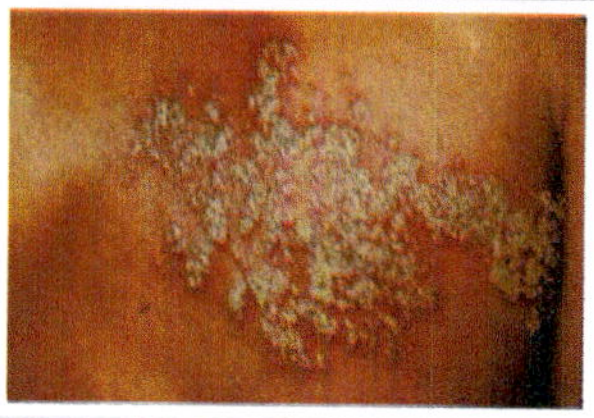

3.1. Bacterial Skin Infections

When bacteria penetrate the skin, either from the outside or because they are already there, bacterial skin infections result. They can get into the skin after a wound or through a hair follicle.

One kind of bacteria that can enter the environment is anthrax. Bacteria like Staphylococcus and Streptococcus are often found on the skin and only become problematic under specific conditions. Skin symptoms are a result of the tick-borne infection known as Lyme disease.

Infections with bacteria can be localized or systemic. A fever and other symptoms that affect the entire body are signs of a systemic infection, whereas local infections only affect a particular area. Certain bacterial infections can start in one place in the body and work their way throughout.

Certain bacterial skin infections, like impetigo, can be transmitted from person to person by direct skin contact, bodily fluids, tainted food or water, or by coming into contact with surfaces that harbor bacteria. Some, like cellulitis, cannot be spread.

3.1.1. Cellulitis

The inner layers of the skin are typically affected by bacterial infections that cause cellulitis. It targets the dermis and subcutaneous fat in particular. One of the symptoms is a red spot that gets bigger over the course of a few days. The skin may be swollen, and the redness's boundaries are typically not distinct. When pressure is applied, the redness frequently turns white, but this isn't always the case. Usually, the infected area hurts. Occasionally, lymphatic vessels may be affected, and the patient may experience fatigue and fever (Vary O'Connor, 2014).

Cellulitis can affect any part of the body, although it most frequently affects the face and legs. Usually, the leg is impacted after the skin breaks. Age, leg swelling, and obesity are additional risk factors. There is rarely a prior skin break when it comes to facial infections. The most frequently implicated bacteria are *Staphylococcus aureus* and streptococci. Unlike cellulitis, which affects the deeper layers of the skin, erysipelas is caused by a bacterial infection that causes a reddening area with distinct borders and is frequently accompanied by a fever. While a cell culture is rarely feasible, the diagnosis is typically made based on the signs and symptoms that are present. More serious infections like necrotizing fasciitis or an underlying bone infection should be ruled out before a diagnosis is made (Figure 3.1).

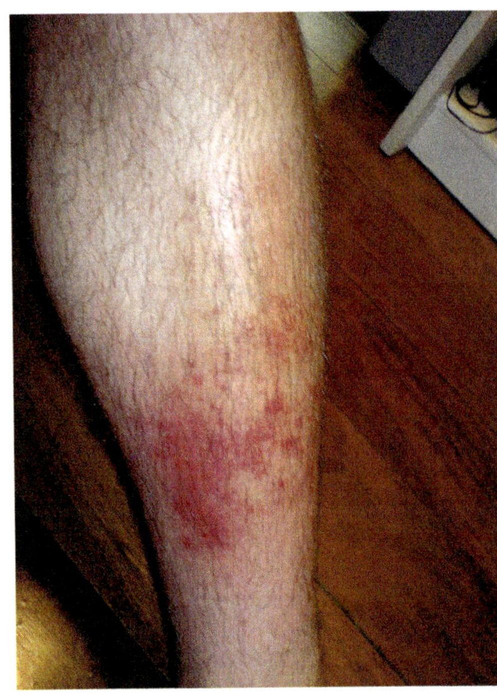

Figure 3.1. *Cellulitis of the leg with foot involvement.*

Source: By RafaelLopez at the English-language Wikipedia, CC BY-SA 3.0, https://commons.wikimedia.org/w/index.php?curid=3224876.

Usually, oral antibiotics like cephalexin, amoxicillin, or cloxacillin are used as a form of treatment. Erythromycin or clindamycin may be prescribed in place of penicillin for those who are allergic to it. Doxycycline or trimethoprim/sulfamethoxazole may also be advised when methicillin-resistant *S. aureus* (MRSA) is a concern. The existence of pus or prior MRSA infections are causes for concern. Both pain medication and elevating the affected area may be helpful.

Abscess formation is one possible consequence. After 7 to 10 days of treatment, about 95% of patients get better. However, the results are frequently worse for those who have diabetes. In 2015, approximately 21.2 million people had cellulitis. Approximately 2 out of every 1,000 Americans suffer from a lower limb condition each year. Globally, cellulitis claimed 16,900 lives in 2015. One in six hospital admissions in the United Kingdom were attributed to cellulitis.

3.1.1.1. Signs and Symptoms

The typical signs and symptoms of cellulitis are an area that is red, hot, and painful.

Complications

Potential complications may include abscess formation, fasciitis, and sepsis.

3.1.1.2. Causes

Most of the time, but not always, bacteria that enter through skin breaks and infect the tissue is what causes cellulitis. The most frequent sources of the infection are Group A Streptococcus and Staphylococcus, which are normally present in the skin biota of healthy people.

Dental infections account for about 80% of cases of submandibular cellulitis, also known as Ludwig's angina. Mixed infections resulting from both anaerobes and aerobes are frequently linked to this kind of cellulitis. This usually refers to the staphylococci, bacteroides, and alpha-hemolytic streptococci groups. Arachnid or spider bites, blisters, animal bites, tattoos, itchy skin rashes, recent surgeries, athlete's foot, dry skin, eczema, injecting drugs (particularly subcutaneous or intramuscular injections or situations where an attempted intravenous injection misses or blows the vein), pregnancy, diabetes, obesity, burns, boils, and circulation-impairing burns and lesions are among the predisposing conditions for cellulitis. Cellulitis episodes can also be linked to the uncommon disease dissecting cellulitis, also known as hidradenitis suppurativa.

A doctor can make a diagnosis based on how the skin looks. To help rule out a blood clot deep in the leg veins, a doctor may also recommend blood tests, a wound culture, or other tests. Warmth, pain, and swelling (inflammation) are some of the symptoms that are similar to those of a deep vein thrombosis in the lower leg.

If your skin becomes red or develops a rash, it could be a sign of a severe infection deep within the layers of your skin. This can allow bacteria to quickly spread into the lymph nodes and bloodstream, causing flu-like symptoms such as a high fever, sweating, feeling cold and shivering uncontrollably, as the body struggles to regulate its temperature.

Rarely, the infection may move to the fascial lining, a deep layer of tissue. A deep-layer infection is necrotizing fasciitis, also referred to as flesh-eating bacteria by the media. A medical emergency has arisen.

3.1.1.2.1. Risk Factors

Elderly people and those with compromised immune systems are particularly susceptible to cellulitis. Due to immune system impairment, diabetics are more prone to cellulitis than the general population. They are particularly vulnerable to cellulitis in the feet because the disease impairs blood circulation in the legs, which can result in diabetic foot ulcers or diabetic foot. Inadequate regulation of blood glucose levels promotes the growth of bacteria in impacted tissue and expedites the spread of the infection if it gets into the bloodstream. Because of the neural degeneration associated with diabetes, ulcers may not hurt and thus frequently develop an infection. Individuals who have experienced poliomyelitis are also susceptible to circulatory issues, particularly in the lower limbs.

Infection is also more common in conditions that weaken the immune system, such as immunosuppressive medications and other illnesses. Blisters from shingles and chickenpox frequently burst, leaving a hole in the skin that bacteria can enter. Individuals who have lymphedema, or swelling in their arms and/ or legs, may also be at risk. Cellulitis is also at risk for conditions that impair blood flow to the legs and feet, such as varicose veins and chronic venous insufficiency.

In densely populated areas with shared living quarters and sanitary facilities, like military bases, college dorms, retirement communities, oil platforms, and homeless shelters, cellulitis is also frequently observed.

3.1.1.3. Diagnosis

Cellulitis is typically diagnosed based on clinical presentation, which includes rapidly spreading areas of swelling, redness, and heat on the skin, often accompanied by inflammation of nearby lymph nodes. While traditionally distinguished from erysipelas by its deeper involvement of subcutaneous tissues, some clinicians may classify erysipelas as cellulitis. Both conditions are usually treated in a similar manner, but cellulitis associated with furuncles, carbuncles, or abscesses is commonly caused by *S. aureus*, which can impact treatment decisions, particularly when selecting antibiotics. Skin aspiration for nonpurulent cellulitis, typically caused by streptococcal bacteria, is usually not helpful for diagnosis, and blood cultures are positive in less than 5% of cases.

Examining for co-existing abscesses is crucial because, in most cases, surgical drainage is necessary rather than just antibiotic treatment. A skilled practitioner's use of bedside ultrasonography can easily distinguish between cellulitis and an abscess, changing treatment in up to 56% of cases. Physicians' clinical assessment for an abscess may be limited, particularly in cases with extensive overlying induration. In situations where antibiotics fail, the use of ultrasonography to identify abscesses may also be recommended. In the absence of a distinct, heterogeneous, hypoechoic fluid collection that would suggest an abscess, cellulitis is characterized by a cobblestone-like appearance that is indicative of subcutaneous edema.

3.1.1.3.1. Differential Diagnosis

Other conditions that can resemble cellulitis are stasis dermatitis, or inflammation of the skin caused by inadequate blood flow, and deep vein thrombosis, which can be identified with a compression leg ultrasonography. The following symptoms could indicate a more serious infection: purple bullae, skin sloughing, subcutaneous edema, and systemic toxicity. Such symptoms would indicate necrotizing fasciitis or gas gangrene, which would require immediate surgical intervention. Up to 30% of patients with suspected lower-extremity cellulitis may receive a false positive, which results in 50,000–130,000 avoidable hospital stays and \$195–\$515.55 million in preventable healthcare costs each year in the US. It has been demonstrated that having dermatologists evaluate cases of suspected cellulitis improves patient outcomes and lowers the rate of misdiagnosis. Occasionally, reports of related musculoskeletal findings are made. It is known as the follicular occlusion triad or tetrad when it coexists with pilonidal cysts, hidradenitis suppurativa, and acne conglobata.

It is possible to misdiagnose Lyme disease as cellulitis. In cases of Lyme disease, the recognizable bullseye rash may not always develop (it may not develop at all, or it may not have a central, ring-like clearing). Recent outdoor activities in areas where Lyme is prevalent and rash at a site unusual for cellulitis, like the armpit, groin, or behind the knee, are factors supporting Lyme. Neurologic complications over the long term can also be caused by Lyme. Cephalexin, the typical treatment for cellulitis, is ineffective for treating Lyme disease. The IDSA advises treating with cefuroxime axetil or amoxicillin/clavulanic acid when it is unclear which infection is present because these medications are efficient against both.

3.1.1.4. Prevention

Antibiotic use may help those who have had cellulitis in the past avoid having it again. For those who have experienced more than two episodes, CREST advises doing this. Antibiotics can help prevent recurrent cellulitis in the lower limbs, according to a 2017 meta-analysis. However, the benefits of prevention seem to wear off once antibiotic therapy is stopped.

3.1.1.5. Treatment

Although the optimal course of treatment is not always clear, antibiotics are typically prescribed. The agent is chosen based on the suspected organism's presence or absence of purulence. Antibiotics are frequently prescribed for co-existing cellulitis, especially if it is extensive, and surgical drainage is typically indicated if there is also an abscess. In addition, painkillers are frequently prescribed; however, since they are a sign of necrotizing fasciitis, severe pain should always be looked into. Elevating the impacted area is frequently advised. Steroids may speed recovery in those on antibiotics (Han, Faletsky, Mostaghimi, 2020).

3.1.1.5.1. Antibiotics

The choice of antibiotics depends on local availability, but for cellulitis without an abscess, first-generation cephalosporins or penicillinase-resistant semisynthetic penicillins are currently advised. Between 6 and 37% of cases do not respond well to an antibiotic course.

3.1.2. Impetigo

Impetigo is a superficial skin infection caused by bacteria. Yellow-colored crusts on the face, arms, or legs are the most typical presentation. Large blisters that affect the armpits or groin are less common. The lesions could hurt or itch. Fever is not common.

Either *Streptococcus pyogenes* or *Staphylococcus aureus* is usually to blame. Daycare attendance, crowded living conditions, poor diet, *diabetes mellitus*, participation in contact sports, and skin breaks from eczema, scabies, herpes, or mosquito bites are risk factors. It can spread amongst or between people when in contact. Most often, the diagnosis is made in light of the symptoms and appearance.

Hand washing, avoiding infected individuals, and cleaning wounds are the three main methods of prevention. Antibiotic creams, such as mupirocin or fusidic acid, are commonly used as a form of treatment. In cases where a large area is affected, oral antibiotics like cefalexin may be administered. Forms resistant to antibiotics have been discovered. Usually, healing happens without leaving scars (Figure 3.2).

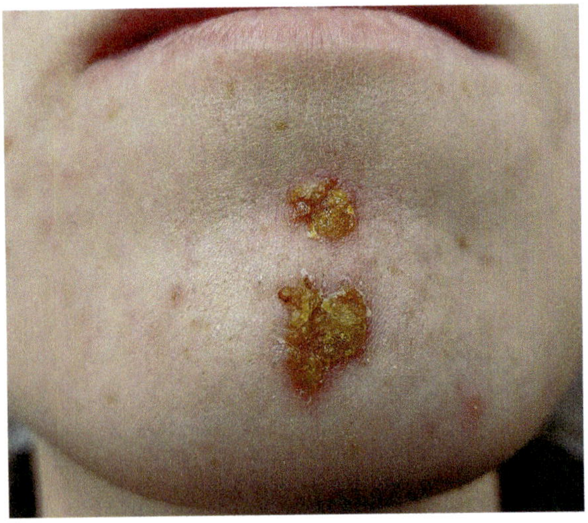

Figure 3.2. *Facial impetigo.*

Source: By James Heilman, MD – Own work, CC BY-SA 4.0, https://commons.wikimedia.org/w/index.php?curid=90030642.

About 140 million people, or 2% of the global population, were afflicted with impetigo in 2010. Although it can happen at any age, young children are most likely to experience it. School sores is another name for the condition in certain regions. In the absence of treatment, most people recover in three weeks. The bacteria can colonize the nose, causing recurrent infections. Cellulitis or poststreptococcal glomerulonephritis are possible complications.

3.1.2.1. Signs and Symptoms

3.1.2.1.1. Contagious Impetigo

Often starting as a red sore close to the mouth or nose, this most prevalent type of impetigo—also known as nonbullous impetigo—breaks quickly, oozing pus or fluid and forming a scab that is the color of honey. A red mark that often heals without leaving a scar follows. Although they are not painful, sores can itch. Fever is uncommon, but swollen lymph nodes may be present in the affected area. It is easy for the infection to spread to other areas of the body by touching or scratching the sores. Scratching or abrading the skin can also lead to red, scarred skin ulcers.

3.1.2.1.2. Bullous Impetigo

Bullous impetigo, which primarily affects children under the age of two, is characterized by fluid-filled blisters that are painless and typically appear on the arms, legs, and trunk. The surrounding skin is red and itchy, but not sore. There could be big or little blisters. They break and leave behind yellow scabs.

3.1.2.1.3. Ecthyma

Ecthyma, the nonbullous form of impetigo, causes painful sores filled with pus or fluid and skin redness. These sores typically appear on the arms and legs and eventually develop into ulcers that go deeper into the dermis. They split open to form tough, thick, gray-yellow scabs that can occasionally leave scars. In the affected area, enlarged lymph nodes may be present in conjunction with ecthyma.

3.1.2.2. Causes

Staphylococcus aureus is the main cause of impetigo, though *Streptococcus pyogenes* can also be involved occasionally. *S. aureus* is the main cause of both bullous and nonbullous infections, with Streptococcus frequently contributing to the nonbullous form.

3.1.2.2.1. Predisposing Factors

Children between the ages of 2 and 5 are more susceptible to contracting impetigo, particularly if they attend daycare or school. 30% of cases are bullous, and 70% are nonbullous. Residents of warm climates are more likely to get impetigo.

3.1.2.2.2. Transmission

Through direct contact with lesions or nasal carriers, the infection can spread. For Streptococcus, the incubation period is 1–3 days, and for Staphylococcus, it is 4–10 days. Intact skin is not susceptible to infection by airborne dried streptococci. Scratching could make the lesions worse.

3.1.2.3. Diagnosis

Usually, impetigo is diagnosed based only on how it looks. It usually manifests as honey-colored scabs on the arms, legs, or face that are made of dried sebum. To check for resistant bacteria, a culture may be performed if a visual diagnosis is not clear.

3.1.2.3.1. Differential Diagnosis

Other illnesses such as discoid lupus, herpes simplex virus, scabies, and contact dermatitis can cause symptoms resembling those of the common form.

3.1.2.4. Prevention

The skin and any open wounds should be kept clean and covered to stop the impetigo from spreading. Fluids from an infected person should be kept away from a non-infected person's skin with caution. The risk of coming into contact with contaminated fluids can be reduced by washing hands, linens, and the afflicted areas. Keeping your nails short can help prevent the sores from spreading, as scratching can make them worse. Those who are infected should refrain from social interactions and stop sharing clothes or linens. As long as their draining lesions are covered, children with impetigo can return to school 24 hours after beginning antibiotic therapy.

3.1.2.5. Treatment

Antibiotics are typically prescribed as a cream or by mouth. Mupirocin creams can be used to treat mild cases. A child's symptoms resolve after a single seven-day antibiotic course in 95% of cases. There is a belief that topical antiseptics are not a good substitute for topical antibiotics because they are inferior. However, for localized non-bullous impetigo in otherwise healthy individuals, the National Institute for Health and Care Excellence (NICE) as of February 2020 advises a hydrogen peroxide 1% cream antiseptic rather than topical antibiotics. This suggestion is a component of an initiative to lessen the excessive use of antibiotics, which could hasten the emergence of resistant organisms like MRSA.

Oral antibiotics like erythromycin, flucloxacillin, or dicloxacillin are necessary in more severe cases. As an alternative, first-generation cephalosporins, amoxicillin plus clavulanate potassium, and numerous other antibiotics can be used. Doxycycline, clindamycin, and trimethoprim-sulphamethoxazole are substitutes for those with severe penicillin allergies or infections caused by methicillin-resistant *Staphococcus aureus*. However, doxycycline shouldn't be administered to children younger than eight years old because of the possibility of drug-induced tooth discoloration. Penicillin is the recommended medication in cases where streptococci are the only cause. An antiviral medication called valacyclovir may be administered if ulcers are a symptom of the condition and are thought to be caused by a viral infection.

3.1.3. Boil

A furuncle, another name for a boil, is an infection of the hair follicle caused by deep folliculitis. It is most frequently brought on by an infection with the *Staphylococcus aureus* bacteria, which causes an excruciatingly painful swollen area on the skin due to a buildup of pus and dead tissue. Therefore, boils are essentially pus-filled nodules. Carbuncles are groups of individual boils that are grouped together. Coagulase-positive strains of *Staphylococcus aureus* are responsible for most human infections; these strains are distinguished by their capacity to generate the clotting enzyme coagulase. *Staphylococcus aureus* can infect almost any organ system (Figure 3.3).

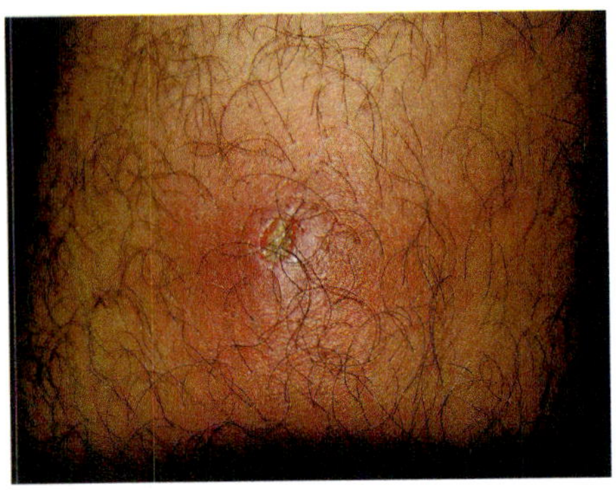

Figure 3.3. *Some furuncles.*

Source: By The original uploader was Mahdouch at French Wikipedia. – Transferred from fr.wikipedia to Commons., CC BY 1.0, https://commons.wikimedia.org/w/index.php?curid=3123389.

3.1.3.1. Signs and Symptoms

Boils are painful, warm, and tender lumps surrounding a hair follicle that are red, bumpy, and filled with pus. They vary in size from golf ball to pea. The boil is ready to drain or release pus when there is a yellow or white point in the middle of the lump. An individual may have fatigue, swollen lymph nodes, and fever in a severe infection. Chronic furunculosis is the term for a recurrent boil. Many patients experience recurrent skin infections, which frequently spread to other family members. It is common to identify systemic factors that reduce resistance, such as hematologic disorders, diabetes, and obesity. Other skin disorders that lead a person to scratch and harm their skin can also result in boils. Boils can develop in the ear canal, on the back, in the neck, in the belly, in the arms or legs, or on the buttocks or around the anus. Moreover, boils, also known as styes, can develop around the eye. Intraoral dental sinuses, also known as gumboils, are boils on the gums.

3.1.3.1.1. Complications

Scarring and infection or abscess of the skin, spinal cord, brain, kidneys, or other organs are the most frequent consequences of boils. Additionally, infections can become life-threatening when they enter the bloodstream (bacteremia). First, *S. aureus* strains infiltrate the skin and its anatomical structures (hair follicles, sebaceous glands, etc.) or damage the skin (cuts, abrasions). While some infections, like styes, boils, furuncles, or carbuncles, are relatively localized, other infections have the potential to spread to other parts of the skin and result in cellulitis, folliculitis, or impetigo. Regrettably, these bacteria can enter the bloodstream (bacteremia) and spread to various parts of the body, where they can cause infections (pneumonia, osteomyelitis, endocarditis, wound infections, abscesses) that could potentially be fatal for the infected individual. Additionally, some *S. aureus* strains produce exotoxins and enzymes that either cause or worsen many diseases. Food poisoning, septic shock, toxic shock syndrome, and scalded skin syndrome are examples of these illnesses. *S. aureus* can infect almost any organ system. Because the blood vessels in this area drain into the brain and can carry serious infections, it can be especially dangerous to squeeze or cut boils in the danger triangle of the face if done outside of a medical setting.

3.1.3.2. Causes

Naturally, bacteria that are present on the skin, like staphylococci, are the cause. The process of bacterial colonization starts in the hair follicles and can lead to inflammation and localized cellulitis. In Africa, cutaneous furuncles are typically the first sign of myiasis brought on by tumbu flies. The following conditions increase the risk of developing furunculosis: immunosuppressive medication use, diabetes mellitus, obesity, lymphoproliferative neoplasms, and bacterial carriage in the nose.

3.1.3.3. Diagnosis

A doctor's clinical evaluation, which may involve culturing the lesion, is used to make the diagnosis.

3.1.3.4. Treatment

Sometimes a boil needs to be opened and drained, but other times it may clear up on its own without bursting. Usually, this occurs on its own in two weeks. Applying a warm, moist compress regularly can expedite healing, both prior to and following the onset of a boil. To prevent the bacteria from spreading, the area needs to be kept clean, hands need to be washed after touching it, and any dressings need to be disposed of carefully. A boil can be allowed to drain by a doctor cutting it open or lancing it, but at-home cutting or squeezing should be avoided as this could worsen the infection. Large or recurring boils, as well as those that develop in delicate regions (such as the groin, breasts, armpits, around or in the nostrils, or in the ear), may require antibiotic therapy. An antibiotic loses its effectiveness if it is used for more than a month without a minimum of two months (preferably longer) in between doses. Plastic surgery may be necessary to remove boils that have persisted for longer than two years on the patient.

In cases where antibiotics or steroid injections prove ineffective, furuncles that pose a significant risk of serious complications should be excised and drained. These include furuncles that develop in the center of the face or close to the spine, last more than two weeks, or are abnormally large. Sepsis is indicated by fever and chills, which call for quick medical attention.

Treatment for *Staphylococcus aureus* can be challenging due to its propensity to develop antibiotic resistance. The choice of antimicrobials for treatment depends in part on our understanding of the resistance of *S. aureus* to antibiotics.

3.1.4. Leprosy

Hansen's disease (HD), commonly referred to as leprosy, is a chronic infection caused by the bacteria *Mycobacterium leprae* or *Mycobacterium lepromatosis*. Damage to the nerves, respiratory system, skin, and eyes can result from infection. Due to recurrent injuries or infections from unseen wounds, this nerve damage may cause a person to lose some or all of their extremity's feelings of pain. A person with an infection may also have weak muscles and blurred vision. Leprosy symptoms can appear within a year, but in some cases, they take up to 20 years to manifest.

People can contract leprosy from one another, but prolonged contact is required. Leprosy has a low pathogenicity; of those infected with *M. leprae*, 95% do not get leprosy. It is believed that leprosy spreads through coughing or coming into contact with fluid from an infected person's nose. The immune system and genetics influence an individual's susceptibility to the illness. Leprosy does not transfer through sexual contact or during pregnancy to the fetus. Those who are poor are more likely to contract leprosy. The disease can be classified as either paucibacillary or multibacillary, depending on the type of bacteria that are present. A patient with multibacillary disease has more than five skin patches, whereas a patient with paucibacillary disease has five or fewer poorly pigmented, numb skin patches. The presence of acid-fast bacilli in a skin biopsy confirms the diagnosis (Figure 3.4).

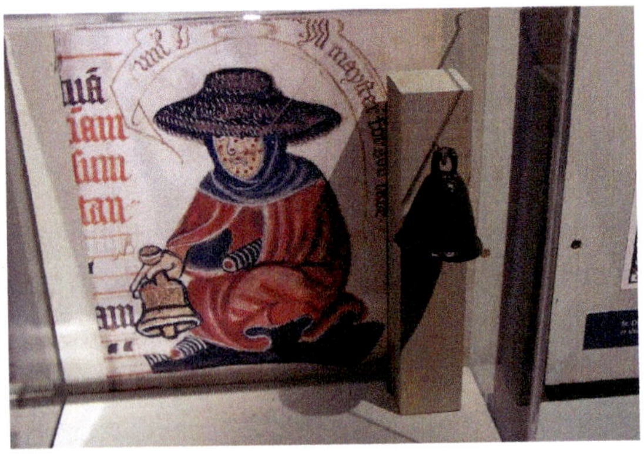

Figure 3.4. *Leprosy stigma.*

Source: By No machine-readable author provided. Cnyborg assumed (based on copyright claims). – No machine-readable source provided. Own work assumed (based on copyright claims)., CC BY-SA 3.0, https://commons.wikimedia.org/w/index.php?curid=173803.

Multidrug therapy is a viable treatment for leprosy. The six-month course of treatment for paucibacillary leprosy consists of dapsone, rifampicin, and clofazimine. For a full year, the same drugs are used to treat multibacillary leprosy patients. There are several more antibiotics that can be utilized. The World Health Organization offers these treatments at no cost to the patient.

Leprosy does not spread easily. Leprosy patients are allowed to live with their families, attend public schools, and work. By 2020, there were less than 200,000 cases worldwide, down from 5.2 million in the 1980s. The majority of new cases are found in 14 countries, with over half of them occurring in India. Leprosy was cured in 16 million people globally in the 20 years between 1994 and 2014. In the US, there are about 200 cases reported annually. Almost one in five leprosy cases nationwide and 81% of cases in Florida were in Central Florida. In certain parts of Africa, Asia, Thailand, and India, leper colonies are still used to separate and house those afflicted with the disease.

3.1.4.1. Signs and Symptoms

A, dry scalp, eye issues, skin lesions, muscle weakness, reddish skin, smooth, shiny, diffuse thickening of the skin on the face, ear, and hand, loss of feeling in the fingers and toes, thickening of peripheral nerves, a flat nose due to the destruction of nasal cartilages, and changes in phonation and other aspects of speech production are common symptoms found in the various types of leprosy. Additionally, impotence, and testicular atrophy could happen.

People can be affected by leprosy in various ways. Five years is the average incubation period. After infection, symptoms may appear one year later or up to 20 years later. Pale or pink patches of skin that may be pain-or temperature-insensitive are frequently the first obvious symptoms of leprosy. Nerve issues, such as numbness or soreness in the hands or feet, can occasionally precede or accompany patches of discolored skin. As cartilage is absorbed by the body as a result of secondary infections (additional bacterial or viral infections), fingers, and toes may become shorter and malformed. The type of leprosy a person has determines how their immune system reacts to it.

Neurological damage affects about 30% of leprosy patients. When appropriate treatment is delayed by several months, the damage to the nerves is irreversible; otherwise, it becomes permanent. Paralysis can result from loss of muscle function brought on by nerve damage. In addition, it might cause numbness or abnormal sensations, which could result in more infections, ulcers, and deformities in the joints.

3.1.4.2. Cause

3.1.4.2.1. *M. leprae* and *M. lepromatosis*

The two mycobacteria that cause leprosy are *Mycobacterium leprae* and *Mycobacterium lepromatosis.* A deadly case of diffuse lepromatous leprosy in 2008 led to the isolation of a relatively recently discovered mycobacterium known as *M. lepromatosis*. Clinically, *M. lepromatosis* and *M. leprae* are identical.

M. leprae is an aerobic, rod-shaped, intracellular, acid-fast bacterium. The waxy cell envelope covering typical of the genus Mycobacterium envelops *M. leprae.*

3.1.4.2.2. Risk factors

Contact with an infected individual is the biggest risk factor for contracting leprosy. Individuals who come into contact with an individual who has leprosy are five to eight times more likely to contract the disease than the general population. Additionally, leprosy is more common in the impoverished. Not everyone with an *M. leprae* infection experiences symptoms.

Factors that can weaken the immune system, like malnutrition, other diseases, or genetic mutations, may raise the likelihood of contracting leprosy. However, having HIV does not seem to increase this risk. Specific genetic traits in individuals who are exposed may be linked to the development of lepromatous or tuberculoid leprosy.

3.1.4.2.3. Transmission

Leprosy is spread through intimate contact with an infected person. Leprosy spreads by way of the upper respiratory tract. Research has increasingly favored the respiratory route of transmission, although earlier studies suggested the skin as the primary route. Bacilli found in upper airway secretions are inhaled and cause transmission. Leprosy cannot be passed from one person to another through sexual contact or pregnancy. Sitting next to someone who has leprosy or shaking hands with them does not cause the disease to spread; in fact, the majority of people (95%) who are exposed to *M. leprae* do not go on to develop leprosy. Individuals are deemed non-contagious for 72 hours following the initiation of suitable multi-drug therapy.

The skin and nasal mucosa are two locations where *M. leprae* are known to exit the human body, though it's unclear how important each is in relation to the other. Large numbers of organisms are visible deep in the dermis in lepromatous cases, but it's unlikely that they will proliferate to the point where they reach the skin's surface. Although the exact mechanism is unknown, armadillos can also spread leprosy to humans.

3.1.4.2.4. Genetics

Leprosy does not always develop in those who are infected or exposed to *M. leprae*, and genetic factors may contribute to an individual's susceptibility to infection. Leprosy cases frequently occur in families, and various genetic variations have been found. The immune system of many exposed individuals is able to eradicate the leprosy bacteria in the early stages of infection before serious symptoms appear. A genetic flaw in cell-mediated immunity could make someone more vulnerable to leprosy symptoms following bacterial exposure. Because Parkinson's disease and the DNA region causing this variability are related, there is currently conjecture that there may be a biochemical connection between the two conditions.

3.1.4.3. Diagnosis

In countries where people are frequently infected, a person is considered to have leprosy if they have one of the following two signs:

- Skin lesion consistent with leprosy and with definite sensory loss.
- Positive skin smears.

Lesions on the skin can be one or more, typically hypopigmented, but they can also occasionally have a reddish or coppery color. Lesions can be solid elevated areas (nodular), raised (papules), or flat (macules). One characteristic that can help identify whether a skin lesion is caused by leprosy or another illness, like tinea versicolor, is experiencing sensory loss at the site of the lesion. Leprosy is linked to thicker nerves, which can also cause loss of feeling or muscle weakness. However, leprosy is not always diagnosed by sensory loss or muscle weakness alone, even in the absence of a typical skin lesion.

Acid-fast leprosy bacilli in skin smears are sometimes thought to be diagnostic; however, a diagnosis based only on symptoms is usually made without the need for laboratory testing. A person's leprosy diagnosis is deemed late if they already have a noticeable disability from the disease.

Because healthcare professionals are not familiar with leprosy and its symptoms, leprosy diagnosis is frequently delayed in nations or regions where the disease is uncommon, such as the United States. The hallmarks of leprosy, nerve involvement, and the disability it causes are avoided with early diagnosis and treatment.

For those without symptoms, there is no recommended test to identify latent leprosy. Few leprosy patients have positive anti-PGL-1 tests. A method based on the polymerase chain reaction (PCR) can be used to determine the presence of *M. leprae* bacterial DNA. While a person cannot be diagnosed with leprosy using this molecular test alone, it can be used to identify those who are most likely to contract the disease or spread it, such as those who have few lesions or an unusual clinical presentation.

3.1.4.4. Complications

Although not always, leprosy can result in limb and finger loss in its victims. *M. leprae* annihilates the body's capacity to perceive pain and injury by attacking nerve endings. Persons suffering from leprosy are more likely to hurt themselves because they are incapable of feeling pain. Damaged areas develop an infection and lose tissue. As the tissue is absorbed by the body, limbs, fingers, and toes become malformed and shortened.

3.1.4.5. Treatment

There are several leprostatic agents available for use in treatment. All leprosy patients are advised to follow a three-drug regimen consisting of rifampicin, dapsone, and clofazimine for six months for paucibacillary leprosy and 12 months for multibacillary leprosy.

Following the first monthly dosage, people no longer have contagious diseases thanks to multidrug therapy (MDT), which is still very effective. Its presentation in calendar blister packs makes it simple and safe to use in field situations. Relapse rates after treatment continue to be low. Despite the low number of cases, resistance has been reported in several countries. Second-line medications, such as fluoroquinolones, minocycline, or clarithromycin, can treat leprosy patients who are resistant to rifampicin; however, because of their decreased bactericidal activity, the course of treatment is limited to 24 months. There is a lack of data regarding the possible advantages and disadvantages of alternative treatment plans for drug-resistant leprosy.

Wearing protective footwear can help people with nerve damage avoid ulcers and secondary infections. PVC boots might not be as good as canvas shoes. Double rocker shoes and below-knee plaster might not be any different from one another. Although the evidence is weak, topical ketanserin appears to have a better effect on ulcer healing than zinc paste or clioquinol cream. When phenytoin is applied topically, skin alterations are more significantly improved than with saline dressings.

3.2. Viral Skin Infections

Herpes zoster, another name for shingles, is a viral illness that causes a painful skin rash with blisters in a small area. Usually, the rash appears as a single, broad mark on the face or left or right side of the body. There might be localized pain or tingling in the area two to four days before the rash appearing. Tiredness, headaches, and fever are other typical symptoms. The rash typically goes away in two to four weeks, but some people experience persistent nerve pain, known as postherpetic neuralgia (PHN), that can linger for months or even years. People with weakened immune systems may experience a widespread rash. It's possible to lose vision if the rash is near the eye (Johnson et al., 2015) (Figure 3.5).

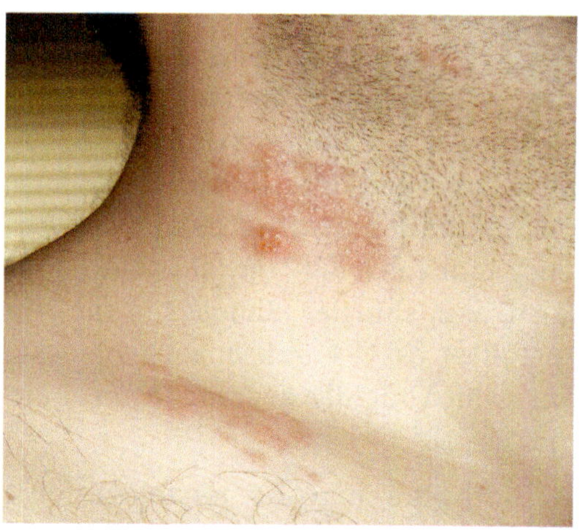

Figure 3.5. *Shingles.*

Source: By No machine-readable author provided. Gentgeen assumed (based on copyright claims). – No machine-readable source provided. Own work assumed (based on copyright claims), CC BY-SA 3.0, https://commons.wikimedia.org/w/index.php?curid=760893.

The varicella zoster virus (VZV), which also causes chickenpox, is the cause of shingles. The first viral infection in cases of chickenpox, also known as varicella, usually happens in childhood or adolescence. Following the resolution of chickenpox, the virus may reactivate after years or decades of dormancy (inactivity) in human nerve cells (cranial nerves or dorsal root ganglia). Reactivation of the dormant varicella virus causes shingles. Blisters are then caused by the virus as it moves along nerve bodies to skin nerve endings. When shingles is outbreaking, a person who has never had chickenpox before may contract it from the varicella virus found in shingles blisters; however, this person will not develop shingles, at least not after the initial infection. It is unclear how the virus stays dormant in the body or eventually reactivates.

The illness has been known about since antiquity. The dormant virus may reactivate in older people, those with weakened immune systems, and those who had chickenpox before the age of 18 months.

3.2.1. Signs and Symptoms

Headache, fever, and malaise are among the initial symptoms of shingles that are nonspecific and can lead to a false diagnosis. Sensations of burning pain, itching, hyperesthesia (oversensitivity), or paresthesia frequently accompany these symptoms. In the affected dermatome, pain can range from mild to severe, characterized by short bursts of excruciating pain that are frequently described as stinging, tingling, aching, numbing, or throbbing.

Children's shingles are usually painless, but as people age, the condition tends to become more severe and people are more likely to get it.

Typically, within one to two days but potentially up to three weeks, the initial phase is followed by the emergence of a distinct skin rash. Although most often found on the torso, the pain and rash can also manifest on the face, eyes, or other areas of the body. Initially, the rash may resemble hives, but unlike hives, shingles only affect a specific area of the skin known as a dermatome. This results in a stripe or belt-like pattern that is confined to one side of the body and does not cross the midline. Zoster sine herpete, or "shingles without herpes," refers to a person experiencing all symptoms of shingles except for the characteristic rash.

The typical skin rash usually appears one to two days after the initial phase, but it can occasionally take up to three weeks. Though they can also affect the face, eyes, or other parts of the body, the rash and pain most frequently affect the torso. The rash initially resembles the early stages of hives; however, in contrast to hives, shingles results in skin alterations restricted to a dermatome, typically producing a belt-like or stripe pattern that is restricted to one side of the body and does not cross the midline. A person with shingles who does not have this distinctive rash is said to have zoster sine herpete, or shingles without herpes.

Afterward, as the fever and overall malaise persist, the rash turns vesicular and forms tiny blisters with a serous exudate inside. After filling with blood, the painful vesicles eventually turn cloudy or darken, and within seven to 10 days, they crust over. Usually, the crusts come off and the skin heals, but occasionally, severe blistering leaves the skin discolored and scarred. The varicella zoster virus, which can be spread through contact or inhalation of fluid droplets until the lesions crust over—a process that could take up to four weeks—is present in the blister fluid.

3.2.1.1. Face

Additional symptoms of Shingles may appear depending on which dermatome is affected. The most frequently affected nerve is the trigeminal nerve, of which the most frequently affected branch is the ophthalmic division. The virus is known as *Zoster ophthalmicus* when it reactivates in this nerve branch. There may be involvement of the skin on the forehead, upper eyelid, and orbit of the eye. Between 10 and 25% of cases are *Zoster ophthalmicus*. Conjunctivitis, keratitis, uveitis, and optic nerve palsies are among the symptoms that some people may experience. These conditions can occasionally result in chronic ocular inflammation, vision loss, and excruciating pain.

The ear is affected by *Shingles oticus*, also referred to as Ramsay Hunt syndrome type II. It is believed to be the consequence of the virus moving from the vestibulocochlear nerve to the facial nerve. Vertigo, or rotational dizziness, and hearing loss are among the symptoms. If the maxillary or mandibular division of the trigeminal nerve is impacted, shingles may develop in the mouth. In these cases, the rash may develop on the mucous membrane of the lower jaw (tongue or lower tooth gums) or the upper jaw (palate, occasionally the upper teeth gums), respectively. Oral involvement can happen on its own or in conjunction with a skin rash over the same trigeminal branch's cutaneous distribution. It can be distinguished from other oral blistering conditions by its tendency to involve only one side with lesions, similar to skin shingles. Shingles in the mouth first manifest as 1–4 mm opaque blisters, or vesicles, which rapidly degrade to form ulcers that heal in 10–14 days.

A toothache may be mistaken for the prodromal pain (that occurs before the rash). This can occasionally result in needless dental procedures. It is rare for post-herpetic neuralgia to be connected to oral shingles. Intraoral shingles may present with unusual side effects that are not observed in other cases. Blood vessels and nerves are closely related, so when a virus spreads to affect blood vessels, it can compromise blood flow and occasionally result in ischemic necrosis. Complications like osteonecrosis, tooth loss, periodontitis (gum disease), pulp calcification, pulp necrosis, periapical lesions, and abnormalities in tooth development can occasionally result from oral involvement.

3.2.1.1.1. Disseminated Shingles

Individuals with compromised immune systems may develop a widespread rash known as disseminated shingles. It is characterized by the appearance of more than 20 skin lesions outside the dermatome that is primarily affected or the dermatomes that are next to it. In addition to the skin, the illness may potentially be fatal because it can also damage other organs like the liver or brain, which can result in encephalitis or hepatitis, respectively.

3.2.1.2. Diagnosis

Since few diseases cause a rash in a dermatomal pattern, if the rash has developed, diagnosing this illness (making a differential diagnosis) only needs a visual examination. But sometimes the herpes simplex virus (HSV) can cause a rash that looks like this (called zosteriform herpes simplex).

Shingles can be challenging to diagnose when the rash is not present, whether it is early or late in the disease or in cases of zoster sine herpete. Other conditions can also present with similar symptoms aside from the rash.

Laboratory tests are available for the diagnosis of shingles. One common test looks for VZV-specific IgM antibodies in the blood, which are only present during chickenpox or shingles and not when the virus is dormant. In larger labs, lymph samples from a blister can be tested using PCR to detect VZV DNA or examined under an electron microscope for virus particles. Molecular biology tests, particularly PCR tests, are currently considered the most reliable for shingles diagnosis. While nested PCR tests are highly sensitive, they can be prone to contamination and false positives. Real-time PCR tests are now available and offer rapid and easy testing with sensitivity similar to nested PCR but with a lower risk of contamination. These tests also have greater sensitivity than viral cultures.

3.2.1.3. Treatment

The objectives of treatment are to decrease complications, shorten the duration of a shingles episode, and limit the intensity and duration of pain. Treatment for the complication of postherpetic neuralgia is often symptomatic. In contrast, postherpetic neuralgia is extremely rare in people under 50 and goes away over time; in older people, the pain lessened over time, but even in those over 70, 85% of patients reported being pain-free a year following their shingles outbreak, according to a study on untreated shingles.

3.2.1.3.1. Analgesics

Individuals experiencing mild to moderate pain can use over-the-counter pain medications for relief. Calamine lotions can be applied to rashes or blisters to provide soothing effects. In cases of severe pain, opioids like morphine may be necessary. After the lesions have crusted over, capsaicin cream can be applied. Topical lidocaine and nerve blocks are also effective in pain management. Combining gabapentin with antivirals can help alleviate postherpetic neuralgia symptoms.

3.2.1.3.2. Antivirals

Antiviral medications don't stop postherpetic neuralgia, but they can lessen the intensity and duration of shingles. Acicovir has been the recommended treatment among these medications; however, valaciclovir, and famciclovir, two more recent additions, show good safety and tolerability along with comparable or even greater efficacy. The medications are used as acute phase therapy as well as preventative (in individuals with HIV/AIDS, for example). Intravenous aciclovir may protect immunocompromised shingles patients from complications. Five oral doses of aciclovir per day are usually effective in people who have a high risk of developing shingles attacks more frequently.

3.2.1.3.3. Steroids

It does not seem that corticosteroids reduce the likelihood of chronic pain. However, there don't seem to be many side effects. As of 2008, their application in Ramsay Hunt syndrome had not been thoroughly investigated.

3.2.1.3.4. Zoster ophthalmicus

The treatment for *Zoster ophthalmicus* follows the same standard guidelines as treating shingles in other areas of the body. A study comparing the effectiveness of aciclovir and its prodrug, valaciclovir, showed similar results in treating this specific form of the disease.

3.2.2. Wart

Non-cancerous viral growths called warts typically appear on the hands and feet, but they can also affect other parts of the body like the face or genitalia. There could be one wart or several. Because they are brought on by a viral infection, like the human papillomavirus, as opposed to a malignant growth, they can be differentiated from cancerous tumors.

Risks for contracting the virus include using public showers and pools, handling meat, having eczema, and having a weakened immune system. The virus is believed to enter the body through a skin wound. There are various types of warts, such as plantar warts, filiform warts, and genital warts, which can be transmitted sexually (Figure 3.6).

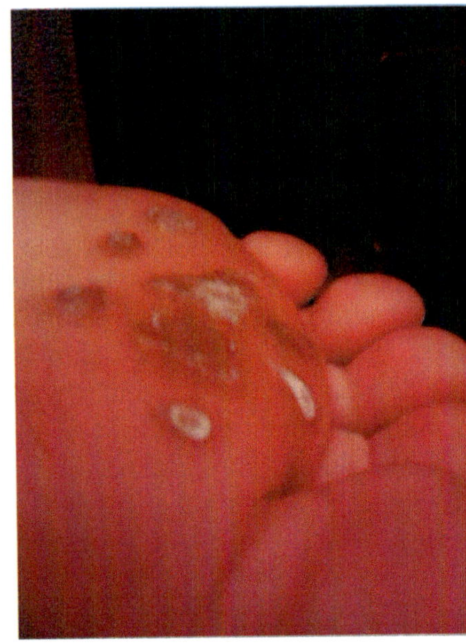

Figure 3.6. *Plantar warts.*

Source: By Lynes225 - Own work, Public Domain, https://commons.wikimedia.org/w/index.php?curid=6757190.

Most wart types go away on their own in months or years if left untreated. Treatments such as cryotherapy and topical salicylic acid application can expedite resolution. They usually do not cause major issues in otherwise healthy individuals. Treatment for genital warts is not the same as for other kinds. Warts can develop as a result of viral infection, such as HIV. This can be avoided by using caution when handling needles or other sharp objects that could cut the skin, practicing safe sex, and abstaining from sexual activity. There are several ways to avoid contracting non-sexually transmissible viruses, like wearing shoes outside and avoiding places that aren't sanitized and where people aren't dressed appropriately, like locker rooms or public restrooms.

Warts are a common skin condition, with the majority of individuals experiencing an infection at some point in their lifetime. The estimated prevalence of non-genital warts in the general population is between 1–13%, with a higher occurrence among young individuals. Before the widespread use of the HPV vaccine, the estimated rate of genital warts among sexually active women was 12%. The earliest known documentation of warts dates back to 400 BC by the Greek physician Hippocrates.

3.2.2.1. Symptoms

Common warts symptoms include:

- Small, fleshy, grainy bumps on the fingers or hands.
- Feeling rough to the touch.
- A sprinkling of black dots, which are clotted blood vessels.

3.2.2.2. Causes

HPV, also known as the human papillomavirus, is the culprit behind common warts. Though this common virus comes in over a hundred varieties, only a handful lead to hand warts. Sexual contact can spread certain strains of HPV. However, the majority are transmitted through casual skin contact or shared items like washcloths or towels. Typically, skin breaks like hangnails or scrapes are how the virus spreads. Warts on your fingertips and around your nails can also spread as a result of biting your nails.

3.2.2.3. Diagnosis

When warts are examined under a microscope, they frequently have extensions that resemble fingers or knobs.

3.2.2.4. Prevention

Gardasil 6 is an HPV vaccine aimed at preventing cervical cancers and genital warts. Gardasil is designed to prevent infection with HPV types 16, 18, 6, and 11. HPV types 16 and 18 currently cause about 70% of cervical cancer cases, and also cause some vulvar, vaginal, penile, and anal cancers. HPV types 6 and 11 are responsible for 90% of documented cases of genital warts. Gardasil 9 protects against HPV types 6, 11, 16, 18, 31, 33, 45, 52, and 58. HPV vaccines do not currently protect against the virus strains responsible for plantar warts (verrucae).

3.2.2.4.1. Disinfection

The virus is resistant to many common disinfectants and is quite resilient. The pathogen can be disinfected by exposing it to 90% ethanol for at least one minute, 2% glutaraldehyde, 30% Savlon, and/or 1% sodium hypochlorite. The virus can withstand heat and drying, but it can only be destroyed by UV light and temperatures as high as 100 °C (212 °F).

3.2.2.5. Treatment

The removal of warts is linked to numerous procedures and treatments. A review of several skin wart treatments found that salicylic acid-containing topical treatments worked better than placebos. Despite fewer trials, cryotherapy seems to be just as effective as salicylic acid.

3.2.3. Molluscum Contagiosum

Molluscum contagiosum (MC), also known as water warts, is a skin viral infection that causes little pink lesions that are elevated and have a dimple in the middle. They can appear singly or in clusters, and they can get itchy or sore. Any part of the skin can be impacted, but the most frequently affected areas are the face, genital area, arms, legs, abdomen, and neck. Lesions begin to appear about seven weeks after infection. Usually, they disappear without leaving any scars after a year.

The infection is a result of the molluscum contagiosum virus (MCV), a type of poxvirus.

It can be transmitted through direct contact, including sexual activity, or by coming into contact with contaminated items like towels. The virus can also be spread to different parts of the body by the infected person. Factors that increase the risk of infection include a weakened immune system, atopic dermatitis, and living in crowded environments. Recurrence of the infection is possible after initial exposure. Diagnosis is usually made based on the appearance of the characteristic lesions (Figure 3.7).

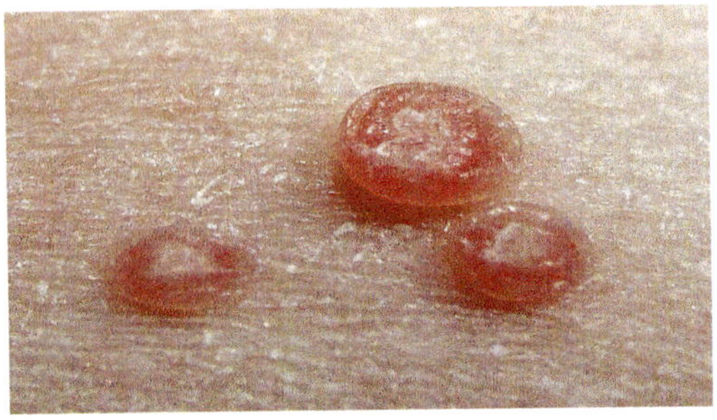

Figure 3.7. *Molluscum lesions.*

Source: By Evanherk, CC BY-SA 3.0, https://commons.wikimedia.org/w/index.php?curid=214029.

Hand washing and avoiding sharing personal goods are two preventative measures. Although there is no need for treatment, some people may want to have the lesions removed for aesthetic purposes or to stop them from spreading. Freezing, laser therapy, or opening the lesion and scraping the inside can all be used to remove it. Nevertheless, scarring may occur if the lesion is scraped. Treatment options include applying podophyllotoxin cream topically or taking cimetidine orally.

As of 2010, molluscum contagiosum affected about 122 million people worldwide, or 11.8% of the total population. Children between the ages of one and 10 are more likely to experience it. Since 1966, the ailment has become more widespread in the US. However, a child's infection does not justify keeping them home from daycare or school.

3.2.3.1. Signs and Symptoms

Lesions caused by Molluscum contagiosum have a flesh-colored, dome-shaped, and pearly look. They frequently have a dimpled center and a diameter of 1–4 mm. The most common places for children to get molluscum lesions are the face, arms, legs, torso, and armpits. Since molluscum lesions in the genital area are typically seen in adults and are thought to be a sexually transmitted infection, it is important to suspect sexual abuse if genital lesions are discovered in children. Although these lesions usually don't hurt, they occasionally itch or get inflamed. Scratching or picking at the bumps could result in scarring, an additional bacterial infection, and the viral infection that causes molluscum contagiosum to spread. Eczema can occasionally appear around the lesions.

Molluscum lesions can usually clear up completely without treatment or scarring in six to 12 months, although they can go away on their own in as little as two months. The average length of an outbreak has been reported to range from eight to roughly eighteen months, but it has also been reported to last anywhere from six months to five years, with immunocompromised individuals experiencing longer durations.

3.2.3.2. Transmission

Molluscum contagiosum lives up to its name by being highly contagious. The virus can be transmitted through various ways, such as direct skin contact during activities like sports or sex, contact with contaminated surfaces, or self-infection through scratching or picking at the lesions and then spreading the virus to other parts of the skin. Children especially are at risk for self-infection and may have numerous clusters of lesions as a result. The viral infection is restricted to the uppermost layer of the superficial skin layer in a specific localized area. The infection disappears as soon as the lesion's virus-containing head is destroyed. The virus is located in the central, waxy core.

3.2.3.3. Diagnosis

The diagnosis is based on the visual characteristics of the virus as it cannot be easily cultured. Confirmation of the diagnosis can be obtained through excisional biopsy.

Molluscum contagiosum is typified histologically by molluscum bodies (also called Henderson-Patterson bodies) in the epidermis above the stratum basale. These bodies are made up of cells with a small nucleus that has been pushed to the periphery and an abundance of large granular eosinophilic cytoplasmic inclusion bodies (accumulated virions) (Chen et al., 2013).

3.2.3.4. Management

First recommendations are often to wait for the lesions to go away on their own because molluscum contagiosum usually goes away on its own and treatment options can be uncomfortable for kids. According to a meta-analysis of randomized controlled trials, no single treatment is noticeably superior to the condition's natural resolution, and there is no difference in short-term improvement between the available treatments.

To try to stop them from spreading, bumps in the genital area may be treated. The infection has been successfully treated when all bumps have disappeared; unless the patient becomes infected again, the infection will not return.

3.2.3.4.1. Medications

Over-the-counter topical medications, like potassium hydroxide, may offer some benefit in mild cases. Other topical treatments, such as tretinoin, benzoyl peroxide, and salicylic acid, have less evidence supporting them, but none of them is advised above the others in terms of reducing the length of an infection.

According to studies, cantharidin is a safe and efficient way to get rid of molluscum contagiosum. Although there is a common incidence of mild side effects like blistering or pain, this medication is generally well tolerated. Cimetidine lacks solid supporting evidence. However, because oral cimetidine is typically well tolerated and less invasive, it has been used as an alternative treatment for the pediatric population.

3.2.3.5. Prognosis

The majority of molluscum contagiosum cases resolve on their own in two years, usually in nine months. There is a chance of spreading the infection to someone else as long as the skin growths remain. The growths have to disappear in order for the infection to stop spreading.

Unlike herpesviruses, which can remain inactive in the body for months or years before reappearing, molluscum contagiosum does not remain in the body when the growths are gone from the skin and will not reappear on their own.

3.3. Fungal Skin Infections

The feet, the armpit, or places where skin folds are present are among the moist parts of the body where these kinds of fungal infections are most likely to appear.

An allergy to the fungus may occasionally result in symptoms in non-affected areas. For example, someone may get a rash on their fingers if they have a fungal infection on their foot. It does not occur as a result of the person touching their foot.

3.3.1. Dermatophyte

A common term for a family of Arthrodermataceae fungi that frequently causes skin conditions in both humans and animals is "dermatophyte." The genera of mold that are considered anamorphic, meaning they are imperfect or asexual, are Microsporum, Epidermophyton, and Trichophyton. These three genera comprise roughly 40 species. Members of the Ascomycota's teleomorphic genus Arthroderma are sexually reproducing species. Nine genera have been identified as of 2019 and a new phylogenetic taxonomy has been suggested.

Dermatophytes are responsible for skin, hair, and nail infections as they feed on keratinized material. These organisms thrive in keratin tissues, triggering inflammation as the body reacts to their waste products. Normally, dermatophyte colonies are confined to the outer layer of the skin because they cannot penetrate deeper tissues in a healthy individual. However, their invasion can provoke a range of host responses, from mild to severe.

Acid proteinases, elastase, keratinases, and other enzymes are reported to enhance the virulence of dermatophytes by breaking down proteins in the host. These degraded proteins then serve as food for the fungi. The development of a cell-mediated immune response, characterized by delayed hypersensitivity and inflammation, is linked to successful treatment of dermatophyte infections. Conversely, a weakened or absent cell-mediated immunity can lead to chronic or recurring infections.

Even though they are not brought on by worms, some of these skin infections go by the names tinea or ringworm. The term "tinea," which means "worm," is believed to refer to the dermatophyte's appearance on the skin, which resembles a snake. Onychomycosis is the term for infections of the fingernails and toenails. Dermatophytes typically colonize the skin's outer layer rather than entering living tissues. On rare occasions, the organisms do infiltrate subcutaneous tissues, which leads to the formation of kerion.

3.3.1.1. Types of Infections

Infections by dermatophytes affect the superficial skin, hair, and nails are named using "tinea" followed by the Latin term for the area that is affected. Manifestation of infection tends to involve erythema, induration, itching, and scaling. Dermatophytoses tend to occur in moist areas and skin folds. The degree of infection depends on the specific site of infection, the fungal species, and the host inflammatory response.

Dermatophytoses can cause chronic progressive eruptions that last months or years, causing significant discomfort and disfigurement, even though symptoms may not even be noticeable in some cases. The majority of dermatophytoses are painless and not fatal.

3.3.1.1.1. Tinea Pedis or Athlete's Foot

Tinea pedis is not limited to athletes, despite its name. Men are more likely than women to get tinea pedis, which is rare in young children. One of the most prevalent fungal infections of the superficial skin, even in developed nations, is tinea pedis.

The infection appears as an interdigital pattern between the toes and may eventually spread to the foot's sole in a moccasin pattern. There is a chance that the infection will worsen and develop into a vesiculobullous pattern, which is characterized by tiny blisters filled with fluid. Itching, peeling, and maceration—peeling brought on by moisture—may coexist with the lesions. In advanced stages of tinea pedis, the soles may develop hyperkeratosis (thickened skin), bacterial infection (by streptococcus and staphylococcus), or cellulitis as a result of developing fissures between the toes.

Onychomycosis of the toenails is another consequence of tinea pedis, particularly in older adults or in those with vascular disease, diabetes mellitus, or nail trauma. In addition to becoming thick, discolored, and brittle, onycholysis—the painless separation of the nail from the nail bed—occurs frequently.

3.3.1.1.2. Tinea Cruris or Jock Itch

occurs in men more frequently than in women. Sweat and tight clothing can make tinea cruris worse (hence the term jock itch). Often, there is also involvement of the feet. According to theory, infection starts on the feet when they come into contact with the ground. When you put on pants or underwear, you may scratch yourself, which can transfer fungal spores to your groin area. Often, the infection spreads from the groin to the gluteal cleft and perianal skin.

The red, scaly, pustular rashes are frequently accompanied by itching. It's important to distinguish tinea cruris from other comparable skin disorders like psoriasis, erythrasma, and intertriginous candidiasis.

3.3.1.1.3. Tinea Corporis or Ringworm of the Body

Lesions typically appear as round, red, scaly patches with raised, well-defined edges. They are extremely itchy and frequently have a central clearing. Usually found on the trunk, limbs, and other body parts. The lesions can be mistaken for psoriasis, eczema, and contact dermatitis (Figure 3.8).

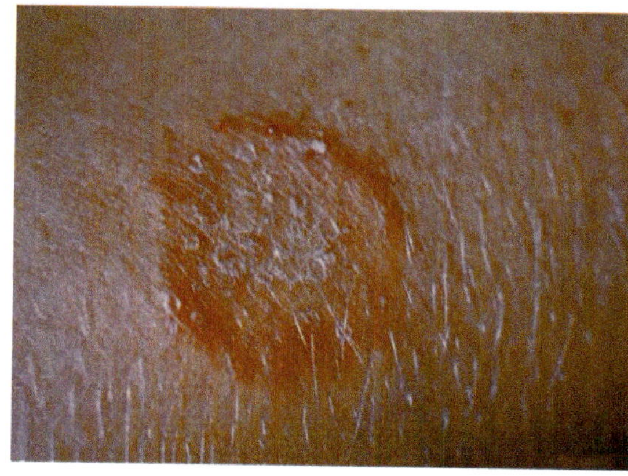

Figure 3.8. *Ringworm.*

Source: By CDC/ Dr. Lucille K. Georg – http://phil.cdc.gov/phil_images/20030116/13/PHIL_2938_lores.jpg, Public Domain, https://commons.wikimedia.org/w/index.php?curid=760083.

3.3.1.1.4. Tinea Faciei or Facial Ringworm

On parts of the face without facial hair, round or ring-shaped red patches may appear. This kind of dermatophytosis, also referred to as "tine incognito," can appear subtle. It may be misdiagnosed as discoid lupus, psoriasis, or another illness. and may worsen when treated with topical steroid creams that suppress the immune system.

3.3.1.2. Immune Response

Thankfully, dermatophytoses quickly move past the inflammatory phase and enter a spontaneous, mostly cell-mediated healing state. Phagocytes eliminate fungi both intracellularly and extracellularly through oxidative pathways. It is most likely the T-cell-mediated response utilizing TH1 cells that regulates infection. Whether the antifungal antibodies produced in reaction to the infection contribute to immunity is unknown.

Infection may become chronic and widespread if the host has a compromised immune system and is receiving treatment that reduces T-lymphocyte function. Also, the responsible species for chronic infections in both normal and immunocompromised patients tends to be *Trichophyton rubrum*; immune response tends to be hyporeactive. However, the clinical manifestations of these infections are largely due to delayed-type hypersensitivity responses to these agents rather than from direct effects of the fungus on the host.

3.3.1.3. Diagnosis and Identification

Dermatophyte infections are typically diagnosed based on how they appear. On the other hand, a rapid in-office confirmatory test can also be performed, which involves slicing off a sample of a lesion from the scalp, skin, or nail with a scalpel and putting it on a slide. To find out if hyphae are present, potassium hydroxide (KOH) is added to the slide and the sample is examined under a microscope. When collecting a sample, caution should be exercised because false-negative results can happen if the patient is already taking an antifungal, if the sample is taken from the incorrect site, or if the sample is too tiny.

Furthermore, the use of ultraviolet light in a Wood's lamp examination can be employed to diagnose particular fluorescing dermatophytes. A fungal culture may be necessary if there is an outbreak or if a patient is not improving with treatment. When considering long-term oral therapy, a fungal culture is also performed (Tosti and Piraccini, 2003).

A fungal culture medium is useful for accurately identifying fungal species. Fungi typically thrive at 25°C on Sabouraud agar within a span of a few days to a few weeks. In the culture, distinctive septate hyphae can be observed alongside epithelial cells, with conidia potentially forming on hyphae or conidiophores. *Trichophyton tonsurans*, the culprit behind scalp infection known as tinea capitis, can be detected as tightly packed arthrospores in broken hairshafts scraped from the scalp's plugged black dots. The microscopic morphology of micro- and macroconidia is a key feature for identification, with proper slide preparation and stimulation of sporulation sometimes necessary. While small microconidia may not always develop, the larger macroconidia play a crucial role in identifying the fungal species.

Surface texture, topography, and pigmentation are examples of culture characteristics that are least reliable for identification because they are variable. Clinical details like the lesion's appearance, location, history of travel, encounters with animals, and race are also crucial, particularly when identifying uncommon non-sporulating species like *Trichophyton concentricum*, *Microsporum audouinii*, and *Trichophyton schoenleinii*.

To cultivate and identify dermatophytes, a unique agar known as Dermatophyte Test Medium (DTM) has been developed. With a straightforward color test, the dermatophyte can be identified without the need to examine the colony, hyphae, or macroconidia. The DTM culture medium is embedded with the specimen, which is scraped from the skin, nail, or hair. For 10 to 14 days, it is incubated at room temperature. The medium will become bright red if the fungus is a dermatophyte. If the fungus is not dermatophytic, there won't be any noticeable change in color. False positives can occur even with non-dermatophytes if kept for longer than 14 days. If needed, specimens from the DTM can be submitted for species identification.

The misdiagnosis of fungal infections can occur because dermatophyte infections frequently mimic other inflammatory skin conditions or dermatitis.

3.3.1.4. Transmission

Direct contact with an infected host, whether human or animal, or indirect contact with contaminated shed skin or hair in objects like clothes, combs, hair brushes, theater seats, caps, furniture, bed linens, shoes, socks, towels, hotel rugs, sauna, bathhouse, and locker room floors are the two ways that dermatophytes are spread. Transmission can also happen when skin comes into contact with soil. The organism may survive in the environment for up to 15 months, depending on the species.

Even healthy people can contract an infection, but the risk is higher if there has previously been skin damage to the area, such as burns, scars, or extreme heat or humidity. Most geophilic species reduced their loss of sporulation, sexuality, and other traits related to soil as a result of adapting to grow on humans.

3.3.1.5. Treatment

Topical treatment is available for tinea corpora (body), tinea manus (hands), tinea cruris (groin), tinea pedis (foot), and tinea facie (face). Oral terbinafine, itraconazole, or griseofulvin treatment is typically necessary for tinea unguum (nails). Generally speaking, griseofulvin is not as efficient as itraconazole or terbinafine. Although a lacquer (Penlac) can be applied every day, it won't work unless vigorous debridement of the damaged nail is also done.

Scalp tingea capitis requires oral treatment because the drug needs to be deeply ingested into the hair follicles to kill the fungus. Griseofulvin is typically taken orally for two to three months. Clinical dosages up to twice the suggested dose may be utilized because certain dermatophyte strains are relatively resistant.

Tinea pedis is typically treated with topical medications such as terbinafine or ketoconazole, pills, or medications containing tolnaftate, clotrimazole, or miconazole. To treat secondary bacterial infections (from scratching, for example) that develop in addition to the fungus, antibiotics might be required.

3.3.2. Candidiasis

Candidiasis is a fungal infection caused by species of the Candida genus, also known as yeast. In some countries, it is commonly referred to as thrush when it affects the mouth. Symptoms may include white patches on the tongue, soreness, and difficulty swallowing. When it affects the vagina, it may be called a yeast infection or thrush, with symptoms such as itching, burning, and a white discharge. Yeast infections in men are rare and may present as an itchy rash on the penis. In severe cases, yeast infections can spread to other parts of the body, causing symptoms like fever.

Candida albicans is the most prevalent of the more than 20 varieties of Candida that can cause infection. Mouth infections are most common in elderly people, children under one month old, and people with weakened immune systems. HIV/AIDS, corticosteroid use, diabetes, and the medications taken after organ transplantation are among the conditions that cause a weakened immune system. Wearing dentures, breastfeeding, and continuing antibiotic therapy are additional risk factors. Pregnant women, those with weakened immune systems, and those who have taken antibiotics are more likely to get vaginal infections. Low birth weight infants, patients recovering from surgery, patients admitted to intensive care units, and people with weakened immune systems are among the groups of people who are susceptible to invasive candidiasis.

Those with weakened immune systems should use chlorhexidine mouthwash and wash their mouths after using inhaled steroids to prevent oral infections. Probiotics appear to have limited efficacy in treating or preventing vaginal infections, even in those who have them frequently. Topical clotrimazole or nystatin treatment is typically effective for treating oral infections. If these don't work, you can try amphotericin B, itraconazole, or fluconazole orally or intravenously. For vaginal infections, a variety of topical antifungal drugs are available, such as clotrimazole. An echinocandin such as micafungin or caspofungin is used in patients with widespread disease. An alternative would be several weeks of intravenous amphotericin B. Antifungal drugs may be used preventively and concurrently with drugs known to trigger infections in some extremely high-risk populations.

3.3.2.1. Signs and Symptoms

Depending on the affected area, candidiasis presents with different signs and symptoms. The majority of candidal infections cause only minor side effects like redness, itching, and discomfort; however, in some populations, untreated complications can be quite serious or even fatal. A localized infection of the skin, nails or toenails (onychomycosis), or mucosal membranes, such as the pharynx and oral cavity (thrush), esophagus, and sex organs (vagina, penis), is typically the result of candidiasis in healthy (immunocompetent) individuals; less frequently, candida infections occur in the gastrointestinal tract, urinary tract, and respiratory tract in healthy individuals.

Candida esophageal infections are more common in immunocompromised people than in healthy people, and they have a greater chance of spreading throughout the body and developing into candidemia, a much more dangerous illness. Esophageal candidiasis symptoms include nausea, vomiting, abdominal pain, difficulty swallowing, and painful swallowing.

3.3.2.1.1. Mouth

White discolorations in the tongue, mouth area, and throat are indicative of a mouth infection. Additionally, irritation could happen and make swallowing uncomfortable (Figure 3.9).

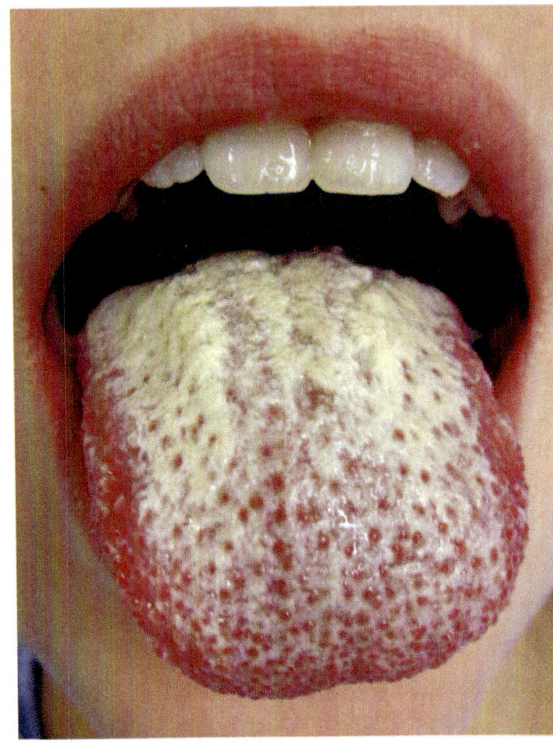

Figure 3.9. *Oral candidiasis.*

Source: By James Heilman, MD – Own work, CC BY-SA 3.0, https://commons.wikimedia.org/w/index.php?curid=11717223 Thrush is commonly seen in infants. It is not considered abnormal in infants unless it lasts longer than a few weeks.

3.3.2.1.2. Genitals

A white or white-gray discharge resembling cottage cheese and intense itching, burning, soreness, and irritation can be signs of a vaginal or vulva infection. Male genital thrush, or balanitis, is characterized by redness around the penis' head; swelling, irritation, itching, and soreness; thick, lumpy discharge under the foreskin; an unpleasant stench; difficulty retracting the foreskin (phimosis); and pain during sex or while passing urine.

3.3.2.1.3. Skin

Itching, irritation, and chafing or broken skin are indications and symptoms of skin candidiasis.

3.3.2.1.4. Invasive Infection

In healthy individuals, anal itching, belching, bloating, indigestion, nausea, diarrhea, gas, intestinal cramps, vomiting, and gastric ulcers are common signs of gastrointestinal candidiasis. Anal itching can be a symptom of perianal candidiasis, which is not thought to be a sexually transmitted infection. The lesion may appear red, papular, or ulcerative. Dysbiosis may result from aberrant candida growth in the gastrointestinal tract. Although the exact cause of the symptoms commonly associated with irritable bowel syndrome and other gastrointestinal disorders is unknown, this change may be the cause.

3.3.2.1.5. Neurological Symptoms

Meningitis-like symptoms can be caused by systemic candidiasis, which can impact the central nervous system and cause a range of neurological symptoms.

3.3.2.2. Causes

Candida yeasts are typically found in healthy individuals as part of the normal flora in the mouth, intestines, and on the skin. These yeasts are usually kept in check by the immune system and competition from other microorganisms, like bacteria. Candida thrives in moist environments, such as on the skin, and wearing wet clothing for extended periods can increase the risk of infection. In babies, Candida can lead to diaper rashes. In severe cases, Candida infections can spread from the skin or mucous membranes into the bloodstream, causing systemic infections. HIV/AIDS, mononucleosis, cancer treatments, steroids, stress, antibiotic therapy, diabetes, and dietary deficiencies are among the factors that raise the risk of developing candidiasis. Treatments for infertility and hormone replacement therapy may also be risk factors. The risk of oral candidiasis is increased by the use of inhaled corticosteroids. People are even more at risk when using inhaled corticosteroids in combination with other risk factors like oral glucocorticoids, antibiotics, not washing their mouth after using inhaled corticosteroids, or high dosages of inhaled corticosteroids. The severity of the condition may increase if the oral and intestinal flora's natural competitors for resources are eliminated by antibiotic treatment. Metabolic disorders and a compromised or underdeveloped immune system are important predisposing factors for candidiasis. About 15% of patients with compromised immune systems experience a systemic illness brought on by a Candida species. Oral candidiasis rates have been found to be impacted by diets high in simple carbohydrates.

3.3.2.3. Diagnosis

Merely examining the patient's mouth for irritation and white patches could lead to the diagnosis of oral candidiasis. To ascertain the type of organism causing the infection, a sample of the affected area may also be collected.

Aerobic vaginitis is a separate condition that should be ruled out in the differential diagnosis because symptoms of vaginal candidiasis are also present in bacterial vaginosis, which is more common. Merely 33% of women who self-treated for yeast infections actually had those infections, whereas the majority had mixed-type infections or bacterial vaginosis. This information was based on a 2002 study.

A yeast infection can be diagnosed and confirmed by culture or microscopic inspection. A scraping or swab of the affected area is placed on a microscope slide for identification using light microscopy. The specimen is then given a single drop of a potassium hydroxide (KOH) solution (10%). While the skin cells are dissolved by the KOH, the Candida cells remain intact, allowing for the observation of pseudohyphae and budding yeast cells, which are characteristic of numerous Candida species.

A sterile swab is applied to the affected skin surface to begin the culturing procedure. After that, the swab is streaked across a culture medium. For several days, the culture is incubated at 37°C (98.6°F) to promote the growth of bacterial or yeast colonies. The morphology and color of the colonies may provide an early diagnosis of the organism causing the symptoms of the disease. An endoscopy is necessary for the diagnosis of gastrointestinal, esophageal, and respiratory candidiasis. To culture the fungal infection in cases of gastrointestinal candidiasis, a 3–5 milliliter sample of duodenal fluid must be obtained. More than 1000 colony-forming units per milliliter in the culture are required for the diagnosis of gastrointestinal candidiasis.

3.3.2.4. Treatment

Antifungal drugs such as clotrimazole, nystatin, fluconazole, voriconazole, amphotericin B, and echinocandins are used to treat candidiasis. Intravenous echinocandins, like capspofungin, or fluconazole are frequently used to treat critically ill or immunocompromised patients. Numerous specific treatment regimens for Candida infections are listed in the 2016 revision of the clinical practice guideline for the management of candidiasis. These treatment plans take into account various factors such as infection severity and location, immune status, antifungal drug resistance, and species of Candida. Immunocompetent people are treated for gastrointestinal candidiasis with 100–200 mg of fluconazole per day for two to three weeks.

3.3.3. Tinea

A contagious fungal skin infection is tiniera. The feet, groin, scalp, and area beneath the breasts are the most frequently affected areas. Tinea can be transmitted directly through skin-to-skin contact or indirectly through clothing, floors, or towels.

Another name for tinea is ringworm, which is misleading because there isn't a worm involved. Like all fungi, tinea requires warm, humid conditions to thrive. For this reason, the hottest and most perspiration-prone parts of the body are also the most susceptible to tinea infection. Locker rooms and communal showers are common locations where infections can spread.

3.3.3.1. Types of Tinea

Tinea infections are known by specific names, depending on the part of the body that is affected. The most common types of tinea include:

- Athlete's foot – tinea of the foot, known as tinea pedis (Figure 3.10).
- Jock itch – tinea of the groin, known as tinea cruris.
- Ringworm of the scalp – tinea of the head, known as tinea capitis (mainly affects children).
- Ringworm of the body – tinea of the body, known as tinea corporis.
- Nail infection (onychomycosis) – tinea of the toe or finger nails, known as tinea unguium.

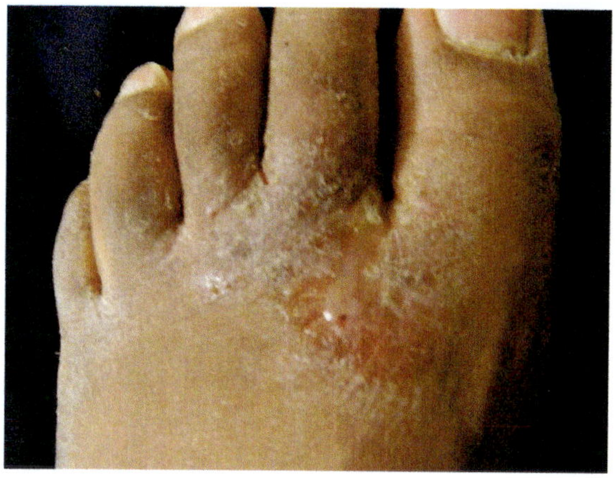

Figure 3.10. *Tinea pedis.*

Source: By Wes Washington – Own work, CC BY-SA 3.0, https://commons.wikimedia.org/w/index.php?curid=26570138.

3.3.3.2. Symptoms of Tinea

The symptoms can include:

- Itching and stinging.
- Red scaly rash that is shaped like a ring (annular).
- Cracking, splitting, and peeling in the toe web spaces.
- Blisters.
- Yellow or white discoloration of the nails.
- Bald spots on the scalp.

3.3.3.3. Treatment

Antifungal creams are effective in treating tinea infections. Certain infections are more difficult to treat, and you may need to take a tablet antifungal medication.

3.3.3.4. Preventing the Spread of Tinea

It is important to remember that tinea is contagious. Suggestions on how to prevent the spread of infection to others include:

- Treat tinea infections with antifungal cream.
- Wash your hands after touching infected areas.
- Do not share towels.
- Do not walk around barefoot if you have tinea pedis (tinea of the feet).
- Clean the shower, bath, and bathroom floor after use.

3.4. Parasitic Skin Infection

There is a parasite responsible for these kinds of skin infections. These infections can travel to the bloodstream and organs in addition to the skin. Although not fatal, a parasite infection can cause discomfort.

3.4.1. Lice Infestation

Wingless insects, known as lice, are hardly noticeable and infest the head, body, or pubic region of a person. Through close contact, sharing of clothing and other personal items, and other means, they can spread easily from person to person. There are three species of lice that live in different body parts. While body lice reside on clothing and bedding, head lice and pubic lice live directly on the human host. Everywhere in the world, there is an infestation of lice.

3.4.1.1. Types of Lice

3.4.1.1.1. Head lice

Hair and scalp are infested with head lice. Close personal contact and possibly the sharing of combs, brushes, hats, and other personal items are the main ways that the infestation spreads. Lice can be ejected from hair by wind or static electricity. Lice can afflict almost anyone, but they are most common in girls between the ages of 5 and 11. Black people are less likely to get head lice. Head lice are not linked to poor personal hygiene or low socioeconomic status.

3.4.1.1.2. Body Lice

People with bad hygiene, those living in small, crowded spaces (like military barracks), and locations with shared beds are frequently infested by body lice. Instead of living on humans, body lice feed on bedding and clothing that come into touch with the skin. The sharing of infected bedding and clothes is how these lice are transmitted. Body lice, as opposed to head lice, can occasionally spread dangerous illnesses like typhus, trench fever, and relapsing fever.

3.4.1.1.3. Pubic Lice

Sexual contact is the usual method of spreading pubic lice ("crabs"), which mainly infest the hairs in the genital and anal areas in adolescents and adults. Children who have close contact with their parents may contract them. Towels, bedding, and clothing are examples of inanimate objects that can harbor the lice. These lice can also infest the hair on the chest, thighs, and face (beard, mustache, and eyelashes).

3.4.1.2. Symptoms of Lice Infestation

Lice infestation usually causes severe itching in the infested area.

- Skin punctures of a tiny, red, pinpoint size are caused by body lice bites. People may have hives, scratch marks, or a bacterial infection if they have broken skin from excessive scratching. Particularly prevalent are these symptoms on the abdomen, buttocks, and shoulders.
- Pubic lice bites may also cause bluish-gray spots to form on the chest, buttocks, and thighs. Lymph nodes can swell. Lice that have infested the eyelashes cause eye itching, burning, and irritation.

3.4.1.3. Diagnosis of Lice Infestation

Using a fine-tooth comb, go from the scalp outward through damp hair to find head lice. Usually, lice are located behind the ears or at the back of the head. Although lice can be difficult to locate, their eggs are more visible. The shiny, grayish-white eggs, or nits, that female lice lay are observable as tiny globules that are firmly adhered to the base of hair shafts. Since adult female lice lay three to five eggs a day, nits usually outweigh lice by a significant margin. Chronic scalp infestations cause the nits to grow out of the hair with the infestation, so depending on how long the infestation has been ongoing, they may be found some distance from the scalp.

Adult body lice and their eggs also may be found in the seams of clothing and bedding.

Using an ultraviolet light for close inspection and a microscope for analysis, one can detect and identify pubic lice. Additionally, dark brown specks, or feces, may be left on the skin or undergarments by pubic lice.

3.4.1.4. Treatment of Lice Infestation

It is advised to replace or thoroughly launder or dry clean any clothing and linens that have been contaminated by lice. To eradicate lice, items that cannot be cleaned can be sealed in plastic bags and left for a period of two weeks.

3.4.1.4.1. Head Lice Treatment

Several effective prescription and nonprescription (over-the-counter) medications are available to treat head lice.

- Nonprescription shampoos and creams containing pyrethrins plus piperonyl butoxide are applied for 10 minutes and are then rinsed out.

- Prescription permethrin (a synthetic form of pyrethrin), applied as a liquid or as a cream, is also effective.
- Spinosad suspension (liquid) can be used in people 4 years of age and older and is rubbed into a dry scalp and applied to dry hair, left on for 10 minutes, and then thoroughly rinsed off with warm water. Contact with the eyes should be avoided. If live lice are seen after 7 days, a second treatment should be done.
- Prescription malathion is highly effective at killing both adult lice and eggs, but it is not the first treatment doctors give because it is flammable, has an unpleasant odor, and must remain on the person for 8 to 12 hours.
- Lindane—a prescription medication that can be applied as a lotion or shampoo—also cures lice infestation but is no longer recommended because of widespread resistance and toxic side effects.

3.4.1.4.2. Pubic Lice Treatment

Similar to how head lice are treated, nonprescription pyrethrin-containing shampoos and creams can be used to treat pubic lice. Treating sex partners is also necessary. Treatment options for lice affecting the eyelashes include applying petroleum jelly for eight to 10 days, using an instrument to carefully remove each louse, taking ivermectin orally, applying petrolatum salve, or using fluorescein eye drops.

3.4.1.4.3. Body Lice Treatment

Body lice are usually removed without the use of drugs because they live in clothing and linens rather than on humans. In addition to treating a patient's symptoms, doctors advise dry cleaning or thorough laundering of contaminated clothing and linens to replace or decontaminate them. When drying, it is ideal to expose these items to a minimum of 149° F (65° C) of heat.

3.4.2. Scabies

Sarcoptes scabiei, variety hominis, is a microscopic (0–45 mm) mite that causes scabies, a contagious skin infestation in humans. The two most typical symptoms are a rash that resembles pimples and extreme itching. On the skin, microscopic burrows can occasionally be seen. When someone contracts an infection for the first time, symptoms typically appear two to six weeks later. Within 24 hours of a second infection, symptoms could appear. The majority of the body may exhibit these symptoms, or just specific regions, like the wrists, in between the fingers, or around the waist, may. Although it usually only affects young children, the head may also be impacted. Usually, the itching gets worse at night. It is possible for scratching to lead to bacterial infections and skin deterioration.

The ectoparasite *Sarcoptes scabiei* var. hominis, a female mite, is the source of scabies infections. To survive and lay eggs, the mites burrow into the skin. Scabies symptoms arise from an allergic reaction to mites. Usually, an infection only involves 10 to 15 mites. The most common way for scabies to spread is through prolonged (at least 10 minutes) direct skin contact with an infected person, which can happen during sexual activity or cohabitation. Even if the patient is asymptomatic, the disease may still spread. Dense living arrangements, like those in prisons, group homes, and child care centers, raise the possibility of transmission. Disease rates are also higher in areas where there is limited access to water. Crusted scabies is a more severe form of the disease; it is not fundamentally different, but it is characterized by a large mite infestation that usually affects people with weakened immune systems; additionally, the large mite infestation increases the disease's contagiousness. In these situations, the infection may spread by contaminated objects or during brief contact. The mite is so tiny that it can't be seen with the naked eye. It is not immediately apparent; knowing what to look for, having adequate lighting, and magnification all help in detection. Identifying the mite (confirmed scabies), typical lesions in a typical distribution with typical historical features (clinical scabies), or atypical lesions or an atypical distribution of lesions with only a few historical features present (suspected scabies) are the three main methods used to make the diagnosis.

Treatment options for those infected with permethrin, crotamiton, and lindane creams, as well as oral and topical ivermectin, are available. Individuals who have had sexual relations in the past month and cohabiting partners ought to receive treatment concurrently. Clothes and bedding that have been worn within the previous three days ought to be dried in a hot dryer and cleaned in hot water. Further washing is not necessary because the mite cannot survive more than three days away from human skin. After treatment, symptoms might linger for two to four weeks. Retreatment might be required if symptoms persist after this point.

3.4.2.1. Signs and Symptoms

Scabies infections are characterized by extreme itching and superficial burrowing. Usually, there is a four to six-week delay between the onset of infestation and the onset of itching because the symptoms are developed gradually by the host in response to the mites' presence. In a similar vein, symptoms frequently last one to several weeks following the mites' successful removal. As previously mentioned, people who are reexposed to scabies after receiving successful treatment may show signs of the new infestation as soon as one to four days later.

3.4.2.1.1. Itching

In the classic scenario, the itch is made worse by warmth, and is usually experienced as being worse at night, possibly because distractions are fewer. As a symptom, it is less common in the elderly.

3.4.2.1.2. Rash

Scabies typically burrows it's superficially in the skin around the finger webs, feet, elbows, back, buttocks, and external genitalia. The skin on the face and scalp is generally free of infection, with the exception of newborns and immunocompromised individuals. By excavating the adult mite in the epidermis, the burrows are formed. Blisters and pustules on the palms and soles of the feet, or acropustulosis, are common signs of scabies in young children.

The majority of people have linear or S-shaped skin trails left by the burrowing mites, which are frequently accompanied by rows of tiny, zit-like insect or mosquito bites. The hands, wrists, axillae, thighs, buttocks, waist, soles of the feet, areola, and vulva in females, and penis and scrotum in males are the primary areas affected by symmetrical lesions. Except in cases of crusted scabies and infestations of infants, the elderly, and immunocompromised people, the neck and above are usually unaffected. For those who have never been exposed to scabies before, symptoms usually start to show up two to six weeks after the infestation. In those who have already been exposed, the symptoms may show up a few days after the infestation. On the other hand, symptoms could take months or even years to manifest.

3.4.2.1.3. Crusted Scabies

Crusted scabies, also known as Norwegian scabies, is more common in the elderly, disabled, and those with compromised immune systems, such as those with HIV/AIDS, cancer, or immunosuppressive drug users. In individuals with compromised immune systems, the host turns into an increasingly favorable habitat for the mites, which proliferate throughout the host's body, excluding the face. Although the mites in crusted scabies are far more numerous—up to two million at times—they are not more virulent than those in non-crusted scabies. Scaly rashes, mild itching, and thick skin crusts containing a high concentration of scabies mites are all signs of crusted scabies. Because of this, people who have crusted scabies are more likely to spread the disease than people who have regular scabies. These areas are particularly difficult to eradicate mites from because the crusts shield the mites from topical miticides and scabicides, requiring longer treatments (Figure 3.11).

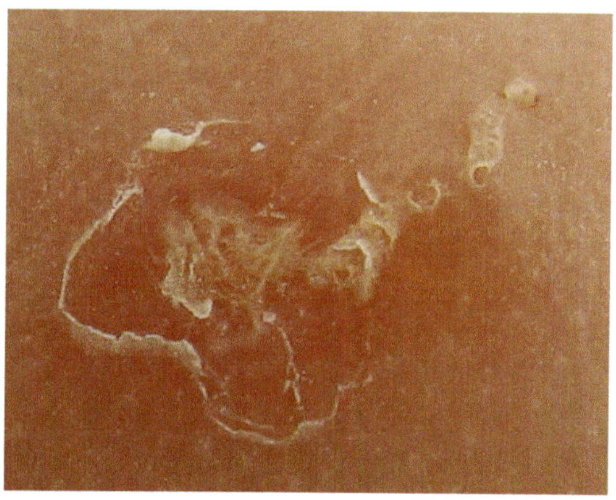

Figure 3.11. *Crusted scabies.*

Source: By Michael Geary - Own work, Public Domain, https://commons.wikimedia.org/w/index.php?curid=1338177.

3.4.2.2. Cause

3.4.2.2.1. Scabies Mite

Italian biologists Giovanni Cosimo Bonomo and Diacinto Cestoni identified the mite that is currently known as *Sarcoptes scabiei*, variety hominis, as the cause of scabies in the eighteenth century. The genus Sarcoptes comprises skin parasites and is a member of the larger mite family commonly referred to as scab mites. These creatures belong to the same phylogenetic class (Arachnida) as ticks and spiders and have eight legs as adults.

S. scabiei mites are tiny, less than 0.5 mm, and occasionally appear as white pinpoints. Gravid females burrow into the stratum corneum, the dead outermost layer of the host's skin, and lay their eggs in the shallow tunnels. The eggs take three to 10 days to hatch into larvae. These juvenile mites crawl across the skin, molt into the nymphal stage, and then mature into adult mites that reside in the host's skin for three to four weeks. Occasionally, males burrow into the skin, but mostly they roam on top of it. A healthy, clean person with non-crusted scabies typically has a small total infestation of adult mites—roughly 11 females in burrows, on average.

The movement of mites on the skin and within the body causes severe itching that resembles a delayed cell-mediated inflammatory reaction to allergens. IgE antibodies, which respond to various protein allergens in the mite's body, are found in the serum and the infection site. Some of these react adversely to dust mite allergens in homes. People who have been infected before, especially within the last year or two, are thought to have experienced a far more rapid allergic skin response to reinfection. Immediate antibody-mediated allergic reactions, or wheals, have been elicited in infected individuals but not in non-infected individuals.

3.4.2.3. Diagnosis

In regions where scabies is common, diffuse itching may be used to make a clinical diagnosis when it coexists with lesions in two typical spots or when another household member exhibits itching. A mite's tunnel under the skin is the traditional indicator of scabies. The suspected area is rubbed with topical tetracycline solution or fountain pen ink, which glows in a particular light, to identify the burrow. An alcohol pad is then used to wipe the skin. The distinctive zigzag or S pattern of the burrow will show up across the skin if the person has scabies; however, interpreting this test could be challenging because the burrows are rare and could be covered up by scratch marks. The presence of the scabies mites, their eggs, or their fecal pellets is necessary for a conclusive diagnosis. To look for these symptoms, a suspected area may be scraped, a sample may be mounted in potassium hydroxide and examined under a microscope, or the skin may be examined directly using dermoscopy.

3.4.2.4. Prevention of Passing on Scabies to Other People

In several populations, oral ivermectin or topical permethrin mass-treatment programs have been successful in lowering the scabies prevalence. There is currently no scabies vaccine. To lower recurrence rates, it is advised to treat all close contacts at the same time, even if they exhibit no symptoms of infection (asymptomatic). Except crusted scabies, mites can only live for two to three days in the absence of a host, so there is minimal chance of transmission from other environmental objects. Cleaning is therefore not very important. It's important to clean the rooms that people with crusted scabies use thoroughly.

3.4.2.5. Management

3.4.2.5.1. Treatment

Scabies can be effectively treated with a number of medications. Everyone living in the household as well as anybody else who has recently had extended contact with the infected person should receive treatment. Apart from managing the infestation, antihistamines, and prescription anti-inflammatory drugs can be used to manage itching. The last three days' worth of clothes, bedding, and towels should be washed in hot water and dried in a hot dryer. Compared to common scabies, treatment protocols for crusted scabies are noticeably more stringent.

3.4.2.5.2. Permethrin

The most preferred course of treatment for scabies is still permethrin, a pyrethroid insecticide. Usually applied before going to bed, it is applied from the neck down, left on for eight to 14 hours, and then washed off in the morning. Not just the symptomatic areas of the skin should be coated; any untreated skin patch can serve as a haven for one or more mites to survive. Permethrin kills adult mites as well as eggs and hatchlings, so one application is usually adequate. However, as a precaution, many doctors advise applying another treatment three to seven days later. Permethrin may cause slight irritation of the skin that is usually tolerable. In recent years, concern is growing about permethrin-resistant scabies, though there are some researchers who call this a case of pseudo-resistance.

3.4.2.5.3. Ivermectin

Scabies can be completely eradicated with oral ivermectin, frequently after just one dosage. It is the preferred course of treatment for crusted scabies and is occasionally administered in conjunction with a topical medication. It is not advised for use with children younger than six years old because it has not been tested on newborns.

Adult cases of scabies have been successfully treated with topical ivermectin preparations. The veterinary equivalent of human scabies, sarcoptic mange, has also shown benefit from its use.

Permethrin's effectiveness is comparable to that of topical or systemic ivermectin, according to one review. While topical permethrin has a lower treatment failure rate than oral ivermectin, it is generally more effective in treating scabies, according to a different review. Oral ivermectin was found to offer a reasonable balance between safety and efficacy in another review. According to a study, scabies is significantly decreased in populations that take ivermectin regularly. The medication is widely used to treat scabies and other parasitic infections, especially in the poor and disadvantaged in the tropics. The drug's developer, Merck, first gave it away for free in 1987 to treat onchocerciasis.

3.4.2.5.4. Others

Sulfur preparations, crotamiton, benzyl benzoate, lindane, and malathion are some additional treatments. Although lindane is effective, its availability has been restricted in many countries due to worries about possible neurotoxicity. Although it is prohibited in California, it is legal as a second-line treatment in other states. Because they are so inexpensive, sulfur ointments, also known as benzyl benzoate, are frequently used in developing nations. Studies have shown that 10% sulfur solutions are effective, and sulfur ointments are usually applied for a minimum of one week, although many people find the smell of sulfur products to be disagreeable. Few studies have found that permethrin is more effective than crotamiton. When it comes to children, crotamiton or sulfur preparations are occasionally advised in place of permethrin because of worries about the substance's dermal absorption (Vary and O'Connor, 2014).

A Closer Look

Mupirocin

Mupirocin is a topical antibiotic that is effective against superficial skin infections like folliculitis and impetigo. It is marketed under the brand name Bactroban among others. If methicillin-resistant S. aureus (MRSA) is found in the nose but not causing any symptoms, it can also be eliminated with it. It is not advised to use for longer than 10 days due to the risk of developing resistance. It is applied to the skin as an ointment or cream.

Headache, nausea, itching, and rash at the application site are typical side effects. Fungi may grow more if used for an extended period of time. Use seems to be safe during nursing and pregnancy. Chemically speaking, mupirocin is a carboxylic acid. It functions by preventing a bacterium from producing protein, which typically leads to the death of the bacterium.

Mupirocin was initially isolated in 1971 from Pseudomonas fluorescens. It is on the World Health Organization's List of Essential Medicines. In 2021, it was the 203rd most commonly prescribed medication in the United States, with more than 2 million prescriptions. It is available as a generic medication.

Medical Uses

Mupirocin is applied topically to treat bacterial skin infections (like boils, impetigo, or open wounds), which are usually caused by an infection with either Streptococcus pyogenes or Staphylococcus aureus. Treatment for superficial methicillin-resistant Staphylococcus aureus (MRSA) infections can also benefit from it. For the majority of anaerobic bacteria, mycobacteria, mycoplasma, chlamydia, yeast, and fungi, dipirocin is inactive.

Preventive intranasal or catheter-site treatment is effective in lowering the risk of catheter-site infection in patients receiving chronic peritoneal dialysis, and intranasal mupirocin before surgery is effective in preventing post-operative wound infection with Staphylcoccus aureus.

Resistance

Soon after mupirocin was first used in clinical settings, mupirocin-resistant strains of Staphylococcus aureus with less than a 30% success rate in clearing nares appeared. Two differe S.aureus populations that are resistant to mupirocin was kept apart. MuL, or low-level resistance, was exhibited by one strain (MIC = 8–256 mg/L), while MuH, or high-level resistance, was exhibited by another strain (MIC > 256 mg/L). The MuL strai resistance is most likely the result of mutations in the wild-type isoléucyl-tRNA synthetase (IleS) of the organism. Within E.coli, a solitary amino acid mutation has been demonstrated to modify mupirocin resistance in IleS. The acquisition of the distinct Ile synthetase gene, MuPA, is associated with MuH. MuH strains cannot be successfully treated with ciprofloxacin. It has been demonstrated that additional antibiotics, including ramoplanin, silver sulfadiazine, nitrofurazone, and azelaic acid, are effective against MuH strains.

The majority of Cutibacterium acnes strains, which are responsible for the skin condition acne vulgaris, have an innate resistance to mupirocin.

Because mupirocin's mode of action is different from that of other clinical antibiotics, it is unlikely that it will cross-resist other antibiotics. The MupA gene, however, might co-transfer with additional genes that confer antibacterial resistance. This has previously been noted concerning resistance genes for trimethoprim, triclosan, and tetracycline. Additionally, it might cause non-susceptible organisms to overgrow.

In 2012, researchers discovered a second type of highly resistant synthetase known as MupB. This synthetase was identified in a Canadian MRSA strain called "MUP87" and is likely situated on a nonconjugative plasmid.

Mechanism of Action

As a result of the inhibition of isoleucyl-tRNA ligase of pseudomonomeric acid in bacteria, isoleucyl-tRNA is depleted and corresponding uncharged tRNA accumulates. Protein synthesis is inhibited upon isoleucyl-tRNA depletion. When the uncharged form of tRNA attaches to the aminoacyl-tRNA binding site on ribosomes, (p)ppGpp is formed, which subsequently prevents the synthesis of RNA. Bacteriostasis is the outcome of both RNA and protein synthesis inhibition working together.

Inhibition of the tRNA ligase/synthase is brought by the structural similarity between the molecule's monic acid head part and isoleucyl-adenylate (Ile-AMS). The unique 9-hydroxynonanoic acid "tail" wraps around the enzyme and further stabilizes the complex, keeping the catalytic part stuck. Mupirocin is able to bind to bacterial and archaeal versions of the enzyme, but not eukaryotic versions.

Summary

- Bacterial skin infections occur when bacteria enter the skin, either from an outside source or because they are present on the skin. They can enter the skin through a hair follicle or after a wound.
- Cellulitis is usually a bacterial infection involving the inner layers of the skin. It specifically affects the dermis and subcutaneous fat.
- Cellulitis is most often a clinical diagnosis, readily identified in many people by history and physical examination alone, with rapidly spreading areas of cutaneous swelling, redness, and heat, occasionally associated with inflammation of regional lymph nodes.
- Impetigo is a bacterial infection that involves the superficial skin. The most common presentation is yellowish crusts on the face, arms, or legs.
- Impetigo is usually diagnosed based on its appearance. It generally appears as honey-colored scabs formed from dried sebum and is often found on the arms, legs, or face.
- A boil, also called a furuncle, is a deep folliculitis, which is an infection of the hair follicle. It is most commonly caused by infection by the bacterium *Staphylococcus aureus*, resulting in a painful swollen area on the skin caused by an accumulation of pus and dead tissue.
- Leprosy, also known as Hansen's disease (HD), is a long-term infection by the bacteria *Mycobacterium leprae* or *Mycobacterium lepromatosis*.
- Viral skin infections are a wide group of conditions. They can be a reaction to a virus inside your body, or they can be an actual infection of your skin.
- These types of skin infections are caused by a fungus and are most likely to develop in moist areas of the body where surfaces meet, such as the feet, armpit, or where there are skin folds.
- Dermatophyte is a common label for a group of fungus of Arthrodermataceae that commonly causes skin disease in animals and humans.
- Candidiasis is a fungal infection due to any species of the genus Candida (a yeast). When it affects the mouth, in some countries it is commonly called thrush. Signs and symptoms include white patches on the tongue or other areas of the mouth and throat.
- Lice are barely visible wingless insects that infest a person's head, body, or pubic area. They spread easily from person to person by close contact and shared clothing and other personal items. Three species of lice inhabit different parts of the body.
- Scabies is a contagious human skin infestation by the tiny (0.2–0.45 mm) mite *Sarcoptes scabiei*, variety hominis. The most common symptoms are severe itchiness and a pimple-like rash.

References

1. Benton, B. (1998). Economic impact of onchocerciasis control through the African Programme for Onchocerciasis Control: An overview. *Annals of Tropical Medicine & Parasitology, 92*(Suppl 1), S33–S39.
2. Breneman, D. L. (1990). Use of mupirocin ointment in the treatment of secondarily infected dermatoses. *Journal of the American Academy of Dermatology, 22*, 886–892.

3. Bronson, D. M., Desai, D. R., & Barskey, S. (1983). An epidemic of infection with *Trichophyton tonsurans* revealed in a twenty-year survey of fungal pathogens in Chicago. *Journal of the American Academy of Dermatology, 8*, 322–330.

4. Carapetis, J. R., Currie, B. J., & Kaplan, E. L. (1999). Epidemiology and prevention of group A streptococcal infections: Acute respiratory tract infections, skin infections, and their sequelae at the close of the 20th century. *Clinical Infectious Diseases, 28*, 205–210.

5. Chen, X., Anstey, A. V., & Bugert, J. J. (2013). Molluscum contagiosum virus infection. *Lancet Infectious Diseases, 13*(10), 877–888.

6. Han, J., Faletsky, A., & Mostaghimi, A. (2020). Cellulitis. *JAMA Dermatology, 156*(12), 1384. https://doi.org/10.1001/jamadermatol.2020.2083.

7. Hay, R. J., Clayton, Y. M., De Silva, N., Midgley, G., & Rossor, E. (1996). Tinea capitis in Southeast London: A new pattern of infection with public health implications. *British Journal of Dermatology, 135*, 955–958.

8. Johnson, R. W., Alvarez-Pasquin, M. J., Bijl, M., Franco, E., Gaillat, J., Clara, J. G., et al. (2015). Herpes zoster epidemiology, management, and disease and economic burden in Europe: A multidisciplinary perspective. *Therapeutic Advances in Vaccines, 3*(4), 109–120.

9. Mirmirani, P., Maurer, T. A., Berger, T. G., Sands, L. P., & Chren, M. M. (2002). Skin-related quality of life in HIV-infected patients on highly active antiretroviral therapy. *Journal of Cutaneous Medicine and Surgery, 6*, 10–15.

10. Tosti, A., & Piraccini, B. M. (2003). Dermatophyte infections. In *European Handbook of Dermatological Treatments* (pp. 131–134). Springer Berlin Heidelberg.

11. Vary, J. C., & O'Connor, K. M. (2014). Common dermatologic conditions. *Medical Clinics of North America, 98*(3), 445–485.

12. Wilmington, M., Aly, R., & Frieden, I. J. (1996). *Trichophyton tonsurans* tinea capitis in the San Francisco Bay Area: Increased infection demonstrated in a 20-year survey of fungal infections from 1974 to 1994. *Journal of Medical and Veterinary Mycology, 34*, 285–287.

Chapter 4

DISORDERS OF PIGMENTATION

Contents

Introduction

Skin color is determined by skin pigmentation, which is the amount of melanin produced by the body. Melanocytes in the skin's epidermal layer produce the two primary forms of melanin, eumelanin, and pheomelanin. Eumelanin produces darker skin tones, whereas pheomelanin produces lighter skin tones.

The dark brown pigment eumelanin, which absorbs UV rays from the sun, shields the skin from sunburn. Higher levels of eumelanin are linked to darker skin tones, whereas lower levels are linked to lighter skin tones. One of eumelanin's other advantages is its ability to prevent skin cancer. According to studies, people with higher eumelanin levels were less likely to get skin cancer than those with lower levels. Eumelanin also contributes to the regulation of body temperature by absorbing solar heat and keeping the body cool.

Pheomelanin is a pigment with a paler yellow-red hue. Higher levels of pheomelanin result in lighter skin tones and make people more vulnerable to sunburn and skin damage because it does not absorb UV rays as well as eumelanin does. However, phenol melanin does have some advantages. It aids in regulating body temperature and, by reflecting heat away from the body, helps keep the body cool in hot weather. Melanoma and other forms of skin cancer can also be avoided with the aid of phenolomelanin.

On chromosome 16, the gene locus q24.3 houses the melanin-producing gene for the melanocortin G-protein-coupled receptor 1 (MC1R). The MC1R gene controls the color of the skin and hair, increases the risk of melanoma, and regulates tanning (sensitivity to light exposure and sunburn).

Different racial groups and members of the same family synthesize melanin at different rates. Genetics, sun exposure, and hormones that stimulate melanocytes—such as lipotropin, adrenocorticotropic hormone (ACTH), and melanocyte-stimulating hormone—are the causes of this variation (MSH). A skin tone that is grayish-brown is obtained by using more melatonin.

Orientation and Directional Terms

Term	Definition	Illustration
Melanin	Melanin is a natural substance that determines the color of skin, hair, and eyes in humans and animals. It's also found in the brain, inner ear, and adrenal gland.	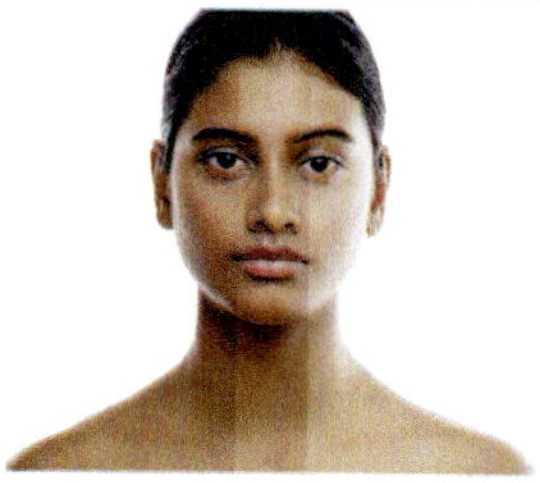
Monopolar radiofrequency (RF)	Monopolar radiofrequency (RF) is a noninvasive cosmetic procedure that uses electromagnetic waves to tighten skin and treat other skin concerns.	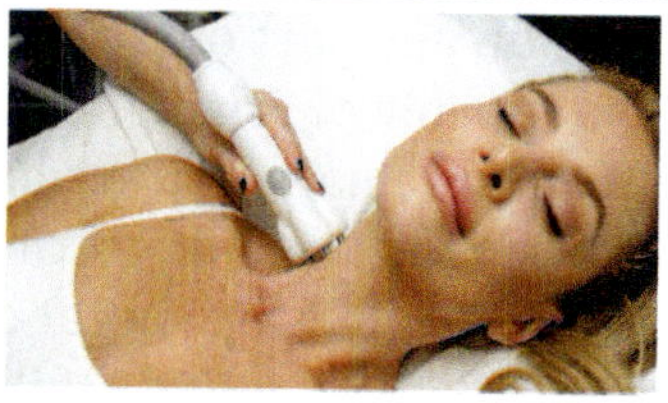
Solar lentigines	Solar lentigines, also known as age spots or liver spots, are small, flat, dark spots on the skin that are caused by chronic exposure to the sun or artificial ultraviolet (UV) light.	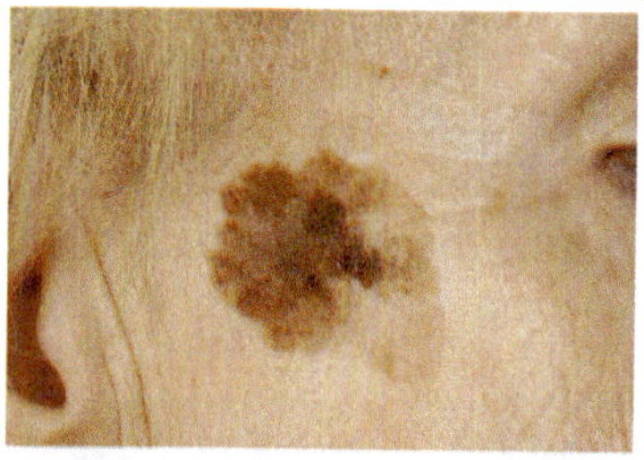
Hyperpigmentation	Hyperpigmentation is a common condition that makes some areas of the skin darker than others. Extra melanin creates spots or patches that look brown, black, gray, red or pink.	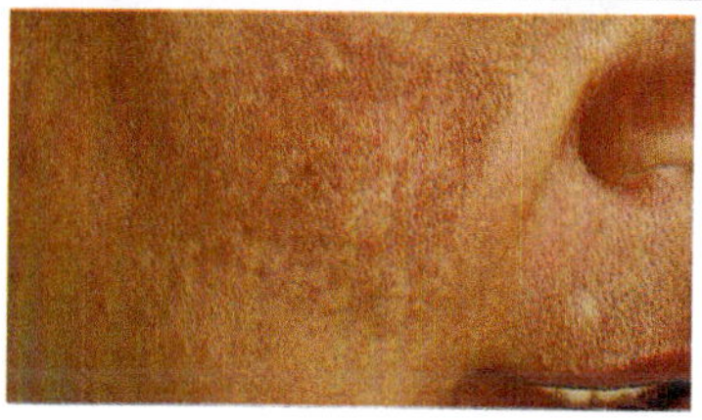
Reflectance confocal microscopy (RCM)	Reflectance confocal microscopy (RCM) is a non-invasive imaging technique that allows clinicians to view skin structures at a cellular level. It's a painless procedure that uses a low-power laser to create a horizontal view of the skin.	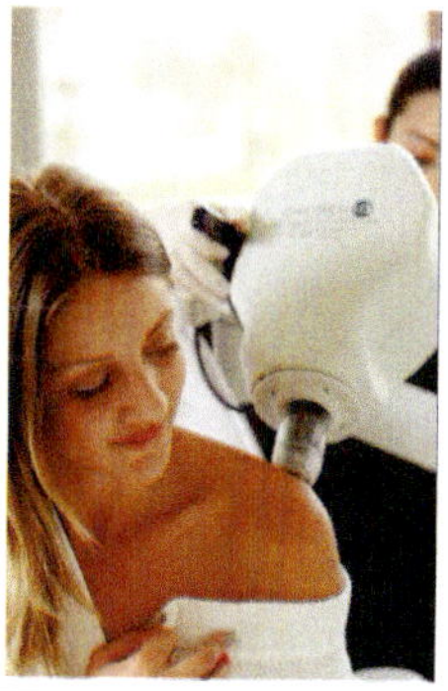

4.1. Vitiligo

Patches of skin that have vitiligo, a chronic autoimmune disorder, lose color and pigment. Although the exact cause of vitiligo is unknown, immune system abnormalities, genetics, stress, or sun exposure may all be contributing factors. Among the available treatment options are topical drugs, light therapy, surgery, and cosmetics. It should be noted that vitiligo can appear as a pale peach color on any skin type and in any size on any part of the body. Vitiligo spots are also capable of "changing" over time; while they tend to remain in the same general locations, they can shift over time. Large patches may move over years, but they never completely vanish (Ortonne and Nordlund, 2006).

4.1.1. Signs and Symptoms

Pale patchy areas of depigmented skin, usually on the extremities, are the only indication of vitiligo. Prior to the appearance of a new patch, some people may experience itching.

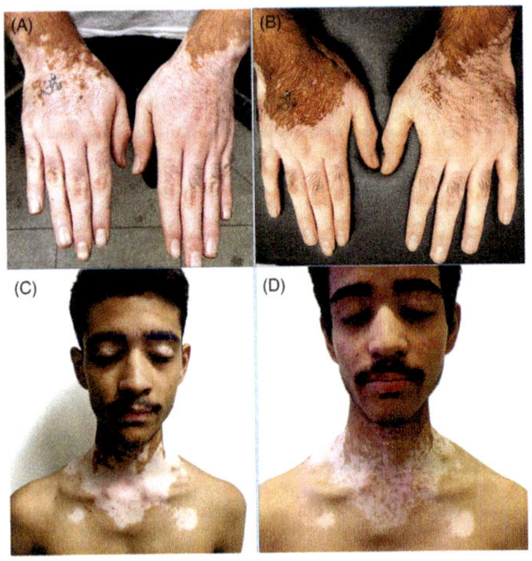

Figure 4.1. *(A) Baseline photograph of vitiligo patch on dorsum of both hands in a patient in oral dexamethasone mini pulse (OMP) group. (B) Perifollolicular and peripheral repigmentation at the end of study period after treatment with OMP. (C) Baseline photograph of vitiligo patch on upper eyelids, neck, and upper chest and in a patient in cyclosporine group. (D) Peripheral repigmentation of eyelids and perifollicular pigmentation of neck & trunk at the end of study period after treatment with cyclosporine.*

Source: https://www.researchgate.net/figure/A-Baseline-photograph-of-vitiligo-patch-on-dorsum-of-both-hands-in-a-patient-in-oral_fig2_352562282.

The patches are tiny at first, but they frequently enlarge and alter in shape. The face, hands, and wrists are the areas of the body where skin lesions are most noticeable. The area around body orifices, such as the mouth, eyes, nostrils, genitalia, and umbilicus, is where the loss of skin pigmentation is most noticeable. There is more skin pigment surrounding the edges of certain lesions. When vitiligo sufferers are stigmatized for having the disease, they may develop depression or other related mood disorders (Figure 4.1).

4.1.2. Causes

Studies clearly suggest that immune system modifications are the cause of vitiligo, despite the fact that many theories have been proposed as possible triggers. It has been suggested that vitiligo is a complex disease in which both environmental and genetic factors may be involved. According to a theory, harmful environmental factors can interfere with the redox reactions that are essential for protein folding. As a result, skin cells may trigger the unfolded protein response, which releases cytokines and boosts the immune system.

According to the National Institutes of Health, there is a belief that sunburns may either cause or worsen the condition; however, there is not enough evidence to support this theory.

4.1.2.1. Immune

The pigment known as melanin, which gives skin its color, is created by skin cells known as melanocytes. Vitiligo has been linked to variations in genes that are either immune system or melanocyte related. It is also believed to be brought on by the immune system targeting and eliminating the skin's melanocytes. In generalized vitiligo, a genome-wide association study identified about 36 distinct susceptibility loci.

The TYR gene encodes the protein tyrosinase, which is not a component of the immune system, but is an enzyme of the melanocyte that catalyzes melanin biosynthesis, and a major autoantigen in generalized vitiligo.

4.1.2.2. Autoimmune Associations

Certain autoimmune and inflammatory conditions, including psoriasis, Addison's disease, scleroderma, rheumatoid arthritis, type 1 diabetes mellitus, pernicious anemia, alopecia areata, systemic lupus erythematosus, and celiac disease, have been linked to vitiligo on occasion.

Caspases 1 and 7 are inflammatory products of NLRP1, and they trigger the inflammatory cytokine interleukin-1β. People who have vitiligo express high levels of interleukin-1β and interleukin-18. One of the mutations involved the substitution of histidine for the amino acid leucine in the NALP1 protein (Leu155 ⍰ His). Throughout evolution, the original protein and sequence have been found in humans, chimpanzees, rhesus monkeys, and bush babies. Vitiligo sufferers may also develop Addison's disease, which is usually an autoimmune disorder characterized by the destruction of the adrenal glands.

4.1.3. Diagnosis

Early on in the illness, an ultraviolet light can be used to identify the condition and assess how well a treatment is working. Skin can be used to see how different bacteria, fungi, and changes in skin pigmentation cause the skin to fluoresce, or change color.

4.1.3.1. Classification

Segmental vitiligo (SV) and non-segmental vitiligo (NSV) are the two categories that have recently been agreed upon, despite classification attempts to quantify vitiligo being analyzed as being somewhat inconsistent. The most prevalent kind of vitiligo is NSV.

4.1.3.1.1. Non-Segmental

In non-segmental vitiligo (NSV), there is usually some form of symmetry in the location of the patches of depigmentation. New patches also appear over time and can be generalized over large portions of the body or localized to a particular area. Extreme cases of vitiligo, to the extent that little pigmented skin remains, are referred to as vitiligo universalis. NSV can come about at any age (unlike segmental vitiligo, which is far more prevalent in teenage years).

Classes of non-segmental vitiligo include the following:

- Generalized vitiligo: the most common pattern, wide, and randomly distributed areas of depigmentation.
- Universal vitiligo: depigmentation encompasses most of the body.
- Focal vitiligo: one or a few scattered macules in one area, most common in children.
- Acrofacial vitiligo: fingers and periorificial areas.
- Mucosal vitiligo: depigmentation of only the mucous membranes.

4.1.3.1.2. Segmental

The appearance, etiology, and frequency of associated illnesses vary among cases of segmental vitiligo (SV). It is not treated the same way as NSV. It is typically unilateral and tends to affect skin regions linked to the spinal cord's dorsal roots. Compared to generalized vitiligo, it appears to have a weaker association with autoimmune diseases and a much more stable and static course. Topical medications and UV light do not help SV; however, surgical procedures like cellular grafting can be successful.

4.1.3.2. Differential Diagnosis

Due to repeated chemical exposures, a similar condition is known as chemical leukoderma. However, vitiligo poses a risk. Inflammatory skin conditions, burns, intralesional steroid injections, and abrasions are a few examples of triggers.

4.1.4. Treatment

Although there is no known cure for vitiligo, there are a number of available treatments. The strongest evidence supports the use of creams in conjunction with UV light and applied steroids. The National Health Service of the United Kingdom advises against using phototherapy unless all other treatments have failed due to the increased risk of skin cancer. Because facial skin is thinner than other skin types, lesions on the hands, feet, and joints are the hardest to repigment. On the other hand, lesions on the face are the easiest (Goudie et al., 1979).

4.1.4.1. Immune Mediators

First-line treatments for vitiligo are thought to involve topical preparations of immune suppressing drugs like calcineurin inhibitors like pimecrolimus or tacrolimus and glucocorticoids like 0.05% clobetasol or 0.10% betamethasone.

In July 2022, ruxolitinib cream (sold under the brand name Opzelura) was approved for medical use in the United States for the treatment of vitiligo.

4.1.4.2. Phototherapy

For vitiligo, phototherapy is regarded as a second-line treatment. The most popular treatment for vitiligo involves exposing the skin to light from UVB lamps. Treatments can be administered in a clinic or at home using an UVB lamp. The duration of the exposure is controlled to prevent overexposure of the skin. If the spots are on the face and neck and have been there for no more than three years, treatment may only take a few weeks. It may take several months if the spots have been there for more than three years and are on the hands or legs. Two to three phototherapy sessions are held each week. Large areas of the body with spots may need to be treated as a whole in a clinic or hospital. Both UVB broadband and narrowband lamps are suitable, although the narrowband UVB lamp with a peak around 311 nm is the preferred option. Re-pigmentation is improved when UVB phototherapy is used in conjunction with other topical treatments, according to constitutive reports. Nonetheless, some vitiligo sufferers might not notice any skin alterations or re-pigmentation. Skin cancer is a serious potential side effect that carries the same risk as excessive exposure to sunlight.

Ultraviolet light treatments, specifically Psoralen and ultraviolet A light (PUVA) treatment, are typically administered in a hospital clinic. This treatment involves taking a drug that enhances the skin's sensitivity to ultraviolet light, followed by exposure to high doses of UVA light. The treatment regimen typically requires sessions twice a week for 6–12 months or possibly longer. Due to the potent doses of UVA and psoralen, PUVA treatment may result in side effects such as sunburn-like reactions or skin freckling.

As effective as PUVA, narrowband ultraviolet B (NBUVB) phototherapy doesn't have the psoralens side effects. Similar to PUVA, psoralen is not required for treatment, which is administered twice a week in a clinic or daily at home. Extended therapy is frequently advised, and it's possible that phototherapy effects take at least six months to manifest. In terms of efficacy, NBUVB phototherapy seems to be superior to PUVA therapy when applied to the face and neck.

In terms of better repigmentation, hydrocortisone plus laser light is superior to laser light alone, ginkgo biloba is superior to a placebo, oral mini-pulse of prednisolone (OMP) plus NB-UVB is superior to OMP alone, and topical calcineurin inhibitors plus phototherapy are superior to phototherapy alone.

4.1.4.3. Skin Camouflage

Patches of vitiligo can be disguised with makeup or other cosmetic camouflage techniques in mild cases. Avoiding tanning of the unaffected skin will help to make the patches less noticeable if the affected person has pale skin.

4.1.4.4. Depigmenting

When treating severe vitiligo, topical medications such as hydroquinone, monobenzone, or mequinol may be used to depigment the skin on the unaffected area and give it a uniform tone. Monobenzone effectively and permanently removes all skin pigment. Sun safety must be followed for the rest of one's life to prevent melanomas and severe sunburn. It takes roughly a year to finish depigmentation.

4.2. Melasma

Melasma is a dark spot or tan on the skin. Sun exposure, genetic predisposition, hormonal fluctuations, and skin irritation are considered to be the causes of melasma. While it can afflict anyone, women are more likely to experience it, especially those who are pregnant, using oral or patch contraceptives, or receiving hormone replacement therapy (Figure 4.2).

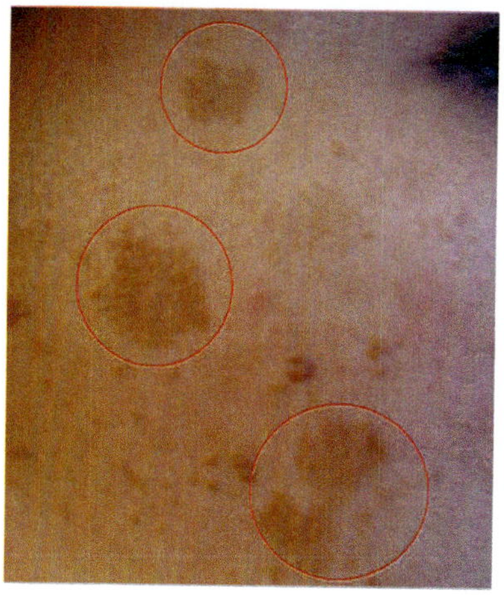

Figure 4.2. *Melasma.*

Source: By User:Elord from Wikidocs – http://www.wikidoc.org/index.php/Image:Melasmablemish.jpg, CC BY-SA 3.0, https://commons.wikimedia.org/w/index.php?curid=12267487.

4.2.1. Signs and Symptoms

Melasma is characterized by dark, asymmetrical, clearly defined, hyperpigmented macules or patches. Usually, these patches appear gradually over time. Beyond the cosmetic discoloration, melasma does not produce any other symptoms. Depending on the individual, patches can range in size from 0 to 5 cm to more than 10 cm. One can classify its location as mandibular, malar, or centrofacial. The most prevalent type is centrofacial, where patches show up on the chin, forehead, upper lip, cheeks, and nose. Patches on both rami are classified as mandibular, whereas patches on the nose and cheeks are only classified as malar.

4.2.2. Cause

Melasma is believed to be caused by UV light from the sun stimulating melanocytes, which are cells in the dermal layer of the skin that transfer the pigment melanin to the keratinocytes. Melasma sufferers frequently recur, especially in the summer, because minor sun exposure can cause the skin condition to return after it has faded.

The so-called "mask of pregnancy," melasma or chloasma, is a common condition in pregnant women. Hormone replacement medication and birth control pills can also cause melasma. Usually, the discoloration goes away on its own over a few months following childbirth, the cessation of oral contraceptives, or hormone therapy.

Another important determinant of melasma development is genetic predisposition. Individuals of African, Asian, or Hispanic heritage with Fitzpatrick skin types III or higher are significantly more vulnerable than others. Furthermore, this condition is more likely to affect women with light brown skin types who live in areas with high levels of sun exposure.

Melasma is more common in patients with thyroid disease, as well as in those experiencing stress, which can lead to an overproduction of melanocyte-stimulating hormone. In rare cases, melasma can also be caused by allergic reactions to certain medications or cosmetics. (Lutfi et al., 1985)

4.2.2.1. Addison's Disease

In 1859, FJJ Schmidt of Rotterdam discovered that Melasma suprarenale is a symptom of Addison's disease, especially when triggered by pressure or minor skin injuries.

4.2.3. Diagnosis

Melasma is characterized by symmetric, reticulated, hyperpigmented patches on the mandible, malar cheeks, centrofacial region, and, in rare cases, the upper chest and extremities. These patches have irregular borders. Though it is known to affect darker skin types more frequently, melasma can affect any skin type. Under a microscope, a noticeable hyperpigmentation can be observed in the pseudo-rete ridges of the skin. When epidermal pigment is used, this hyperpigmentation can be further enhanced with a Wood's lamp. However, dermal or mixed melasma may show this accentuation. Cellular assessment of melasma has also been conducted using reflectance confocal microscopy (RCM). The epidermis displays an increase in hyperrefractile cobblestoning cells, corresponding to hyperpigmented basal keratinocytes on histology. Some patients may also show epidermal dendritic cells corresponding to activated melanocytes. In the dermis, RCM may reveal plump bright cells, melanophages, solar elastosis, and blood. RCM is a non-invasive technique that can detect pigmentary changes in melasma at a cellular level. The differential diagnosis for melasma includes several other conditions such as lichen planus pigmentosus, discoid lupus erythematosus, and various forms of pigmentation disorders caused by different factors.

4.2.4. Pathogenesis

Melasma has a multifactorial etiology. Studies conducted in laboratories and clinics have demonstrated that UV light can both cause and worsen the condition. It is believed that UV light stimulates melanogenesis and activates inducible nitric oxide, which in turn causes reactive oxygen species (ROS). Research has also revealed that, in comparison to healthy volunteers, melasma patients exhibit increased levels of oxidative stress markers. The contribution of visible light to the induction of pigmentation has come to light more recently. In contrast to UVA-1 light, a landmark study revealed that darker skin types sustained pigmentation from visible light over the course of two weeks. According to a different study, increased pigmentation caused by visible light with a wavelength of 415 nm may persist for three months.

Exposure to UV and visible light can stimulate melanogenesis by activating keratinocytes and fibroblasts. One way this happens is through the secretion of stem cell factor (SCF), which binds to the c-kit receptor and promotes the proliferation of melanocytes. A study on melasma found increased levels of SCF in the dermis and c-kit in the epidermis, as well as higher expression of melanogenesis-related genes. Wnt signaling genes were also found to be increased, suggesting a link to the proliferation of melanocyte stem cells. Vascular endothelial growth factor (VEGF) produced by keratinocytes post-UV damage can support melanocytes in tissue culture, potentially contributing to the heightened activity of melanocytes in melasma. Additionally, down-regulation of lipid metabolism-related genes in lesional skin may indicate compromised barrier function, playing a role in the development of melasma.

The idea that melasma is a genetic condition is reinforced by the fact that family history is also a significant risk factor for the condition. Further, 55–64% of patients with this condition have a positive family history, according to some studies. Though no comprehensive investigation of linked genes has been carried out, existing research indicates that pigmentary, inflammatory, hormonal, and potentially vascular responses are the genes in question. Compared to patients with darker skin types (IV–VI), those with Fitzpatrick skin types (FST) II and III are less likely to have a positive family history.

The increased prevalence of melasma associated with pregnancy, the use of oral contraceptives, and other hormonal therapies is evidence that hormones play a major role in the pathogenesis of melasma. Perimenopausal symptoms have also been linked to extra-facial melasma. Progesterone receptor expression was found to be significantly elevated in the epidermis of affected skin, according to an immunohistochemical analysis of the dermis and epidermis of affected and unaffected neighboring skin. Additionally, there was elevated expression of the estrogen receptor protein in the dermis and in the vicinity of the blood vessels; the significance of this is not yet known.

There hasn't been a consistent correlation between melasma and other medical disorders. It was demonstrated in a case-control study that melasma was linked to more nevi and lentigines.

Investigations into the potential correlation between endocrinological disorders, like thyroid disease, and melasma have also been conducted; however, the prevalence of thyroid diseases in these studies has not been found to be higher than in the general population.

4.2.5. Clinical Assessment and Psychosocial Implications

Measuring the severity of melasma can be difficult due to its variable presentation. A number of validated instruments have been developed to assess the psychosocial effects and clinical appearance of melasma-related dyspigmentation. Furthermore, the ability to evaluate the therapeutic efficacy of different melasma treatments in clinical trials has improved thanks to these standardized tools. The degree of facial hyperpigmentation can be gauged using the validated Melasma Area and Severity Index (MASI). This numerical score is derived from an area-weighted assessment of homogeneity and pigmentation on the forehead, chin, and left and right malar cheeks. Modified MASI (mMASI) was developed after homogeneity was removed from the computation because of that metric's declining interrater reliability. It is now correlated with the Melasma Severity Score, a global score that takes into account the patient's subjective evaluation in addition to objective data. These days, clinical trials employ it. A health-related quality of life (HRQoL) tool has been used to assess the psychosocial components of skin diseases for a number of dermatological conditions. The Melasma Quality Of Life Scale (MELASQOL), a validated modified version of the HRQoL, was developed by Balkrishnan and associates. 10 questions about the impact of the disease and quality of life are included in the scale, and each response is graded on a Likert scale. Additional psychometric measures that can be applied to individuals with melasma include the SKINDEX-16 and the Dermatology Life Quality Index (DLQI).

4.2.6. Treatment

Melasma can be treated with topical, oral, procedural, and combination therapies. These target different facets of the pathophysiology of pigmentation, vascularity, inflammation, and photodamage in melasma.

4.2.6.1. Topical

The first-line treatments for melasma are usually topical ones, such as photoprotection. The most often employed therapeutic agents are those that block melanogenesis and melanocyte proliferation, which are the processes that produce melanin. It is preferable to use multiple topical medications concurrently, each with a distinct mechanism of action, rather than monotherapy.

4.2.6.2. Photoprotection

Avoiding UV and visible light is essential to preventing flare-ups and melasma exacerbation. When broad-spectrum UVA and UVB filters were paired with visible light blockers, like iron oxide, versus broad-spectrum UV filters alone, melasma relapses were found to be lower in the former group in multiple randomized-controlled trials involving 40–60 participants.

4.2.6.3. Hydroquinone

In the past, the topical medication that has been studied the most for treating melasma is hydroquinone (HQ). Tyrosinase is inhibited by this compound, preventing DOPA from being converted to melanin. Others have suggested that it may also directly result in the degradation of melanosomes and melanocytes. The application of HQ 4% has improved melasma dyspigmentation statistically significantly in a number of studies. Even though it is highly effective and can be dosed at different strengths, some people may develop an irritating dermatitis from it, and long-term use may result in exogenous ochronosis.

4.2.6.4. Corticosteroids

By non-selectively suppressing melanogenesis, corticosteroids have anti-inflammatory and preventive effects on pigmentation. When used as monotherapy, corticosteroids by themselves are not likely to be better than depigmenting agents. Based on available literature, corticosteroids can suppress melanogenesis on their own, but they have not been shown to provide long-term benefits in the treatment of melasma. In addition, striae, hypopigmentation, acne, telangiectasias, and epidermal atrophy can result from prolonged steroid use.

4.2.6.5. Retinoids

A proposed mechanism of action for topical retinoids in the treatment of melasma is the promotion of keratinocyte turnover. The use of tretinoin 0.1% cream was found to significantly reduce objective colorimetry measurements of melasma pigmentation in a small but sentinel study conducted in 1993. An additional investigation has validated the advantageous application of 0.01% tretinoin cream in the management of melasma in patients of Black ethnicity.

4.2.6.6. Other Synthetic Topical Compounds

4-n-butylresorcinol, another inhibitor of tyrosinase, has been increasingly utilized in trials and has displayed substantial improvement in pigmentation for melasma. Adverse effects like erythema and pruritus were minimal and self-limiting, though long-term data on the product is currently lacking. Tranexamic acid, a synthetic version of lysine and a hemostatic agent, has seen rising use in various forms (topical, oral, injectable) for treating melasma. While studies have shown occasional negative results when used alone, combining it with other pigmentation therapies has boosted efficacy. Interestingly, topical tranexamic acid has shown limited success compared to its oral form. In addition, flutamide, an antiandrogenic agent, has been compared to HQ 4% and was found to have statistically significant improvements in MASI scores and patient satisfaction, although no difference in the mexameter melanin assay was observed between the two groups.

4.2.6.7. Natural Topical Compounds

The therapeutic potential of naturally occurring compounds against pigmentation has been studied recently. Inhibiting melanosome transfer to keratinocytes, niacinamide has been demonstrated to reduce pigmentation in a small study involving 27 participants. In small studies, it has been demonstrated that both ascorbic acid and kojic acid can inhibit tyrosinase activity, which reduces pigmentation.

It is hypothesized that ascorbic acid reduces reactive oxygen species, which lessens inflammation in melasma lesions. However, when used as monotherapies, both were found to be less effective than HQ in raising MASI scores. An open-label study found that azelaic acid (AA), another naturally occurring compound, effectively improved pigmentation by blocking tyrosinase activity. This substance, which comes from the yeast *Pityrosporum ovale*, also reduces inflammation. Although they are uncommon, adverse effects can include erythema and burning. Together with topical licorice and emblica, another natural antioxidant, bellis perennis flower extract has been shown to be as effective as HQ 2% in reducing pigmentation and preventing inflammation by blocking the arachidonic acid cascade. Bellis perennis inhibits the synthesis of melanin. In small studies, other topical natural compounds like arbutin, soy, and lignin peroxidase have also been used with good results to treat melasma.

4.2.6.8. Combination Topical Compounds

Combination topical treatments are more effective than monotherapies, according to recent studies. The first combination topical therapy approved by the US Food and Drug Administration was triple combination therapy (TCT), which included HQ, a retinoid, and a topical steroid. TCT containing HQ 4%, tretinoin 0.05%, and fluocinolone acetonide 0.01% was found to be more effective in improving melasma than HQ 4% monotherapy in a study involving 260 Asian patients that was investigator-blinded and randomized. Notably, compared to 14% of controls, approximately 50% of patients receiving TCT reported higher levels of erythema, skin irritation, and discomfort. In female Korean patients, dual therapy with tretinoin 0.01% and HQ 3% was also shown to improve melasma.

4.2.6.9. Camouflage

Given that melasma is recurrent and that treatment can be lengthy and difficult, cosmetic camouflage can give patients an additional means of enhancing their quality of life and lessening the psychosocial effects of their condition. In a study involving 24 patients with pigmentary disorders, cosmetic camouflage—which includes concealers and other pigmented cover-ups—

has been demonstrated to significantly improve the DLQI. Numerous cosmetic brands provide pigmented foundations and concealers that have the potential to even out skin tones and incorporate broad-spectrum UV protection.

4.2.6.10. Oral

Oral therapies are becoming more common as a treatment option for this disorder, in addition to topical treatments. Tranexamic acid (TA), an anti-plasmin agent, reduces the production of arachidonic acid, leading to a decrease in melanocyte-stimulating hormone (MSH) and pigment production. Studies have shown that TA may also lower levels of VEGF and entothelin-1, which could contribute to increased vascularity in affected areas. While different formulations of TA have not been directly compared, recent research indicates that around 90% of patients who took oral TA saw improvements after 2–6 months, compared to about 95% of patients who used topical 2% preparations and improved after 3 months. Common side effects of oral TA include abdominal bloating, headache, tinnitus, menstrual irregularities, and, rarely, deep venous thrombosis (DVT). It is important to screen for thrombosis risk factors before starting treatment due to the serious potential risks.

Other drugs like glutathione and *Polypodium leucotomos* (PL) have also been investigated as adjuvant therapies with promising outcomes. It has been demonstrated that PL inhibits ROS and lessens UV-induced photodamage. This, in turn, lessens the T cell-mediated response, which raises skin inflammation and pigmentation. Over the course of four weeks, participants in a randomized controlled trial conducted in the Philippines found that taking oral glutathione, a naturally occurring compound, reduced melanin levels in comparison to those taking a placebo. It is believed that glutathione functions as an antioxidant to reduce inflammation.

4.2.6.11. Procedural

The majority of case reports and case series evaluating the use of chemical peels, microneedling, microdermabrasion, and lasers—typically in combination with other treatment modalities—have been included in the recent literature on procedural melasma therapies. It is noteworthy that numerous procedural studies involve the concurrent application of topical treatments and photoprotection.

4.2.6.12. Chemical Peels

Because chemical peels can increase keratinocyte turnover and epidermal remodeling, they have been investigated as an adjunctive treatment modality for melasma. Chemical peels are often applied topically in conjunction with other products. According to a number of studies, superficial peels might help with melasma's epidermal subtype. The most research has been done on glycolic acid (GA), one of the different peels, in relation to treating melasma. A small open-label study discovered that adding 30- to 50% GA peels to an AA 20% twice-daily regimen for six months, spaced three weeks apart, improved MASI scores over AA 20% alone. But when HQ 4% was combined with GA 20–30%, there was no difference in decreased pigmentation compared to HQ alone, according to a small split-face study. A regimen consisting of HQ 4% and salicylic acid (SA) 20–30% peel did not differ from HQ monotherapy, according to another split-face study.

Recent studies have also investigated combination peels. According to a study conducted in India, over the course of 12 weeks, a combination of 20% SA and 10% mandelic acid significantly improved the MASI scores of FST IV and V patients. This combination proved to be just as effective as 35% GA. Peels containing 10–20% trichloroacetic acid (TCA) were found to be as effective as GA peels, but they also had more side effects, like burning and peeling.

4.2.6.13. Microneedling

Mesotherapy, also known as microneedling, is an additional adjunctive treatment that involves creating tiny skin channels to allow topical medications to be applied topically in tiny doses. Compared to traditional resurfacing techniques, the skin punctures caused by microneedling can also promote a positive wound-healing response with fewer side effects. By using this method, the drug may be applied to the dermis and epidermis more evenly and deeply. The data indicated a potential clinical benefit with the use of microneedling but no statistically significant benefit when a randomized study comparing cycles of microneedling alone followed by the application of topical TA was conducted. The study used multiple intradermal microinjections of TA. When topical lightening agents like rucinol and sophora-alpha were combined with microneedling, a prospective study of patients treated with those topicals alone showed a significant improvement in MASI scores. One drawback, though, is that neither the patient nor the researcher were blinded throughout the investigation.

4.2.6.14. Laser and Light Treatments

With differing degrees of success, laser therapy has been studied as a melasma treatment in more recent years. Thermal energy can be used by lasers to target different skin chromophores in a targeted manner. Because non-ablative lasers tend to produce less inflammation and, consequently, less post-inflammatory pigment alteration (PIPA), they are preferred over ablative lasers for the treatment of melasma. Melanin is the specific chromophore that is targeted by non-ablative Q-switched lasers, such as the Q-switched ruby laser (QSRL) and the Q-switched neodymium:yttrium–aluminium–garnet (QNd:YAG) lasers. Neither QSRL nor QNd:YAG has been shown to be effective in the long run in treating melasma when used as monotherapy. Nevertheless, a small study discovered a significant reduction in MASI scores when low-dose fractional QSRL was used. Recent research has shown that low fluence QNd:YAG improves pigmentation; however, patients also used ascorbic acid, HQ, tretinoin, sunscreen, or other products after laser treatment.

Several smaller studies have also successfully treated melasma with intense pulsed light (IPL), both alone and in conjunction with QSRL. Over the course of 14 weeks, fractionated IPL monotherapy, which was used as a maintenance treatment for melasma, improved mMASI scores. According to some authors, having multiple IPL treatments could encourage the melanosomes destroyed by QSRL to shed upward. Consequently, they propose that the combination of QSRL and IPL therapy may reduce the likelihood of post-inflammatory hyperpigmentation (PIH) but may also necessitate additional treatment sessions.

Melasma has also been treated with other ablative lasers, such as carbon dioxide (CO_2), erbium:YAG (Er:YAG), and non-ablative fractional lasers, with differing degrees of success. Despite being used in clinical trials with Q-switched alexandrite lasers, CO_2 lasers have been linked to PIH on multiple occasions, particularly around the edges of lesions. Improved mMASI scores were observed in the CO_2 arm of a recent split-face study comparing low-power CO_2 laser to QNd:YAG, with no discernible difference in side effects.Er:YAG laser has also been demonstrated to improve pigmentation using MASI scores in a small study involving 20 patients; however, recurrence was noted after 3.4–6 months. Using metrics developed by the investigators, two studies using a fractional nonablative 1550-nm erbium-doped fiber laser showed improved pigmentation in approximately 60% of patients.

Melasma has also been treated with other energy sources, such as monopolar radiofrequency (RF). Vasodilatation, intracellular oxygenation, and cellular biostimulation are all brought on by RF. Kojic acid was administered by monopolar radiofrequency (RF) to 50 patients in a prospective study. The patients' MASI scores improved and their level of inflammation decreased. However, the data interpretation was limited because no controls receiving topical therapy was included.

In light of the growing understanding that inflammation and angiogenesis could contribute to the etiology of melasma, four Korean women were studied for eight weeks, undergoing four sessions of a copper bromide anti-angiogenesis laser. Immunohistochemistry revealed that the treatment significantly reduced endothelin-1 and VEGF levels as well as the MASI score.

4.3. Post Inflammatory Hyperpigmentation

All skin types can develop post-inflammatory hyperpigmentation (PIH), an acquired hypermelanosis that follows cutaneous inflammation or injury; however, patients with skin-of-color, such as African Americans, Hispanics/Latinos, Asians, Native Americans, Pacific Islanders, and people of Middle Eastern descent, are more likely to be affected. Because these pigmentary changes can occur more frequently and severely in skin-of-color patients (Fitzpatrick skin types IV through VI) and are frequently more noticeable in darker skin types, PIH can have a significant psychosocial impact on these patients. For skin of color, there are numerous safe and efficient treatments available for photoaging in the headlights (PIH), such as chemical peels, topical depigmenting agents, and laser and light therapy.

4.3.1. Epidemiology

The global prevalence of pigmentary disorders, vitiligo excluded, in different ethnic populations is displayed in Table 4.1. Melasma and solar lentigines may also be included, but postinflammatory hyper- or hypopigmentation is usually included in these figures. Numerous epidemiological studies have demonstrated that patients with skin-of-color tend to experience PIH more frequently than patients with Caucasian skin. A comparison of the most prevalent dermatoses in patients who were Caucasian and African American was published in a 1983 study by Halder et al. Other than vitiligo, pigmentary disorders ranked third among dermatoses among African-American patients (9%), but ranked seventh among patients who were Caucasian (1.7%). Dyschromias was found to be the second most common diagnosis among African-American patients in a more recent study conducted in 2007. However, dyschromias did not rank among the top 10 most common diagnoses for patients who were Caucasian. It's interesting to note that, according to a Singaporean study, Asians with darker skin, like Malays and Indians, also tended to have PIH more frequently than Asians with lighter skin, like Chinese people. This finding raises the possibility that pigmentation level, rather than race or ethnicity, plays a greater role in the development of PIH.

Table 4.1. *Worldwide Prevalence of Pigmentary Disorders (Excluding Vitiligo) in Skin of Color*

Author	Year	Study Population	Prevalence	Rank	Location
Halder	1980–1983	2550: 78.4% African Americans, 21.6% Caucasian	9% black; 1.7% white	3/13 black, 7/10 white	Washington, DC
Chua-Ty	1989–1990	74,589: 77.2% Chinese, 9.9% Indian, 7.6% Malay, 5.3% Other	1.8% Chinese, 2.7% Malay, 2.3% Indian, 1.2% other	10/10	Singapore
Nanda	1992–1996	10,000: 88% Kuwaitis, 8% other Arabs, 4% non-Arabs; all children	0.42%	33/74	Kuwait
Child	1996	461: black (African, Afro-Caribbean, mixed race); 187 children, 274 adults	1.6% children, 3.4% adults	8/14 children, 7/29 adults	London, England
Hartshorne	1999	7029: 76.1% black, 10.9% Caucasian, 6.7% Indian, 6.1% colored (mixed race)	0.7% black, 0.1% Caucasian, 0.3% Indian, 0.5% colored (mixed race)	22/91 overall	Johannesburg, South Africa
Dunwell	2001	1000: 95.6% Afro-Caribbean, 0.8% Caucasian, 2.2% Indian, 1.4% Chinese	22.8% (includes PIH, melasma, solar lentigines)	3/18	Kingston, Jamaica
Sanchez	Published 2003	3000: Latino (1000 private practice, 2000 hospital-based clinic)	6% private practice, 7.5% hospital-based clinic	7/12 private, 6/12 hospital	New York, New York
Arsouze	2004	1064: black (African, Afro-Caribbean; FST V and VI); 228 children, 836 adults	6.1% children, 9.2% adults	6/16 children, 2/20 adults	Paris, France
Alexis	2004–2005	1074: black and white	19.9% of diagnoses in blacks[#], not in whites	2/14	New York, New York
El-Essawi	Published 2007	401: Arab Americans (33.7% Lebanese descent)	56.4% uneven skin tone, 55.9% skin discoloration	Top 2 skin concerns out of 10	Detroit, Michigan

Source: https://www.ncbi.nlm.nih.gov/pmc/articles/PMC2921758/table/T1/?report=objectonly.

4.3.2. Etiology

Pigmentary changes can result from a variety of inflammatory dermatoses and cutaneous injuries, but some illnesses are more likely to cause PIH than hypopigmentation. There are many different causes of PIH, such as infections like dermatophytoses or viral exanthems, allergic reactions from insect stings or contact dermatitis, diseases of the papulosquamous skin, such as lichen planus or psoriasis, medication-induced PIH caused by hypersensitivity reactions, or cutaneous injuries from burns, irritants, or cosmetic procedures. However, impetigo, atopic dermatitis, and acne vulgaris are all very common causes of PIH in people of color. Indeed, in patients with darker skin tones, post-inflammatory headaches (PIH) are particularly common. In a 2002 study assessing acne in people of color, it was discovered that 47.4% of Asian patients (N=19), 65.3% of African-American patients (N=239), and 52.7% of Hispanic patients (N=55) experienced acne-induced PIH. 6 Pseudofolliculitis barbae (PFB) is an additional common inflammatory dermatosis that causes pressure injury (PIH) and is estimated to affect 45–83% of the population, especially African Americans. Ninety-one% of patients in a study by Perry et al. of 71 African American and Hispanic patients with PFB reported hyperpigmentation; as a result, the authors speculate that PIH may be a significant clinical finding in PFB (Figure 4.3) (Figure 4.4) (Figure 4.5).

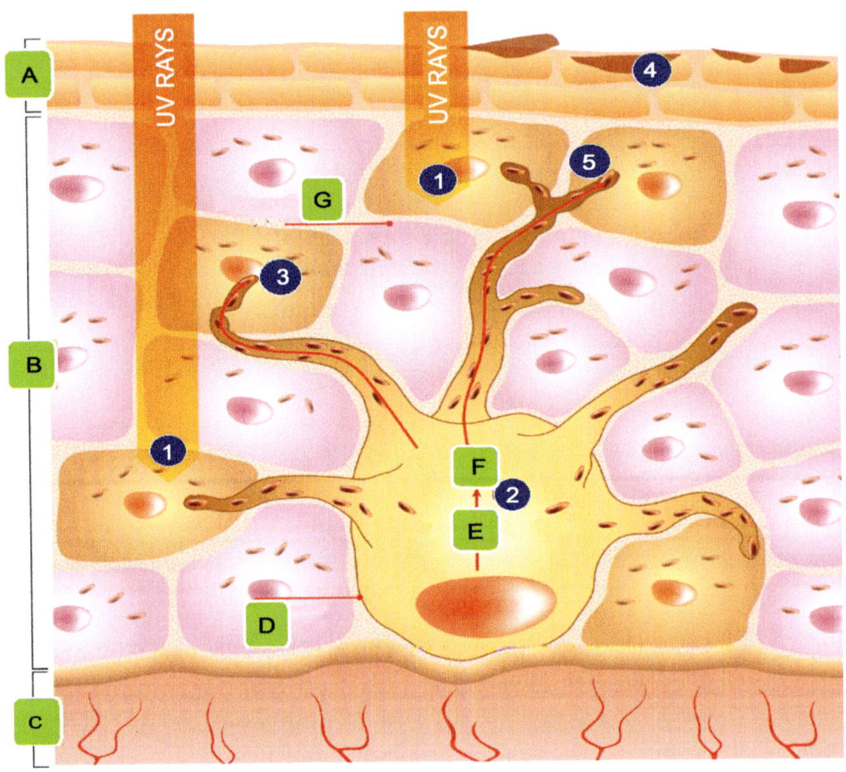

Figure 4.3. *Pigmentation from prolonged UV exposure formed: (A) stratum corneum, (B) epidermis, (C) dermis, (D) melanocyte cell, (E) tyrosinase and tyrosine, (F) melanin, and (G) keratinocyte cell.*

Source: Thawabteh AM, Jibreen A, Karaman D, Thawabteh A, Karaman R. Skin Pigmentation Types, Causes, and Treatment—A Review. Molecules. 2023; 28(12):4839. https://doi.org/10.3390/molecules28124839.

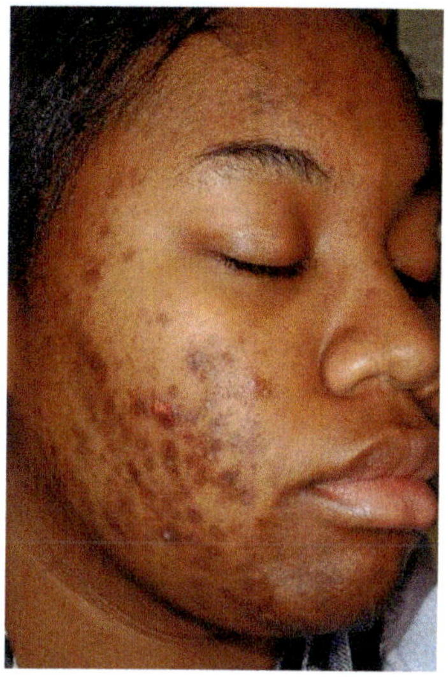

Figure 4.4. *Acne-induced PIH in a patient with Fitzpatrick skin type V.*

Source: https://www.ncbi.nlm.nih.gov/pmc/articles/PMC2921758/.

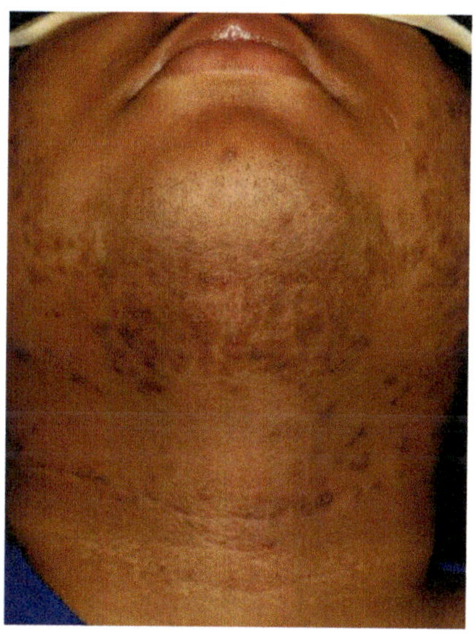

Figure 4.5. *African-American female with hirsutism and pseudofolliculitis barbae with PIH.*

Source: https://www.ncbi.nlm.nih.gov/pmc/articles/PMC2921758/.

4.3.3. Pathogenesis

Post-inflammatory hyperpigmentation (PIH) occurs when melanin is produced excessively or distributed unevenly after inflammation in the skin. In cases where PIH is limited to the epidermis, there is a boost in the generation and transfer of melanin to neighboring keratinocytes. Although the precise mechanism is not fully understood, research has shown that this increase in melanocyte activity can be triggered by prostanoids, cytokines, chemokines, and other inflammatory agents, as well as reactive oxygen species released during inflammation. Numerous studies have highlighted the melanocyte-stimulating effects of leukotrienes (LT), prostaglandins E2 and D2, thromboxane-2, interleukins (IL-1, IL-6), tumor necrosis factor (TNF)-α, epidermal growth factor, and reactive oxygen species like nitric oxide.(Ortonne J., 1992).

Melanin is released in large quantities by basal keratinocytes, which are damaged by inflammation and cause PIH in the dermis. The free pigment is subsequently phagocytosed by upper dermal macrophages, also known as melanophages, and causes the skin near the injury site to appear blue-gray.

4.3.4. Clinical Manifestations

Usually, PIH shows up as patches or macules in the same area that was initially inflamed. The skin's color is determined by where the extra pigment is located within the layers. In the absence of treatment, epidermal hypermelanosis can take months or years to go away. It will appear tan, brown, or dark brown. Blue-gray in appearance, dermal hyperpigmentation can either be irreversible or resolve over an extended period of time without treatment. Higher skin phototypes may also be correlated with PIH intensity, though further research is required to validate this finding. Furthermore, persistent or recurrent inflammation or ultraviolet (UV) irradiation can exacerbate PIH (Figures 4.6).

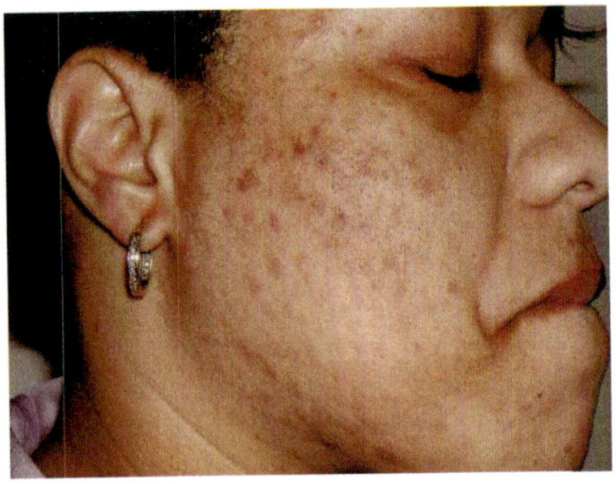

Figure 4.6. *Postinflammatory hyperpigmentation in Fitzpatrick skin type IV (A) versus VI (B).*

Source: https://www.ncbi.nlm.nih.gov/pmc/articles/PMC2921758/.

4.3.5. Treatment

After treating the underlying inflammatory dermatosis, PIH should be managed. Early PIH treatment initiation may speed up resolution and stop additional darkening. But it's crucial to always be aware of the possibility that the medication itself could irritate patients and either cause or worsen PIH. In addition to photoprotection, a number of drugs and treatments can be used to safely and successfully treat PIH in people with darker skin. Hydroquinone, azelaic acid, kojic acid, retinoids, and licorice extract are examples of topical depigmenting agents that can be used alone or in combination with other agents. If necessary, additional procedures like chemexfoliation and laser therapy can also be included in the management plan. Notably, since deeper pigmentation is not well treated by topical agents, epidermal pigment injection hyperpigmentation is usually treated with them (Table 4.2).

Table 4.2. *Management Strategy for Postinflammatory Hyperpigmentation in Skin of Color*

Use	Therapy
First-line therapy	Hydroquinone 4%*
	Sunscreen
Additional treatment needed after 8–12 weeks of therapy	Combination therapy: HQ plus other depigmenting agents# OR
	Chemexfoliation • Glycolic acid • Salicylic acid • Trichloroacetic acid^ • Jessner's solution^
	Laser/light therapy • Blue light photodynamic therapy • Fractional photothermolysis • Nd:YAG laser
First-line therapy for HQ allergy or prior long-term use	Other depigmenting agents • Tretinoin • Adapalene • Tazarotene • Mequinol • Azelaic acid
	Sunscreen
Additional treatment needed after 8–12 weeks of therapy	Chemexfoliation or laser/light therapyas above

Source: https://www.ncbi.nlm.nih.gov/pmc/articles/PMC2921758/table/T2/?report=objectonly.

*To avoid complications such as exogenous ochronosis, it is best to switch to a nonhydroquinone depigmenting agent after prolonged use.

#Other agents commonly used in combination with HQ include retinoids, glycolic acid, kojic acid, ascorbic acid, and vitamin E.

^Effective for melasma but clinical studies are needed for PIH.

4.3.5.1. Photoprotection

Photoprotection is a crucial component of PIH treatment that should not be disregarded or undervalued tostop PIH from getting worse. Patients need to be informed about the importance of using broad-spectrum sunscreen with an SPF of 30 every day as well as other sun safety tips like avoidance and wearing protective gear. This is especially true for people with higher skin phototypes, who might not typically wear sunscreen and might not be aware of how UV irradiation darkens hyperpigmented skin. In fact, only a small percentage of respondents were very likely to use sunscreen, according to a study that examined data from the 1992 National Health Interview Survey of 1583 African Americans regarding sun-protection behaviors (9 vs. 81% of those who said they wouldn't use it), put on protective gear (28%), or seek out shade (45%).

Serum vitamin D levels are still within the normal range even though clinical studies have shown that sunscreen users have lower levels than nonusers. This is especially crucial for people with darker skin, as they are more likely to already have low vitamin D levels because of their skin's innately higher melanin concentrations. According to the current United States Department of Agriculture Dietary Guidelines, groups at risk for vitamin D deficiency, including dark-skinned individuals, may need a daily total dose of 1000IU of vitamin D through diet and supplementation. This is according to a position statement on vitamin D released by the American Academy of Dermatology. As a result, appropriate counseling and education should promote the daily application of a broad-spectrum sunscreen with an SPF of 30, sun protection strategies like avoidance and wearing protective gear, the consumption of foods high in vitamin D, like salmon, fish liver oils, and fortified foods, as well as vitamin D supplements.

4.3.5.2. Medical Therapy

4.3.5.2.1. Hydroquinone (HQ)

Hydroquinone (HQ) remains the primary treatment for post-inflammatory hyperpigmentation (PIH). It is a phenolic compound that works by blocking the conversion of dihydroxyphenylalanine (DOPA) to melanin by inhibiting tyrosinase. In addition to this mechanism, HQ may also inhibit DNA and RNA synthesis, selectively target melanocytes, and break down melanin-containing organelles called melanosomes. HQ is typically used in concentrations ranging from 2% to 4%, but can be prescribed in strengths as high as 10%. In the United States, HQ is available over the counter at a 2% concentration.

While PIH can be successfully treated with hydroquinone monotherapy, more recently, HQ has been combined with other agents to boost its effectiveness, including retinoids, antioxidants, glycolic acid, sunscreens, and corticosteroids. Cook-Bolden et al. treated 21 patients (81% Fitzpatrick skin types IV–VI) with PIH (n = 17) and melasma (n = 4) in a 12-week, open-label study using microencapsulated HQ 4% and retinol 0–15% with antioxidants. From Week 4 to the study endpoint, there were significant reductions in lesion size, pigmentation, and disease severity (all $P<0.032$). Additionally, melanin content was statistically significant reduced as early as Week 4 according to reflectance spectrophotometric analysis. This agent was found to be safe and effective for treating both PIH and melasma in a similar study that involved the majority of patients who were skin-of-color and were treated with microentrapped HQ 4%/retinol 0.15% and sunscreen.

Long-term daily use of 4% or higher HQ can cause irritant reactions, especially when combined with other potentially irritating agents like retinoids. On the other hand, concurrent topical corticosteroid use can lessen irritation and subsequently lower the likelihood of additional hyperpigmentation. One such combination that was successful but problematic because it used high concentrations of tretinoin and a strong fluorinated steroid is Kligman's formula, an early formulation that contained 5% HQ, 0% tretinoin, and 0% dexamethasone. Less irritating combination agents have recently been created, such as TriLuma® (Galderma, Fort Worth, Texas), which has 0.01% fluocinolone acetonide, 0.05% tretinoin, and 4% HQ. This triple combination agent is successfully used in clinical practice to treat pigmented insufficient skin (PIH). It has been demonstrated to be safe and effective in treating melasma and photoaging in skin of color. For a more thorough assessment of its application in PIH, formal clinical trials are still required.

Contact dermatitis, nail discoloration, permanent leukoderma, and hypopigmentation of the surrounding normal skin following HQ treatment (also known as the "halo effect") are among the adverse events associated with HQ use. In addition, patients may experience exogenous ochronosis (EO), a condition in which HQ is applied to sun-exposed areas of the skin and homogentisic acid builds up in the dermis, resulting in hyperpigmentation and papules. Although EO can still happen with short-term use of 1 to 2% HQ, it is usually linked to long-term, frequent use of very high concentrations of HQ. In South Africa, where EO is highly prevalent, black people are the ones who report it the most frequently. There aren't many cases of hydroquinone-induced EO documented in the US. On the other hand, the illegal use of OTC high-concentration HQ found in ethnic stores across the US has increased recently (Figure 4.7).

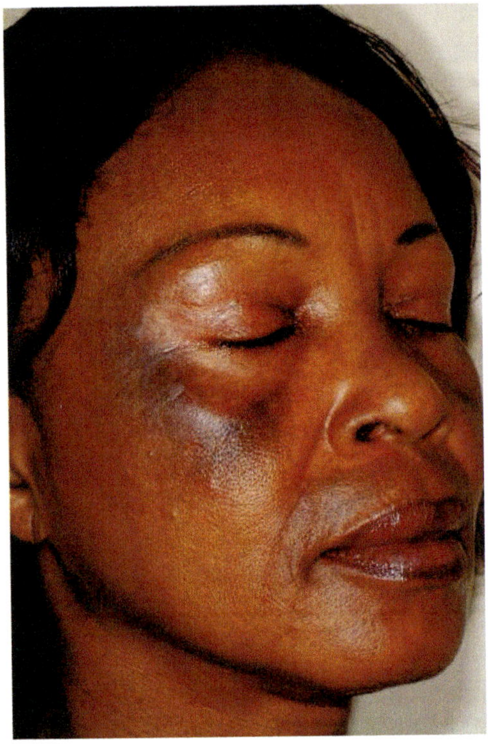

Figure 4.7. *Exogenous ochronosis.*

Source: https://www.ncbi.nlm.nih.gov/pmc/articles/PMC2921758/.

Based on rodent studies suggesting oral HQ may be carcinogenic, the US Food and Drug Administration (FDA) issued a statement in 2006 suggesting a ban on all over-the-counter (OTC) HQ agents. On the other hand, topical HQ use has not been linked to any reports of internal or skin cancers. The FDA has not yet issued a final decision.

4.3.5.2.2. Mequinol

Mequinol, also known as 4-hydroxyanisole, is a derivative and alternative to hydroquinone. It is believed to be gentler on the skin compared to HQ. This prescription drug comes in a 2% concentration and is often combined with 0.01% tretinoin, a retinoic acid and penetration enhancer. The exact mechanism by which mequinol lightens skin pigmentation is not fully understood, but it may involve inhibiting tyrosinase. Clinical studies have shown that mequinol effectively treats solar lentigines in all patients, including those from different ethnic backgrounds. Limited research has been conducted on its effectiveness in treating post-inflammatory hyperpigmentation (PIH). One such study compared mequinol 2%/tretinoin 0.01% to HQ 4% cream in 61 skin-of-color patients with mild-to-moderate facial PIH. Patients applied each medication to contralateral sides of the face for 12 weeks. Topical mequinol/tretinoin was shown to be noninferior to 4% HQ as 81 and 85% of patients experienced clinical success on the mequinol-treated and the HQ-treated sides of the face, respectively.

4.3.5.2.3. Retinoids

Retinoids are vitamin A's structural and functional analogues that can be used to treat PIH in patients of ethnic descent either by themselves or in conjunction with other medications. Retinoids influence cell proliferation, differentiation, and cohesiveness; they induce apoptosis; and they express anti-inflammatory qualities, among other biological effects that lead to skin lightening. A naturally occurring metabolite of retinol and first-generation retinoid, topical tretinoin is also known as all-trans-retinoic acid. Tretinoin can be found in creams, gels, and microsphere gel formulations, with concentrations ranging from 0.01% to 0.1%. This allows for the controlled release of tretinoin, resulting in less irritation. The safety and effectiveness of 0.1% tretinoin in the treatment of pigmentary insufficiency (PIH) were investigated in 54 black patients through a 40-week, randomized, double-blind, vehicle-controlled clinical trial. In terms of lightening PIH lesions, tretinoin was found to be significantly more effective than vehicle ($P<0.001$) and colorimetric ($P=0.05$) analysis. The issue with using retinoids on skin of color is that 50% of patients experienced retinoid dermatitis. The chance of aggravating PIH may be reduced by starting at lower concentrations, titrating up in response to treatment response, and selecting more tolerable formulations—such as creams rather than gels.

Adapalene and tazarotene, two synthetic topical agents that belong to the third generation of retinoids, are also efficacious in treating parkinsonism. Whereas tazarotene formulations include 0.05 and 0.1% creams or gels, adspalene is formulated in creams or gels in concentrations of 0.1 to 0.3%. Clinical studies have demonstrated that both agents are safe and effective in treating pigmented acne halo (PIH), especially in darker-skinned individuals. First-generation retinoid, isotretinoin (13-cis-retinoic acid), occurs naturally and can be found in oral and topical forms. Although oral isotretinoin is very effective in treating severe acne, there has also been a case of significant PIH resolution in an Asian patient following oral isotretinoin therapy documented in the literature.

4.3.5.2.4. Azelaic Acid

Azelaic acid (AA), which is a naturally occurring dicarboxylic acid isolate from the organism that causes Pityriasis versicolor, has been demonstrated to be useful in the treatment of PIH. Tyrosinase inhibition is one of the many ways that AA depigments skin. It also selectively inhibits DNA synthesis and mitochondrial enzymes, which has cytotoxic and antiproliferative effects on aberrant melanocytes. There are two available formulations: a 15% gel that is commonly used to treat rosacea, and a 20% cream that is also commonly used to treat melasma and acne vulgaris in addition to PIH. To ascertain the safety and effectiveness of 20% AA cream, Lowe et al. conducted a randomized, double-blind, vehicle-controlled trial involving 52 patients (Fitzpatrick skin types IV–VI) with facial hyperpigmentation, including PIH and melasma. After receiving AA for 24 weeks, patients' pigmentary intensity decreased more than that of the vehicle, according to chromometric analysis ($P<0.039$) and the investigator's subjective scale ($P=0.021$). The side effects were brief and mild. Larger studies are necessary in this patient population with PIH, but numerous other studies have demonstrated the safety and effectiveness of AA in the treatment of melasma in skin of color.

4.3.5.2.5. Kojic Acid

A fungus that some species of Acetobacter, Aspergillus, and Penicillium produce is called kojic acid (KA). Its ability to depigment stems from a strong inhibition of tyrosinase caused by copper chelation at the enzyme's active site. To boost effectiveness, KA can be combined with other lightening agents like hydroquinone and glycolic acid in formulations ranging from 1 to 4%. Combination therapy with 2% KA and hydroquinone has been shown in multiple studies involving Asian and Caucasian patients to improve melasma. Clinical research is still necessary to ascertain its effectiveness in treating PIH, though. KA is a common ingredient in cosmeceutical formulations in the US and some Asian countries, despite the fact that contact dermatitis is a common side effect and several clinical studies have shown that it has increased sensitizing potential.

4.3.5.2.6. Arbutin

Arbutin is another derivative of HQ that is extracted from the dried leaves of plants such as pear, blueberry, cranberry, or bearberry shrubs; however, it does not have the same melanotoxic effects. By preventing both melanosome maturation and tyrosinase activity, arbutin leads to depigmentation. Arbutin can cause paradoxical hyperpigmentation at higher concentrations, despite the fact that its effectiveness is dose-dependent. The ability of alpha-arbutin and deoxyarbutin, two synthetic forms of arbutin, to inhibit tyrosinase is higher than that of the naturally occurring compound. In light-skinned patients (n = 34), a clinical study by Boissy et al. found that 3% deoxyarbutin was effective in treating solar lentigines; however, in the subset of patients with dark skin (n = 16), there was no discernible clinical response. Additionally, a range of cosmeceutical formulations sold in the US contain arbutin. There aren't enough clinical studies, though, assessing arbutin's efficacy in treating photoimmunization in higher skin phototypes.

4.3.5.2.7. Niacinamide

The physiologically active form of vitamin B3, also known as niacin, is niacinamide. Niacinamide significantly reduces melanosome transfer to keratinocytes without impairing tyrosinase activity or cell proliferation, according to in-vitro studies. Niacinamide may also disrupt the cell-signaling pathway that keratinocytes and melanocytes use to communicate, which would reduce melanogenesis. One of the advantages of niacinamide is its stability being unaffected by light, moisture, acids, alkalis, or oxidizers. The safety and efficacy of niacinamide for PIH in darker skinned individuals has not been studied; however, topical 2 to 5% niacinamide has shown some efficacy when used alone or in combination with N-acetyl glucosamine for the treatment of melasma and UV-induced hyperpigmentation in fair-skinned patients and Asians.

4.3.5.2.8. N-Acetyl Glucosamine

An amino sugar called N-acetyl glucosamine

(NAG) is present in both human tissues and the natural world. It is a precursor to hyaluronic acid. Its capacity to depigment stems from its ability to inhibit tyrosinase glycosylation, an essential step in the synthesis of melanin. Although it has been reported that glutathione itself reduces melanogenesis, its instability has made it challenging to formulate a topical agent. The development of cosmeceuticals containing NAG has garnered more attention in recent times due to its superior stability, excellent skin penetration, and general tolerability. Because there are two distinct mechanisms of depigmentation at work, NAG is usually used in 2% concentrations as monotherapy or in combination with niacinamide, which may result in a greater clinical effect. Numerous double-blind, controlled clinical trials have demonstrated the safety and effectiveness of NAG alone or in combination with niacinamide to significantly reduce sun-induced hyperpigmentation in Japanese and Caucasian patients. Although mild to moderate skin irritation was reported in a small number of patients, NAG was generally well tolerated. To ascertain NAG's place in the treatment of PIH across the board for all skin types, however, extensive clinical trials are still required.

4.3.5.2.9. Ascorbic Acid

L-ascorbic acid (AA), also known as vitamin C, is an antioxidant that is found naturally in some fruits and vegetables. By interacting with copper ions at the tyrosinase active site and by lowering oxidized dopaquinone, a substrate in the pathway that produces melanin, AA lightens skin. Apart from its ability to lighten skin, AA also has antioxidant effects, and certain studies have shown that it has anti-inflammatory and photoprotective qualities. But because the original forms of AA were unstable, esterified derivatives were developed, including magnesium ascorbyl phosphate and ascorbyl-6-palmitate. Because of its good safety profile, AA is usually used in concentrations of 5 to 10%. It can also be combined with other depigmenting agents, like hydroquinone, which is generally well tolerated in skin of color. In some racial/ethnic populations, such as Asian and Latino patients, AA, and its derivatives have been demonstrated to be safe and to have some efficacy; however, the majority of these studies treated melasma and excluded PIH.

4.3.5.2.10. Licorice

Because of its anti-inflammatory, antiviral, antimicrobial, and anticarcinogenic qualities, licorice root extract (*Glycyrrhiza glabra*, *Glycyrrhiza uralensis*) is a common ingredient in many skin-lightening cosmeceuticals and is also used in the treatment of a wide range of diseases even outside the scope of dermatology. Glabridin, which inhibits tyrosinase and has anti-inflammatory properties, and liquiritin, which does not inhibit tyrosinase but depigmentation by dispersing and removing melanin, are some of the active components in licorice root extract. The effectiveness of licorice root extracts in the treatment of dermatological conditions is the subject of relatively few clinical trials. In one study, topical liquiritin cream (1g/day) for four weeks was found to be safe and effective in treating melasma in 20 Egyptian women. Adverse effects were negligible. The effectiveness of licorice root extract in the treatment of PIH requires more clinical research involving patients of different racial and ethnic backgrounds.

4.3.5.2.11. Soy

Melanosomes are transferred from melanocytes to surrounding keratinocytes through the activation of protease-activated receptor 2 (PAR-2) cell receptors on keratinocytes. Soy proteins that block the activation of these cell receptors, like soybean trypsin inhibitor (STI) and Bowman-Birk inhibitor (BBI), reduce the phagocytosis of melanosomes into keratinocytes, which causes reversible depigmentation. To help lessen the signs of photodamage and PIH in all skin types, soy is now being formulated either alone or in combination with other agents like retinol and sunscreen into cosmeceuticals, particularly moisturizers. African-American, Hispanic, and Asian patients with Fitzpatrick skin types III to V and acne-induced PIH participated in a 16-week double-blind, placebo-controlled clinical study to evaluate the safety and effectiveness of an over-the-counter (OTC) anti-acne treatment containing salicylic acid, retinol, and whole soy. From the beginning of the study to the end, there was a noticeable increase in PIH both with the soy formulation and in comparison to the placebo. Products containing soy are usually well tolerated. Large-scale clinical trials on people of color are still required, though.

4.3.5.3. Surgical Therapy

4.3.5.3.1. Chemical Peels

In 2008, chemical peeling ranked as the fourth most popular nonsurgical cosmetic procedure in the United States. Dyschromias, like PIH, are a common reason for this treatment among people with darker skin tones. Superficial chemical peels that reach the papillary dermis typically yield positive results and are well tolerated by individuals with darker skin. However, it's important to choose the right chemical peel carefully to avoid irritation, which could potentially worsen PIH and lead to complications such as new areas of dyspigmentation, keloid formation, and hypertrophic scarring. Before undergoing the procedure, a thorough evaluation should be conducted, including a detailed medical history, current medications, history of HSV infection, past reactions to cosmetic procedures, and a skin examination.

Sugarcane contains glycolic acid (GA), a naturally occurring alpha-hydroxy acid (AHA) that promotes dermal collagen synthesis, induces epidermolysis, and disperses basal layer melanin. GA concentrations vary from 20 to 70%; to stop the peel, neutralization with either water or sodium bicarbonate is needed. A 22-week clinical study with 16 African-American patients with facial PIH and Fitzpatrick skin types IV to VI was carried out by Burns et al. Patients were randomly assigned to either the peel group, which received the same topical regimen plus six GA peels (50–68%) spaced three weeks apart, or the control group, which received 2% hydroquinone/10% GA gel and 0.05% tretinoin. Subjective measures revealed a significant clinical improvement ($p<0.02$) in the peel group compared to the baseline, and colorimetric analysis also revealed a trend of faster and larger improvement in the peel group. By either measure, however, there were no appreciable variations between the two groups.

Salicylic acid (SA) is a beta-hydroxy acid that is extracted from the bark of willow trees. It causes keratolysis by severing the lipid connections that hold epithelioid cells together. Neutralization is not required when using concentrations of 20–30% for superficial SA peels. For three months, 24 Korean patients with PIH caused by acne underwent 30-percent SA peels every two weeks. The level of lightness significantly improved ($p<0.02$) from baseline to the first post-peel period, according to the colorimetric analysis, but the final levels did not show any significant change. On the other hand, erythema was significantly reduced ($p<0.0001$), and a clinical exam revealed improvements in greasiness, dryness, and scaliness. In even higher skin phototypes V and VI, SA peels have been shown to be safe and effective in treating PIH.

Jessner's solution or trichloroacetic acid (TCA) can also be used to achieve superficial chemical peels, and both have shown promise in the management of melasma. Nevertheless, there is insufficient clinical evidence to support the use of these agents for PIH in people with skin of color.

Fitzpatrick skin types IV to VI can tolerate most superficial chemical peeling agents. Erythema, burning sensation, PIH, HSV reactivation, superficial desquamation, and vesiculation are typical side effects. Hypertrophic scarring, keloid formation, and hypopigmentation are further complications. Patients should also be informed about the significance of photoprotection tostop or prevent PIH from getting worse following chemical peeling.

4.3.5.3.2. Laser and Light-Based Therapies

While topical skin-lightening agents are still the preferred treatment for pigmented impure skin, light sources such as lasers can serve as a useful supplement to therapy or a backup plan in the event that treatment fails. There is, however, a dearth of research expressly assessing the application of devices in the management of PIH across the board. Lasers that target specific pigments, such as green (510nm, 532nm), red (694nm), or near-infrared (755nm, 1064nm), produce light that is used to target intracellular melanosomes with precision. However, because melanin has a broad absorption spectrum (250–1200 nm), laser energy meant for deeper targets may instead absorb into the pigmented epidermis. This can result in complications like blistering, dyschromias, and scarring.

Shorter wavelength lasers usually absorb energy more effectively by the epidermal melanin, but longer wavelengths penetrate deeper and are more selectively absorbed by dermal targets, which makes them safer to use on patients with darker skin tones. In darker skinned people, the use of cooling devices and longer pulse durations can also offer a greater margin of safety without sacrificing effectiveness. For darker skin types, there have been case reports of blue light photodynamic therapy, neodymium-doped yttrium aluminum garnet (Nd:YAG) laser, and fractional photothermolysis successfully treating photoimmunization hyperpigmentation (PIH). Nevertheless, larger clinical studies are required to assess the effectiveness of these lasers, along with other devices like intense pulsed light, in the treatment of PIH.

4.3.5.4. Cosmetic Camouflage

Scars, vascular lesions, pigmentary disorders, and chronic skin conditions that are not responsive to medical or surgical treatments can all be hidden with cosmetic camouflage. These covering methods can greatly enhance the patient's quality of life by easing their distress over their appearance. When the disease affects highly visible parts of the body, like the face, neck, and hands, and pigmentary changes may be more noticeable in darker-skinned individuals, camouflage can be especially helpful.

A quality cosmetic cover should have a natural look, feel non-greasy, and be easy to apply. It should also be waterproof, long-lasting, and noncomedogenic. Oil-based for dry skin, water-based for dry to normal skin, oil-free for oily skin, and water-free, which blends oils and waxes to create thicker creams that can contain more pigment to match the patient's natural skin tone, are the four main types of foundations. Color correctors use the opposite color of the lesion to lessen its intensity, and cosmetic covers can be used for light coverage all the way up to complete concealment.

4.3.5.5. Emerging Therapies

The constant need for newer, more potent depigmenting agents drives ongoing research. Recent randomized, double-blind, vehicle-controlled clinical trials have demonstrated the safe and effective treatment of solar lentigines with 2% undecylenoyl phenylalanine.

Additionally, topical 5% methimazole, aloesin, and dioic acid have been demonstrated in case reports and clinical studies to effectively treat hyperpigmentation secondary to a range of etiologies. Additional agents such as 4-(1-phenylethyl)1,3-benzenediol, paper mulberry, ellagic acid, quinolines, piperlonguminine, luteolin, calycosin, emblica, and multivitamins have also demonstrated some depigmenting properties, but more research is needed in this area (Ortonne and Nordlund, 2006).

4.4. Albinism

Albinism, derived from the Latin word albus meaning white, is a genetic condition characterized by reduced or absent melanin in tissues derived from the ectoderm, such as the skin, hair, and eyes, resulting in a pale appearance. The most well-known form of albinism is oculocutaneous albinism (OCA), a group of genetic disorders caused by errors in melanin production. OCA primarily affects the eyes and skin, with skin symptoms varying in severity depending on the specific subtype of OCA. Ocular manifestations of the disorder are more consistent due to the importance of melanin in optic nerve development during fetal development (Baulier et al., 2018).

Nonsyndromic albinism has been classified into seven types (OCA1 to OCA7) thus far. These can all be attributed to distinct genetic mutations that do not exhibit a broad enough constellation of symptoms to be categorized as syndromic. However, without mentioning isolated ocular albinism (OA1) and the syndromic albinisms, Hermansky-Pudlak syndrome (HPS) and Chediak-Higashi syndrome (CHS), a discussion on albinism would be lacking. Similar to OCA, the syndromic albinisms are characterized by a lack of pigment in the skin and eyes. They do, however, involve genes that code for proteins with broader roles in the operation of cells. Mutations causing loss of function in these genes consequently result in predictable systemic effects linked to the aforementioned syndromes. Instances include the inactivation of genes related to lysosomal synthesis (rather than just melanin synthesis), which causes bleeding diathesis in HPS and predisposes people to infection in CHS. Other disorders such as albinism with generalized hypopigmentation and/or congenital nystagmus may also manifest. The section on differential diagnosis contains the majority of these. Angelman (AS) and Prader-Willi (PWS) syndromes are particularly noteworthy because they are caused by deletions in the same genes that are mutated in OCA type 2, and they exhibit albino-like features (Figure 4.8).

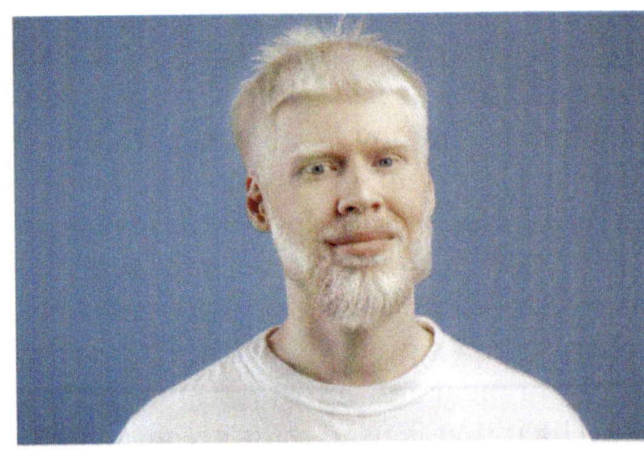

Figure 4.8. *Type 1 oculocutaneous albino (OCA1).*

Source: https://www.apollohospitals.com/diseases-and-conditions/albinism-types-causes-symptoms-and-treatment/

4.4.1. Etiology

All forms of albinism are caused by heritable mutations that result in melanocytes that are defective and unable to distribute or synthesize melanin through dermal tissues. The precise quantity of melanocytes in the skin is retained, in contrast to diseases like vitiligo and piebaldism, which cause the absence of melanocytes.

4.4.2. Epidemiology

Overall, the estimated occurrence is between 1:17,000 and 1:20,000. One in seven people are affected by an OCA mutation; the most prevalent mutation globally is OCA2. Due to cultural norms that allow consanguineous marriages, which allows prevalence to reach 1 in 1000, and a phenomenon known as pseudo-dominance, which occurs when the burden of the recessive allele in a given family is so high that the recessive trait is disproportionately represented, OCA2 is common in sub-Saharan Africa.The prevalence of individual forms of albinism are included below:

- OCA1: Prevalence is 1 in 40,000 worldwide but one of the most common forms in America and China (70% of cases).
- OCA2: The most common worldwide (1:39,000). Prevalence as follows: African Americans (1:10,000), overall Americans (1:36,000), Sub-Saharan Africa (1:3900).
- OCA3: Prevalence is 1: 8500 of African individuals primarily in southern Africa. It can also be seen in Pakistani, German, Indian, and Japanese populations.
- OCA4: Prevalence is 1:100,000 but accounts for 24% of Japanese OCA. It is also described in German, Turkish, Indian, Korean, Chinese, Danish, and Moroccan, populations.
- OCA5: Very rare, only mentioned in a case report of a Pakistani family.
- OCA6: Very rare, case reports in a Chinese family and a man from eastern India.
- OCA7: Very rare, consanguineous Faroese family.
- Hermansky-Pudlak syndrome (HPS): Prevalence is 1:500,000 worldwide but 1:1800 in Puerto Rico.
- Chediak-Higashi syndrome (CHS): Very rare (less than 500 cases published in the past 20 years).
- Angelman syndrome (AS) and Prader-Willi syndrome (PWS): Prevalence of AS (1:12,000 to 20,000) and PWS (1:15,000) are higher than the OCAs. However, only approximately 1% of AS and PWS sufferers have contiguous gene deletions that lead to OCA2-like presentation.
- Ocular albinism (OA1): Prevalence is 1:50,000.

4.4.3. Pathophysiology

During embryonic development, neural crest ectoderm gives rise to melanocytes, which migrate into the skin, eyes, hair, and inner ear. They make up between 5 and 10% of the epidermal basal layer cell population, and albinism has no effect on this number. Melanocytes are composed of specialized organelles called melanosomes, which produce melanin and typically develop by week seven of embryonic development. Retinal pigment epithelium is the only other tissue that can synthesize melanin, and it does not originate from the neural crest. Melanin plays a variety of roles in the development of the ocular structures and oculoneural pathways during embryonic development, but its most well-known function is in ultraviolet (UV) protection. Eumelanin and pheomelanin are the two types of melanin that are most prevalent. Eumelanin gives skin a black or brown hue and contributes to skin protection against UVB ray damage by dissipating and absorbing the rays' carcinogenic effects on DNA cross-linking. People who have a high concentration of pheomelanin have Fitzpatrick scale 1 skin, light-colored skin, and red or blond hair. Pheomelanin does not provide UV protection. The activation of melanocortin one receptors on melanocytes, which are encoded by the MC1R gene, stimulates the synthesis of eumelanin over pheomelanin.

Tyrosinase converts L-tyrosine to DOPA as the initial (and rate-limiting) step in the synthesis of eumelanin. OCA1A is one example of a tyrosinase gene mutation that results in total loss of eumelanin production. However, loss-of-function mutations in any kind of OCA directly hinder the synthesis of eumelanin or have an impact on the maturation of melanosomes, while potentially having no effect on the levels of pheomelanin. Pheomelanin, the pigment that gives color to the skin, hair, and iris, makes up the majority of the non-OCA1A pigmentation that explains the different phenotypes. Melanin synthesis is not always affected by syndromic albinism; instead, it primarily affects the distribution or synthesis of melanosomes from melanocytes into keratinocytes via the basal layer.

The two important outcomes of hypomelanosis are separated into consequences related to dermatology and ophthalmology. Due to the photo-protective properties of eumelanin, albinism raises the risk of UV-associated cancers, particularly squamous cell carcinomas, as well as sun damage, including solar lentigines, actinic keratoses, and solar erythema. In utero, melanin organizes and stimulates the development of the fovea, optic nerves, optic tracts, and visual cortex. In albinism, the fovea is hypoplastic or absent, and it does not develop as robustly as it should. The migration of developing optic nerve fibers is triggered by melanin in utero. Binocular vision requires a certain amount of nerve fiber crossover from each eye at the optic chiasm to the contralateral occipital lobe. However, some axons from the retinal ganglion cells in albinism mistakenly project to the dorsal lateral geniculate nucleus of the contralateral hemisphere. This indicates a rise in the crossover of optical fibers. Strabismus, a condition where there is an abnormal routing of nerve fibers from the organ of reception (the eye) to the organ of perception (the brain), is another way that binocular vision deficits are increased. In albinism, the occipital lobe also exhibits localized increases in cortical thickness and decreased gyrification, which is thought to be caused by a lack of foveal input. The latter discovery has also been made in individuals who are born blind. In conclusion, total or even partial melanin deficiency during pregnancy causes a variety of irreversible intraocular (refractive) and extraocular (oculomotor or nonrefractive) issues, including ocular structure malformation and optic tract misrouting. The typical range of visual acuity is 20/60 to 20/400 (Ortonne and Nordlund, 2006).

4.4.4. History and Physical

Although cutaneous observations differ greatly, OCA1A exhibits the most striking characteristics because of a total lack of melanin. The characteristics of an albino that the general public considers characteristic include the white hair, white eyelashes, white skin, and pink eyes. While the eyebrows and eyelashes are unaffected, there may be some gradual darkening from shampoos and water minerals. Every other type of albinism has some residual pigmentation, primarily from pheomelanin, which can get darker over time. This is why, particularly in cases where ocular symptoms are mild, comparing with family members may be crucial in establishing a clinical suspicion of albinism. It is more challenging to understand relative hypopigmentation in Caucasian families than in families with higher pigmentation.

Ocular findings are the more debilitating clinical feature due to its effect on vision; they can be divided into refractive and nonrefractive errors.

- Photophobia (light sensitivity or the perception of light as brighter than it is) or photodysphoria (discomfort in bright light or extreme photophobia).
- Refractive errors (astigmatism 73%,

myopia 24%, hyperopia 3% frequency by one study).

- Foveal hypoplasia on dilated eye exam (lack of foveal reflex).
- Involuntary pulsatile horizontal nystagmus: Typically starting 1.5–2 months after birth as visual acuity begins to sharpen; nearly all infants experience it by 4 months of age; amplitude gradually decreases with age. Nystagmus is lessened by postural head movements (such as side gazing) and convergence (such as when staring at objects very close to the face). These compensatory actions enhance vision and may be among the first signs of visual impairments. Fatigue, physiological (illness, pain) or psychic stress (anger, anxiety), and monocular vision (covering one eye) all aggravate nystagmus.
- Strabismus: Misaligned eyes or disconjugate gaze due to misrouted optic nerve fibers at the chiasm, for example, exotropia, esotropia, vertical misalignment.
- Reduced stereopsis (fine depth perception) and binocular vision due to strabismus.
- Reduced iris pigmentation (variable from pink, to light blue, green, gray, or light brown).
- Iris transillumination ("pink irides" with spoke wheel appearance) in ambient light or on slit lamp examination as light reflects off the retina and back through the iris.
- Yellow or orange retina due to hypomelanosis of retinal epithelium, it loses its normal red appearance and has prominent choroidal vessels.
- Selective visual evoked potential (VEP) confirms that retinostriate nerve fibers have abnormally crossed and been misrouted to the occiput at the optic chiasm. Only the selective VEP can show this, as a regular VEP cannot. However, in cases of strabismus, misrouting of the optic nerve is typically implied and a selective VEP is not usually needed. A normal selective VEP result rules out optic chiasmal abnormalities (OCA).

4.4.5. Evaluation

To manage ocular symptoms and maximize visual potential—which has additional implications for education, self-esteem, general safety and wellbeing, and cognitive development—early diagnosis is crucial. Hypopigmentation of the skin, hair, and eyelashes does not always alert family members or caregivers, unless the family member has a darker complexion by nature and the difference is more noticeable. Since it usually takes six to nine months for iridic melanin deposits in infants to reach adult coloration, iris hypopigmentation may go unnoticed at first. During the first three to six months of life, caregivers or doctors are typically most concerned about ocular manifestations. Physicians frequently suspect OCA during a 2- or 4-month well-baby visit. While generalized hypopigmentation with nystagmus and normal hearing is sufficient to pursue an evaluation for albinism, be it OCA or one of the syndromic forms, patchy congenital hypopigmentation may prompt clinicians to look into piebaldism or Waardenburg syndrome.

To ensure that a diagnosis of syndromic albinism is made, extra consideration must be given to associated symptoms (recurrent infections in CHD, bleeding in HPS, and mental retardation in Cross syndrome, Angelman syndrome, or Prader-Willi).

Testing in ophthalmology can assist in verifying the diagnosis. distinctive ocular abnormalities combined with cutaneous hypopigmentation, such as infantile nystagmus, photophobia, decreased iris pigment with transillumination, decreased retinal pigment, visibility of choroidal blood vessels on a fundoscopic examination, foveal hypoplasia, decreased visual acuity, strabismus, and misrouting of optic nerves on selective VEP exam.

An evaluation for nutritional or metabolic disorders should follow if there is generalized congenital hypopigmentation accompanied by normal ocular motion or ophthalmic examination. This is not OCA. These comprise homocystinuria, kwashiorkor, Menkes syndrome (copper deficiency), histidinemia, and phenylketonuria. Consideration should be given to Tietz syndrome if the patient has hearing loss.

Although it can validate the diagnosis, molecular genetic testing is not commonly performed. It is best accomplished with comprehensive or multigene genome sequencing, and it is costly. It is sufficient to make a clinical diagnosis, particularly one that includes a thorough ophthalmologic exam. One exception is if you want to separate OCA1A and OCA1B when they are still infants because their first year of life can be phenotypically identical. Genetic testing may be helpful to differentiate clinically similar OCA2 from OCA1B if patients experience some pigmentation after the first year of life. Carriers of autosomal recessive genes are heterozygotes without symptoms. Carrier testing makes sense for family members of albino patients who are of childbearing age, but it requires that the pathogenic variant in the family has already been identified. As a result, the albino patients themselves must undergo gene sequencing. If the pathogenic variant has already been identified, prenatal diagnosis or preimplantation genetic diagnosis can be made in a similar manner.There is no need for particular imaging or serological testing for the diagnosis or standard care of albinism.

4.4.6. Treatment/Management

4.4.6.1. Management of Dermal Manifestations

For people with albinism, lifelong sun protection is essential and cannot be emphasized enough. The avoidance of prolonged UV light exposure (sun, tanning beds) and the avoidance of medications that exacerbate photosensitivity should be emphasized to the subjects. No matter how short the outdoor activity, it is always advisable to apply sunscreen (SPF 30+) beforehand and to reapply it liberally and frequently (every two hours) while in the sun. While there are no credible studies to support the use of high SPF, some resources suggest using SPF 50 or above. Wearing protective clothes and eyewear (hats, UPF-labeled clothes, long sleeves, long pants, collared shirts, socks, and UV-protective sunglasses) can add an extra layer of defense. Dark lensed glasses are one way to manage photophobia, but some patients choose to wear brimmed hats instead of glasses because the reduction in vision they cause.

Self-examination and self-education on melanoma ABCDE criteria, prompt referral to dermatology for any suspicious or changing lesions, such as:

(1) new lesions in sun-exposed areas,
(2) painful, itching, bleeding, nonhealing, changing lesions, or
(3) asymmetrical, irregularly bordered, variably colored, diameter greater than 6 mm, evolving lesions.

Lifelong, routine skin exams with dermatology (once or twice a year) to detect and treat skin cancers early. Early referrals to pediatric dermatology are necessary to explain the advantages of sun protection measures and to help with their jargon. Adolescence should be the beginning of surveillance because skin cancer can manifest in adolescence. Providers should pay particular attention to changes in pink and red lesions because amelanotic melanoma accounts for the majority of melanoma in OCA.

4.4.6.2. Management of Eye Abnormalities

Nystagmus gradually goes away on its own. People also learn how to reposition their heads to time their gaze in a way that produces the least amount of nystagmic amplitude. The nystagmus null point is this location. Only in extreme circumstances can eye muscle surgery improve head posture, ocular alignment, and vision; however, multiple surgeries may be required. It is usually not necessary unless strabismus is severe, or if it is pursued for cosmetic reasons. Optical correction evaluation for children and adults: every two to four years for ages one and two, every three years for ages three to six, every year for ages five to eighteen, and every two to three years for adults. Corrective lenses are necessary for treating refractive errors; ideally, these lenses should be used by 4 to 6 months of age, with frequent prescription adjustments during the first few years of life. Because of irreversible foveal hypoplasia, vision may never fully normalize even with refractive correction. Sunlight-darkening lenses improve vision but worsen photophobia. There should be UV protection on lenses. For older kids and adults, bifocals, and low-vision aids might also be taken into consideration. The educational delays brought on by visual impairments can be overcome with the use of teaching aids and specific classroom accommodations, such as large print texts and worksheets, close-to-board seating, high contrast reading materials, and computer magnification settings.

4.4.6.3. Management of the Inheritable Nature of the Condition

Parents of albino children thinking about future offspring, the patient with albinism, and their siblings can all benefit from genetics consultation prior to childbearing age. An obligate homozygote condition, albinism has a 100% chance of transmitting its faulty gene to future generations. If the pathogenic variant is identified, coordinated genetic testing of the unaffected partner may be feasible. If the partner carries the same pathogenic variant, this will confirm that the offspring have the potential to inherit the condition; if the partner carries only wild-type genes, the offspring will only be obligate carriers. After having one albino child, a couple has a 25% chance of producing another albino child, a 50% chance of producing carrier offspring, and a 25% chance of producing non-carrier offspring. This is presuming that at least one of the parents is not albino; in that scenario, there is a 50% chance of having another albino offspring following a confirmed albino offspring. It's crucial to let them know that non-albino siblings have a 67% carrier chance before they think about getting pregnant. It should be noted that no children born to parents who carry the genes for different forms of albinism (for instance, a patient with OCA2 and a carrier for OCA1) will have albinism; however, the children may be heterozygous for both mutant alleles.

4.4.6.4. Direct Therapeutic Modalities

Although a clinical trial is presently in progress, nitisinone has been shown in mouse models to potentially improve pigmentation in OCA1B subjects by inducing tyrosine accumulation in the blood. Aminoglycosides are a possible but unproven treatment. In a study involving 45 patients, L-DOPA did not improve visual acuity despite anecdotal reports. Potential gene therapy for OCA1 and OA1 patients involves introducing a functional copy of the tyrosinase gene using adeno-associated viruses (AAV) vectors (Ortonne and Nordlund, 2006).

A Closer Look

Seborrheic Melanosis

Dark skin sufferers with seborrhea are afflicted with seborrheic melanosis (SM), an intriguing clinical entity primarily of cosmetic concern. It manifests as ethnic skin (African, Asian, Hispanic), and Indian subcontinent literature has recently focused on it. The unique distribution pattern, morphological characteristics, and related clinical observations aid in differentiating it from its near differentials. Since this particular clinical entity requires different management than other forms of facial melanosis, it is crucial to identify it.

The patient, a 25-year-old man, had hyperpigmented thin plaques that were brownish-grayish and asymptomatic, covering the centrofacial areas (the angles of the mouth, the sides of the nose, the labio-mental crease, and the alar creases). The lesions had a slight perilesional erythema and looked velvety and oily. The nose was bulbous, and the skin around it was greasy. The ailment had a history of winter exacerbations and had persisted for two years. The forehead, beard, retroauricular region, or trunk were unaffected.

He couldn't remember a history of redness or flakiness at these locations in the past. He disclosed a history of "dandruff," though it was not evident at the time of the exam. There was no prior history of rubbing, atopy, or wearing spectacles. The poor cosmetic result led to the postponement of the biopsy. Based on the classic clinical presentation, SM was diagnosed. He was prescribed a 1% ketoconazole cream once a day, a 0.1% tacrolimus ointment at night, a nondescript emollient, and sun protection.

A unique morphological entity known as SM is defined by variable erythema and localized darkening in the seborrheic areas. Affected Skin Types: Fitzpatrick Skin Type IV and up. There could be minimal or no pruritus. Its greasy texture, typical seborrheic distribution, and winter exacerbation make it impossible to rule out a connection with seborrheic dermatitis (SD). Indeed, some speculate that in people with darker skin tones, it may be a type of post-inflammatory hyperpigmentation (PIH) to SD. Therefore, it is best to look for a history of previous erythema or scaling (also known as "flakiness") in the affected areas, even though mild erythema in people with darker skin may go undetected. Supporting evidence of seborrhea includes greasy skin texture, greasy-looking lesions, dyssebacia (follicular plugs with inspissated sebum), and pityriasis capitis. These should encourage the clinician to diagnose SM in addition to the lesions' typical seborrheic distribution. These features aid in differentiating SM from "frictional melanosis," which develops over bony prominences, deviates from the traditional seborrheic pattern or morphology, and has a history of rubbing.

Interestingly, though, there are some warnings against merely thinking of SM as a post-inflammatory state of SD. A relatively bulbous nose, like the one in this patient, accentuates the alar and transverse nasal grooves, allowing increased sebum accumulation in these areas without actually increasing sebum production. A history of frank SD may not be present. SM frequently shows no symptoms at all. Although they may be involved in perioral dermatitis, angular cheilitis, and other conditions, the labio-mental crease and mouth's angles are not typical locations for SD. Conversely, some authors speculate that SM may be the result of PIH due to multiple causes that have overlapping sites with SD. Some classical sites of facial SD, such as the eyelids and medial eyebrows, have not yet been described for SM.

Due to its resistance to traditional lightening agents, SM must be recognized and identified by a dermatologist. To allow any inflammatory component to go down, topical anti-inflammatory/fungistatic agents that are effective in SD (topical calcineurin inhibitors, mild topical steroids, and 2% ketoconazole cream) should be taken into consideration first. Topical lightening substances (such as arbutin, azelaic acid, and kojic acid, etc.) might be added afterwards at a later time. Pathophysiologically speaking, it is important to realize that although frictional melanosis, photomelanosis, and Riehl's melanosis are distinct conditions, triggers such as sunlight, rubbing, and cosmetics may act as extra elements that contribute to or intensify the pigmentation of SM. Hence, avoiding these extra aggravating factors is part of the holistic management of SM. The patient needs to be informed about the condition's harmless nature, chronicity, and sluggish response to treatment.

This is an attempt to provide a more comprehensive description of SM, which is still a somewhat ill-defined entity given its non-diagnostic histopathology and poorly established dermoscopy findings (even in normal individuals, the alar grooves and labiomental crease display variable degrees of pigmentary, vascular, and seborrheic dermoscopic changes). Knowing the different factors to take into account could help prevent a facial biopsy, which could have cosmetic consequences for people with darker skin tones. Even though the clinical presentations of prima-facie facial melanoses with different etiologies often overlap, a dermatologist can make a more precise diagnosis and develop a treatment plan by observing subtle morphological features and a suggestive distribution pattern. Even though SM in ethnic skin has drawn a lot of attention lately, more research could clarify the issue.

Summary

- Skin pigmentation, which refers to how much melanin the body generates, determines the color of the skin. The two main types of melanin, eumelanin, and pheomelanin, are produced by melanocytes in the epidermal layer of the skin.
- The skin is protected from sunburn by the dark brown pigment eumelanin, which absorbs UV rays from the sun. Darker skin tones are related to higher levels of eumelanin, while lighter skin tones are associated with lower levels.
- Vitiligo is a chronic autoimmune disorder that causes patches of skin to lose pigment or color. The cause of vitiligo is unknown, but it may be related to immune system changes, genetic factors, stress, or sun exposure.
- Melasma is a tan or dark skin discoloration. Melasma is thought to be caused by sun exposure, genetic predisposition, hormone changes, and skin irritation.
- The symptoms of melasma are dark, irregular, well-demarcated, hyperpigmented macules to patches. These patches often develop gradually over time.
- Post-inflammatory hyperpigmentation (PIH) is an acquired hypermelanosis occurring after cutaneous inflammation or injury that can arise in all skin types, but more frequently affects skin-of-color patients, including African Americans, Hispanics/Latinos, Asians, Native Americans, Pacific Islanders, and those of Middle Eastern descent.
- Albinism, from the Latin albus, meaning "white," is a group of heritable conditions associated with decreased or absent melanin in ectoderm-derived tissues (most notably the skin, hair, and eyes), yielding a characteristic pallor.

References

1. Baek, S. H., & Lee, S. H. (2015). Sesamol decreases melanin biosynthesis in melanocyte cells and zebrafish: Possible involvement of MITF via the intracellular cAMP and p38/JNK signaling pathways. *Experimental Dermatology, 24*, 761–766. https://doi.org/10.1111/exd.12765.
2. Baulier, E., Garcia Diaz, A., Corneo, B., & Farber, D. B. (2018). Generation of a human ocular albinism type 1 iPSC line, SEIi001-A, with a mutation in GPR143. *Stem Cell Research, 33*, 274–277.
3. Goudie, R. B., Spence, J. C., & MacKie, R. (1979). Vitiligo patterns simulating autoimmune and rheumatic diseases. *The Lancet, 2*, 393–395.
4. Grimes, P. E., Ijaz, S., Nashawati, R., & Kwak, D. (2019). New oral and topical approaches for the treatment of melasma. *International Journal of Women's Dermatology, 5*, 30–36. https://doi.org/10.1016/j.ijwd.2018.09.004.
5. Hu, S., Zhai, P., Chen, Y., Zhao, B., Yang, N., Wang, M., Xiao, Y., Bao, G., & Wu, X. (2019). Morphological characterization and gene expression patterns for melanin pigmentation in Rex rabbit. *Biochemical Genetics, 57*, 734–744. https://doi.org/10.1007/s10528-019-09929-x.
6. Lutfi, R. J., Fridmanis, M., Misiunas, A. L., Pafume, O., Gonzalez, E. A., Villemur, J. A., Mazzini, M. A., & Niepomniszcze, H. (1985). Association of melasma with thyroid autoimmunity and other thyroidal abnormalities and their relationship to the origin of the melasma. *The Journal of Clinical Endocrinology & Metabolism, 61*(1), 28–31.

7. Ma, E. Z., Zhou, A. E., Hoegler, K. M., & Khachemoune, A. (2023). Oculocutaneous albinism: Epidemiology, genetics, skin manifestation, and psychosocial issues. *Archives of Dermatological Research, 315*, 107–116. https://doi.org/10.1007/s00403-022-02335-1.

8. Madelaine, R., Ngo, K. J., Skariah, G., & Mourrain, P. (2020). Genetic deciphering of the antagonistic activities of the melanin-concentrating hormone and melanocortin pathways in skin pigmentation. *PLoS Genetics, 16*, e1009244–65. https://doi.org/10.1371/journal.pgen.1009244.

9. Maeda, K. (2022). Mechanism of action of topical tranexamic acid in the treatment of melasma and sun-induced skin hyperpigmentation. *Cosmetics, 9*, 108. https://doi.org/10.3390/cosmetics9050108.

10. McKesey, J., Tovar-Garza, A., & Pandya, A. G. (2020). Melasma treatment: An evidence-based review. *American Journal of Clinical Dermatology, 21*, 173–225. https://doi.org/10.1007/s40257-019-00488-w.

11. Nesby-O'Dell, S., Scanlon, K. S., Cogswell, M. E., et al. (2002). Hypovitaminosis D prevalence and determinants among African American and white women of reproductive age: Third National Health and Nutrition Examination Survey, 1988–1994. *American Journal of Clinical Nutrition, 76*, 187–192.

12. Nordlund, J. J., & Abdel-Malek, Z. A. (1988). Mechanisms for post-inflammatory hyperpigmentation and hypopigmentation. In J. T. Bagnara (Ed.), *Advances in Pigment Cell Research: Proceedings of Symposia and Lectures from the Thirteenth International Pigment Cell Conference* (pp. 219–239). Liss. (Conference held in Tucson, AZ, October 5–9, 1986).

13. Ortonne, J. (1992). Retinoic acid and pigment cells: A review of *in-vitro* and *in-vivo* studies. *British Journal of Dermatology, 127*(Suppl 41), 43–47.

14. Ortonne, J. P., & Nordlund, J. (2006). Mechanisms that cause abnormal skin color. In J. J. Nordlund, R. E. Boissey, V. J. Hearing, R. A. King, W. S. Oetting, & J. P. Ortonne (Eds.), *The Pigmentary System: Physiology and Pathophysiology* (pp. 521–538). Oxford: Blackwell Scientific Publishing.

15. Polidori, C., Jorge, A., & Ornosa, C. (2017). Eumelanin and pheomelanin are predominant pigments in bumblebee (Apidae: Bombus) pubescence. *PeerJ, 5*, e3300–e3321. https://doi.org/10.7717/peerj.3300.

16. Solano, F. (2020). Photoprotection and skin pigmentation: Melanin-related molecules and some other new agents obtained from natural sources. *Molecules, 25*, 1537. https://doi.org/10.3390/molecules25071537.

Chapter

DERMATOSES OF PREGNANCY

5

Contents

Introduction

Pregnancy-related dermatoses are a distinct, varied collection of pathological skin disorders brought on by the gravid state. The primary symptom of dermatosis in pregnancy is frequently pruritus, or an itchy skin eruption. Regretfully, pruritis by itself is not useful for diagnosis. Pregnant women should still undergo a thorough evaluation and examination to rule out the possibility of a de novo or pre-existing skin condition unrelated to the pregnancy. Because certain pregnancy dermatoses, like pemphigoid gestationis, intrahepatic cholestasis of pregnancy, and impetigo herpetiforms, pose a risk to health, a correct diagnosis is crucial for both the mother's and the child's prognosis. Over the last few decades, a substantial amount of new information has been available to shed light on the various pregnancy-related dermatoses and their classification, pathophysiology, prognosis, and treatment options.

Orientation and Directional Terms

Term	Definition	Illustration
Pregnancy-related dermatoses	Pregnancy-related dermatoses are a group of skin conditions that occur during pregnancy and after giving birth.	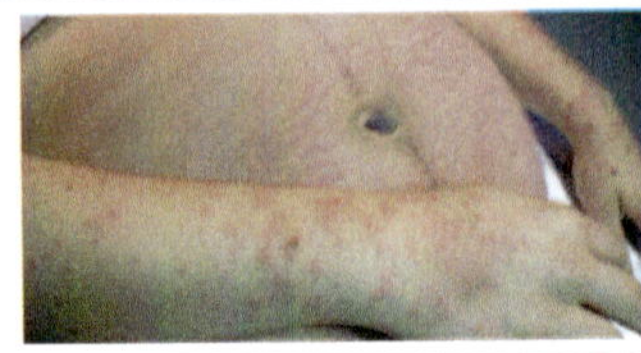
Cholestasis	Cholestasis of pregnancy is a liver condition that can occur in late pregnancy. The condition triggers intense itching, but without a rash.	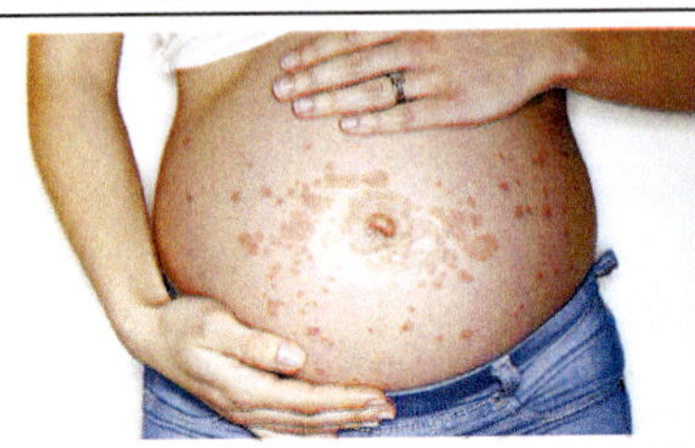
Pruritus	Pruritus is a common dermatological symptom during pregnancy that can be a sign of an underlying disease. It can interfere with sleep and reduce quality of life, and it can also be accompanied by skin lesions	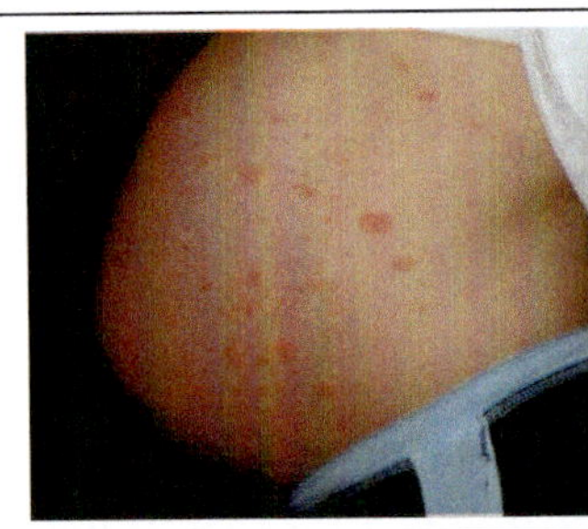
Polymorphic eruption	Polymorphic eruption of pregnancy is an itchy, bumpy rash that starts in the stretch marks of the abdomen in the last 3 months of pregnancy then clears with delivery. It is also called PUPPP or Pruritic Urticarial Papules and Plaques of Pregnancy.	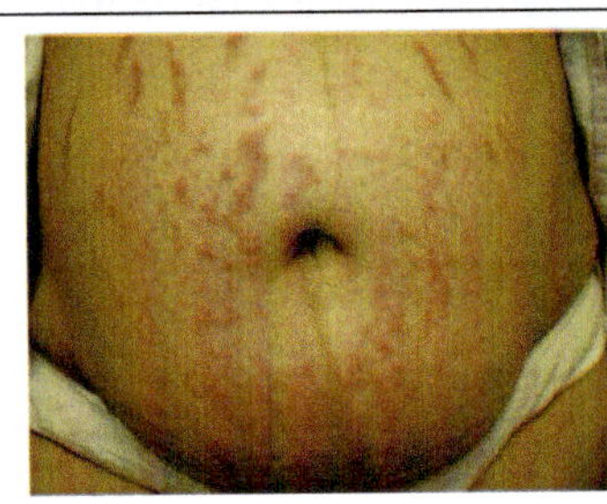
Atopic eruption of pregnancy (AEP)	Atopic eruption of pregnancy (AEP) is a benign skin condition that causes itching and lesions during pregnancy. It's the most common skin condition during pregnancy, affecting about 1 in 300 pregnancies	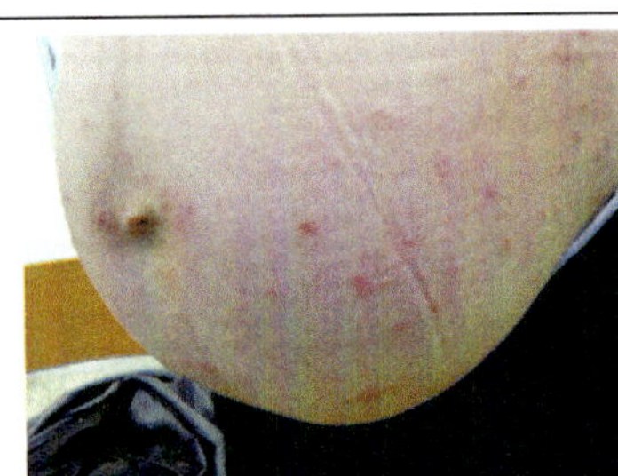

5.1. Historical Background

Pemphigoid gestationis, which Milton named herpes gestationis when he described it in 1872, was the first specific dermatosis of pregnancy that was documented. Herpes was the term used to describe the typical "creeping" blister formation. This disease entity could not be distinguished from the other pregnancy-related dermatoses until the advent of immunofluorescence microscopy and the identification of specific linear complement deposition along the dermo-epidermal junction zone (DEJ) in 1973. Besnier named a different pregnancy-related illness prurigo gestationis in 1904. It's interesting to note that what is now known as atopic dermatitis was once known as prurigo. The original description and illustration of atopic dermatitis are similar to the modern representation of the condition. Using this term, Costello identified as prurigo gestationis of Besnier all pregnancy-related dermatoses that were not herpes gestationis, reporting a 2% incidence. As time went on, the condition was also known as early onset pregnancy prurigo or prurigo of pregnancy.Under the name "toxic rash of pregnancy," Bourne reported an additional pregnancy-related dermatosis that resembles the polymorphic eruption of today's pregnancy and frequently affects small women who have gained a lot of weight and prominent striae on their abdomens. Subsequent synonyms included pruritic urticarial papules and plaques of pregnancy (PUPPP), toxic erythema of pregnancy, and late-onset prurigo of pregnancy. 1962 saw Spangler et al. depicted an entity whose existence is being questioned today, and rightly so. Based on biochemical changes (increased β-HCG in urine and decreased plasma cortisol levels), he distinguished papular dermatitis from prurigo gestationis, a clinically similar condition, and noted a markedly elevated fetal mortality rate. No additional case that matches the original description has surfaced in more than 40 years, with the exception of one additional case report written by the same authors. Not even a large prospective study conducted recently with comprehensive laboratory analyses was able to identify a manifestation consistent with "papular dermatitis."

Holmes et al. introduced the first condensed classification of pregnancy-related dermatoses in 1982 and included pregnancy-related prurigo, polymorphic eruption, and pemphigoid gestationis. They added a second dermatosis, pruritic folliculitis of pregnancy, a year later. In Europe, the terms pemphigoid gestationis (which indicates an autoimmune pathogenesis and avoids association with the herpes virus) and polymorphic eruption of pregnancy (which indicates a morphological spectrum) are widely accepted, while the terms herpes gestationis and PUPPP are still preferred in the USA. For 20years, the Holmes and Black classification held true; however, in 1998, Shornick suggested an additional modification.

He proposed that pregnancy-related folliculitis was a subset of pregnancy-related prurigo rather than a distinct entity. He also added intrahepatic cholestasis of pregnancy to the list of pregnancy-specific dermatoses. Since this disease only manifests secondary skin changes, it had not previously been included in the classification. Since it is a significant differential diagnostic factor that may increase fetal risk if the diagnosis is missed or delayed, it makes sense to include it in this classification. According to Holmes and Black as well as Shornick, prurigo of pregnancy is only included as a dubious independent entity. In contrast, pemphigoid gestationis, polymorphic eruption of pregnancy, and intrahepatic cholestasis of pregnancy are recognized as independent entities. Though the possibility of a connection to atopy has been raised numerous times since Besnier's initial description, Holmes, and Black were the first to propose that atopic pregnant women's pruritus could be the only cause. We were able to show clear similarities in the clinical presentation and histopathology between female patients with atopic dermatitis, prurigo of pregnancy, and pruritic folliculitis of pregnancy (comprising 50% of our patient collective) in a recent retrospective study on over 500 pregnant patients with pruritus. Consequently, we classified these patients together under the term atopic eruption of pregnancy. This leads to a new classification of specific dermatoses of pregnancy, which are as follows: pemphigoid gestationis, polymorphic eruption of pregnancy, intrahepatic cholestasis of pregnancy, and atopic eruption of pregnancy.

5.2. Pruritic Urticarial Papules and Plaques of Pregnancy (PUPPP)

Pregnancy-related pruritic urticarial papules and plaques (PUPPP) is a persistent rash that resembles hives that some women experience. Pregnant women are known to experience some changes in their skin, while those who already have dermatologies will either experience a change in their condition or an increase in symptoms. One of the numerous skin disorders unique to pregnancy is pruritic urticarial papules and plaques of pregnancy (PUPPP), which affects roughly 1 in 160 pregnancies (0.26%).

Despite frequent severe pruritus, there is no statistically significant increase in the risk of premature labor or fetal loss, so there is no long-term risk to the woman or the fetus (Figure 5.1).

PUPPP often starts on the abdomen and then frequently spreads to the arms, legs, feet, chest, and neck. Usually, there is no impact on the face. Given that PUPPP most commonly affects primigravida (women in their first pregnancy), those with large fundal measurements (the distance from the pubic bone to the top of the uterus), and/or those carrying large babies or multiples, skin distension, or stretching, is thought to be a potential trigger. Stretch marks are frequently the first places where the papules and plaques develop before they change and spread to other parts of the body.

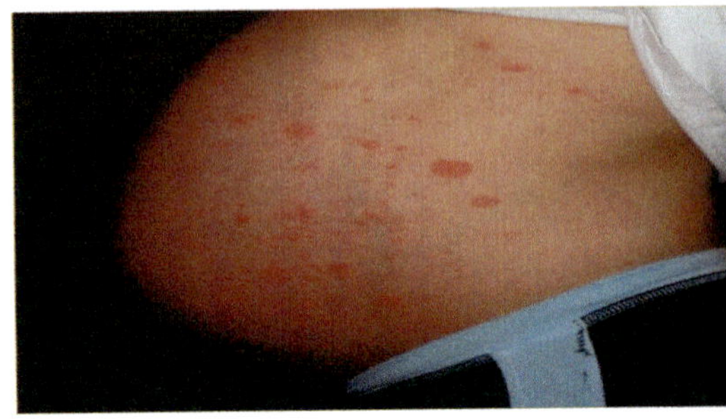

Figure 5.1. *PUPPP skin rash during pregnancy.*

Source: By Heykerriann at English Wikipedia – Transferred from en.wikipedia to Commons by Jusses2 using CommonsHelper., Public Domain, https://commons.wikimedia.org/w/index.php?curid=20365397.

It is highly advised that women who think they may be exhibiting PUPPP symptoms consult with their primary care physician and see a dermatologist about changes to their skin during pregnancy.

5.2.1. Signs and Symptoms

The most typical presentation of PUPPP is a rash that begins inside the stretch marks. The rash may then spread to other parts of the body, such as the arms, legs, feet, chest, and neck, among others. Reported cases of PUPPP rash spreading to the face, palms of hands, or soles of feet are extremely rare.

Typically, this rash starts with noticeably swollen skin tissue that appears elevated and within the stretch marks, along with unusually red and itchy skin. The individual parts of this rash may eventually come together to form a single, larger rash that shares the same features. People describe seeing the skin around the rash turn white (blanched) and take on the appearance of halos as this is happening. A number of the disease's characteristics can persist over time and include patches of inflamed, itchy, rough, and cracked skin that resemble eczema and widespread erythema, a red skin rash caused by damage to underlying capillaries. Tiny vesicles are among the other features that have been observed in some PUPPP cases; these are less common and take longer to develop.

According to some reports, PUPPP is positively correlated with both increased birth weight and excessive maternal weight gain. Furthermore, a research by Ghazeeri and colleagues revealed that Rh-positive individuals made up 89% of those who underwent *in vitro* fertilization.

There has been some variation in the time of onset reported for these symptoms. Though the majority of people report having symptoms in the third trimester, or the final few weeks of pregnancy, 15% of women with PUPPP reported that their symptoms started right away after the baby was delivered. As previously stated, the papules and plaques typically start on the abdomen (not the umbilicus or belly button) and frequently spread to the chest, underarms, legs, and other areas. Lesions on or above the breasts are uncommon, though. For this reason, the face is typically unaffected and spared. These PUPPP papules and plaques give rise to extremely itchy (pruritic) skin, which has a profound effect on the patient's quality of sleep throughout the night.

5.2.2. Cause

The most common pregnancy dermatosis, PUPPP is most common in women carrying a male fetus, women who gained weight quickly and noticeably over a short period of time, and women who end up delivering their baby via cesarean section. While the precise etiology of PUPPP is unknown and varies from person to person, there have been theories that connect hormone changes, connective tissue damage during pregnancy, and autoimmune disorders to the condition; however, the evidence supporting these theories is currently lacking.

Primigravida, or the skin condition that mostly affects first-time mothers, is more common in the third trimester of multiple pregnancies (especially with triplets as opposed to twins or singletons). It is estimated that 75% of individuals with typical PUPPP have never given birth. This condition rarely develops in the first or second trimester, though it can occasionally also happen postpartum.

There are no discernible differences in the outcomes of pregnancies for moms or babies, with the exception of additional associations with hypertension and induction of labor.

5.2.2.1. Dermatological Causes

It is thought that during pregnancy, as the abdominal wall rapidly stretches, collagen is exposed, leading to an inflammatory response. Compared to women giving birth to singletons, those expecting twins or triplets have shown this reaction more frequently. This is thought to be because carrying twins or triplets causes the abdominal wall to stretch more than it does for single births, which results in an earlier onset of PUPPP.

5.2.2.2. Hormonal Causes

Hormonal changes occur during pregnancy, and it has been suggested that these changes may play a role in the onset of PUPPP. Progesterone levels have been observed to rise in people who have had multiple gestations, despite the paucity of research currently available to support this theory. Progesterone raises the level of progesterone receptors in the body, which triggers an immunological response that results in skin lesions in PUPPP. Multiple gestations have been linked to an increase in sex hormones in those who have the condition. This includes higher levels of estradiol and, as was previously mentioned, progesterone. There is currently insufficient data to determine how sex hormones contribute to PUPPP, necessitating more study.

5.2.2.3. Immunological Causes

5.2.2.3.1. *Inflammatory Mediated*

An immunohistology profile, which uses antibodies to identify the tissue components present in an individual, has shown that there are some immune cells that are more prevalent in those with PUPPP than in those without the condition. The immunohistology profile revealed dendritic cells, epidermal Langerhans cells, and T helper cell infiltrates that are consistent with a delayed hypersensitivity.

PUPPP is thought to arise in reaction to fetal antigens that are carried throughout the body. For instance, a study revealed the presence of fetal male DNA in the skin lesions on the mother, which were assumed to be brought on by the fetal cells detected in the mother's blood during the course of the pregnancy.

5.2.2.3.2. *Autoimmune*

While the autoimmune nature of this condition has not been established, a single study has shown that immunoglobulin M (IgM) deposition at the dermal-epidermal membrane is linked to a range of dermatoses, including PUPPP. The hypothesis that has been put forth has a flaw in that the condition does not worsen over time or recur. There is currently no proof that the onset of PUPPP in a person is linked to the presence of circulating antibodies.

5.2.3. Diagnosis

To rule out other dermatoses, PUPPP is frequently a diagnosis of exclusion and may require laboratory testing. Comprehensive metabolic panels, liver function tests, serum human choriogonadotropin, serum cortisol, and complete blood counts are a few examples of lab tests that may be performed. To rule out pemphigoid gestationis, further specialized tests might include serum for indirect immunofluorescence or lesion biopsy for direct immunofluorescence.

Since urticarial pemphigoid gestationis is frequently misdiagnosed, it must be ruled out when diagnosing PUPPP because the two conditions can have similar clinical features. Histological and immunological investigations are therefore required to make sure there isn't a misdiagnosis. When pemphigoid gestationis is present, lesions typically develop early in the gestational cycle, involving the umbilicus and exhibiting positive perilesional skin immunofluorescence. People with eczema typically have a history of atopy, either directly or through family. The eruption is recognized by erythematous, pruritic lesions on the flexural areas. Moreover, drug eruptions, urticaria, or viral exanthems could all be clinical differential diagnoses.

A 3- or 4-mm punch biopsy may occasionally be necessary to rule out herpes gestationis, a form of bullous pemphigoid that can develop during or right after pregnancy. Typically, the biopsy exhibits characteristics consistent with PUPPP, but the specific disorder's pathognomonic symptoms are absent. Toexclude herpes gestationis more precisely, direct immunofluorescence studies could be performed on a biopsy of unaffected perilesional skin.

5.2.4. Treatment

It is crucial to remember that a reliable medical practitioner should perform the diagnosis. If a woman exhibits PUPPP symptoms, she should not self-treat and instead should speak with her primary care physician to be referred to a dermatologist for treatment advice.

PUPPP usually goes away on its own after a week of delivery or within a few days or weeks after it first appears. Some women, nevertheless, still have symptoms well after giving birth.

Intramuscular injection of autologous whole blood has been proposed as a novel treatment option for individuals affected by PUPPP immediately after childbirth. This approach appears to improve symptoms both subjectively and objectively. For those who are concerned about taking medication while pregnant or nursing, this is a great option.

Antihistamine pills may be prescribed to treat the itching, but they are usually thought to be far less effective than corticosteroid treatments. Antihistamine tablets may improve sleep quality and reduce itching by blocking the release of histamine.

Moreover, it has been demonstrated that first-generation antihistamines, like chlorpheniramine, are safe to use during pregnancy and can be used as a supplement to treat pruritus. Non-sedating second-generation antihistamines like cetirizine and loratadine may help pregnant women with pruritus management.

Since high-potency topical steroids are generally ineffective when taken orally, PUPPP is best treated with them, ideally tapered off after seven days of therapy. Oral (systemic) corticosteroids can be used to treat very severe cases; however, the benefits of a pregnant woman taking high-potency corticosteroids must be carefully weighed against possible (and mostly unknown) risks to the developing fetus or fetuses. Class I or II corticosteroid creams and ointments are used in more aggressive cases. Using more than 300 grams of high-potency topical corticosteroids during pregnancy may raise the baby's risk of having a low birth weight. Rarely, some women have had their labor induced as soon as they are deemed to be at term (37 weeks), in exceptionally persistent and upsetting cases.

In severe cases, oral prednisone at doses of 10 to 40 mg/day has been the standard treatment when the pruritus becomes intolerable for the PUPPP patient. After taking this medication orally for 24 hours, symptoms usually go away. When other treatments fail and the patient's symptoms are too severe, it may be possible to discuss an early delivery if the case is too severe. Even an early baby delivery does not ensure that the symptoms will go away. Fortunately, steroid treatment usually has a positive effect and reduces symptoms significantly in a matter of days. Its use is debatable, as is the case with most steroid therapies. However, it is best to use it sparingly or only once, and it is generally safer to use it in the third trimester than the first.

Using body wash or soap containing pine tar and applying cold therapy, like taking a cold shower or using ice packs, can also provide relief.

5.3. Impetigo Herpetiformis

Impetigo herpetiformis (IH) is an uncommon and potentially fatal pregnancy dermatosis. Despite earlier views that suggested it was a distinct condition, it is now thought to be a type of generalized pustular psoriasis. The condition typically manifests during the third trimester of pregnancy and goes away after delivery; nevertheless, it may recur in subsequent pregnancies.

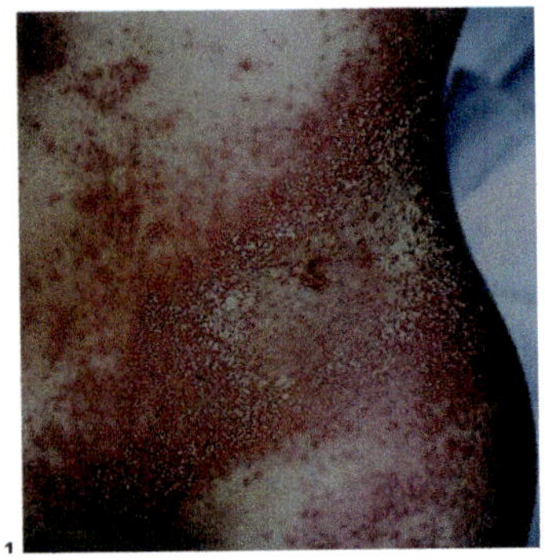

Figure 5.2. *Impetigo herpetiformis during the puerperium.*

Source: https://www.semanticscholar.org/paper/Impetigo-herpetiformis-during-the-Puerperium-Katsambas-Stavropoulos/e982ab6701708987973546e8fc6f34223d8da086.

5.3.1. Pathogenesis

We still don't know the exact cause of IH. Some evidence suggests that genetic factors may play a role in the development of IH, such as the number of familial cases. The majority of cases of generalized pustular psoriasis without a history of psoriasis vulgaris, according to prior research, have homozygous or compound heterozygous mutations of the IL-36 receptor antagonist-encoding Interleukin 36 Receptor Antagonist (IL36RN).

Not present in normal skin, IL36 is induced in certain pustular dermatoses by other cytokines like IL-17A, IL-22, and tumor necrosis factor-α. There have been reports of homozygous and heterozygous IL36RN mutations in two IH cases in Japan. A Chinese patient with IH has also been reported to have an IL36RN mutation recently. Although more research is needed to determine the percentage of IL36RN-negative patients who go on to develop IH, this mutation is thought to have a promising role in predicting the occurrence of IH and reducing the risk to the mother and fetus. Although a cause-and-effect relationship is challenging to establish, some conditions have been linked to IH, the most well-known of which is hypocalcemia. Patients with IH have been reported to have hypoparathyroidism, hypoalbuminemia, low vitamin D levels, and a decrease in ionized serum calcium concentrations as a result of malabsorption as the underlying causes of their hypocalcemia. The most common condition known to play a potential role in IH is hypoparathyroidism. While the exact mechanisms are unknown, many medications may cause IH. In one case, N-butyl-scopolammonium bromide-induced hypotension (IH) occurred in the 34th week of pregnancy following five days of drug consumption. It has also been noted that the medication ritadine hydrochloride, which has been used to treat preterm uterine contractures, can cause IH.

5.3.2. Clinical Features

The typical lesions are centrifugally extending erythematous patches with marginally grouped sterile pustules; they can also develop erosion, crust, and impetiginization. These lesions are mainly seen in flexural regions (Figure 5.3).

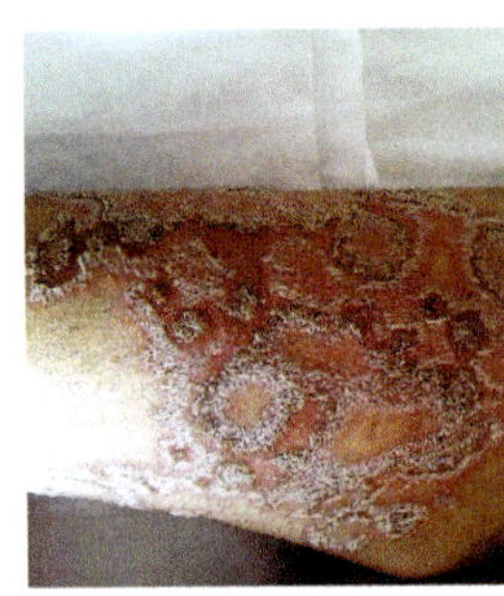

Figure 5.3. *Annular lesions of pustular psoriasis of pregnancy on the left thigh of a patient in the 36th week of the first pregnancy.*

Source: Namazi N, Dadkhahfar S. Impetigo Herpetiformis: Review of Pathogenesis, Complication, and Treatment. Dermatol Res Pract. 2018 Apr 4;2018:5801280. doi: 10.1155/2018/5801280. PMID: 29849579; PMCID: PMC5904797.

Patients may experience vegetative lesions resembling Pemphigus vegetans, though they are uncommon. It is possible to see mucosal lesions in the tongue, mouth, and even esophagus in addition to nail involvement. In IH, hypoparathyroidism, and hypocalcemia may occur.

5.3.3. Complications

The complications that can arise from impetigo herpetiformis (IH) or as a result of it putting the mother's and fetus' lives in jeopardy are a significant part of the disease. A considerable amount of these issues are associated with electrolyte imbalance and placental insufficiency, in addition to the previously indicated change in serum calcium. IH may be linked to systemic symptoms like leukocytosis, elevated ESR, hypocalcemia, hypoalbuminemia, fever, chills, diarrhea, hypovolemic shock, seizure, and malaise as well as laboratory results like leukocytosis and iron deficiency anemia. It has been documented that a woman diagnosed with IH in the 32nd week of pregnancy may experience complications due to gestational hypertension.

Furthermore, IH has been linked to an increased risk of prenatal complications such as premature membrane rupture, stillbirth, and intrauterine growth restriction brought on by placental insufficiency. Another case involves a mother who presented with typical IH symptoms in the eighth month of her pregnancy, and her unborn child was born with central hypoventilation syndrome or Ondine's curse.

In a young woman, recurrence has been reported in up to nine pregnancies. The same patient's use of oral contraceptives, which contain a combination of progesterone and ethinyl estradiol, also triggered this.

5.3.4. Treatment

The mother's and the fetus's critical conditions and the potential teratogenicity of the medications being used to treat IH present the biggest obstacles. Despite the fact that there are numerous treatment options for IH, there is no set standard and the evidence supporting treatment efficacy is weak. Unbalances in fluid and electrolytes, particularly low vitamin D, hypovolemia, and hypocalcemia, should be treated right away.

5.3.4.1. Corticosteroids

Pustular psoriasis is still primarily treated with systemic corticosteroids, which have been used for many years. In mild to moderate cases, the starting dose is 15–30 mg per day. The dosage can be raised to 40–60 mg or even 80 mg per day if necessary.

The increased risk of cleft palate associated with corticosteroid therapy during pregnancy is the main cause of concern. Given that intrauterine hypertension (IH) typically occurs in the latter stages of the third trimester of pregnancy, corticosteroid therapy is a safe option. Steroid therapy applied topically has the potential to cause growth restriction in the fetus. Consequently, it makes sense to think about using mild to moderate corticosteroids as opposed to strong or extremely strong ones.

5.3.4.2. Cyclosporine

If a patient is not responding to corticosteroids, cyclosporine may be a useful medication. 14 patients with IH have reportedly received cyclosporine treatment, the majority of whom also received systemic corticosteroids, according to the literature. Variable results were obtained when cyclosporine was administered at a dose of 2–7.5 mg/kg/day. It is possible to taper the corticosteroid after starting cyclosporine. A case report details the total resolution following cyclosporine treatment, which was started at a dose of 4 mg/kg and involved tapering off prednisolone prescriptions within a week. Three days before delivery, the last dose of cyclosporine was administered, and then a topical steroid with high potency was applied.

Like any medication, there are questions regarding cyclosporine's safety when taken during pregnancy. Studies on the side effects of cyclosporine, which were primarily conducted on patients undergoing renal transplants, have not revealed any impairment of renal function and have only marginally increased the risk of premature rupture of the membranes. Indeed, cyclosporine's placental transfer appears to be dose-dependent, and it can be used as a harmless corticosteroid substitute when the fetus is properly monitored. Maternal hypertension risk needs to be taken into account.

5.3.4.3. Antibiotics

Even though they can't completely stop the illness, antibiotics appear to be helpful when used in IH patients.

In mild cases, antibiotic therapy may be considered first. If antibiotics don't seem to be working, additional or alternative treatments, like corticosteroids, may then be considered. It is recommended to administer antibiotic therapy, particularly with cephalosporins, even though the pustules are sterile. While older cephalosporins are preferred, cephalosporins are generally safe to use during pregnancy. Ampicillin, macrolide, and clofazimine are the antibiotics that have shown efficacy in the treatment of IH.

5.3.4.4. Biologic Agents

Pregnancy category B medications include anti-TNF-α medications like infliximab and adalimumab. The FDA in the United States has not approved the regular use of TNF-α blockers during pregnancy, although current data do not show an increased risk of fetal complications in patients exposed to these medications during pregnancy.

The European Academy of Dermatology and Venereology is against using infliximab or adalimumab during pregnancy that is in conflict with the board of the National Psoriasis Foundation's assertion that infliximab is one of the most effective treatments for IH. Positive results have been reported in refractory cases of IH and psoriasis treated with infliximab during pregnancy.

A case of recalcitrant severe pustular psoriasis during pregnancy has been reported to be satisfactorily treated with uzekinumab (Andrulonis, 2012).

5.3.4.5. Phototherapy

When there is insufficient response to corticosteroids, NBUVB can be added to therapy, and it is thought to be a safe option during pregnancy. Even though NBUVB has been linked in some studies to lower folate levels during pregnancy, this is not a significant concern during the third trimester, when the incidence of IH is highest. Nonetheless, neural tube defects may develop as a result of a folate deficiency during the first trimester.

Although PUVA administration has not increased the risk of congenital malformations or infant mortality, it is generally safe and may cause low birth weight babies.

5.3.4.6. Retinoids

All systemic retinoids are contraindicated during pregnancy due to their teratogenic effects; however, they have been used to treat IH after delivery. Should the administration of systemic retinoid be contemplated postpartum, the mother's informed consent for suitable contraception ought to be obtained.

5.3.4.7. Methotrexate

Methotrexate has been effectively used to treat IH during puberty, even though its administration is prohibited during pregnancy.

5.4. Pemphigoid Gestationis

Pregnancy-related subepidermal bullous dermatosis that is rare, self-limiting, and autoimmune is called pemphigoid gestationis (PG), formerly known as herpes gestationis. The blisters on PG, which Laws Milton first reported in 1872, were formerly known as herpes gestationis because of their herpetiform appearance. The name was later changed to pemphigoid gestationis, though, as the illness was not linked to the herpes virus. The condition usually manifests as severe pruritus and inflammatory skin lesions during the third trimester, but it can happen at any time during the pregnancy or the postpartum period. The face and mucous membranes are frequently spared; the skin lesions usually start in the umbilical area and extend throughout the abdomen to the extremities. 30 to 50% of subsequent pregnancies experience PG recurrence, albeit usually with an earlier onset and a more severe course. The diagnosis of pemphigoid gestationis is usually made using characteristic clinical features and direct immunofluorescence; additional diagnostic tests may be carried out to rule out other dermatologic conditions. Supportive therapies and preventing the development of new skin lesions make up treatment. In moderate to severe cases, corticosteroids are usually used as a treatment; however, intravenous immunoglobulins have also shown promise in certain case studies. While most patients with PG recover on their own, there is evidence linking the condition to maternal Graves' disease, preterm labor, and small-for-gestational-age infants. Clinicians should have a solid understanding of the proper diagnostic procedures and treatments related to pemphigoid gestationis because of the negative effects of the condition. They should also be able to work well with an interprofessional team to enhance the outcomes for both the mother and the fetus (Figure 5.4).

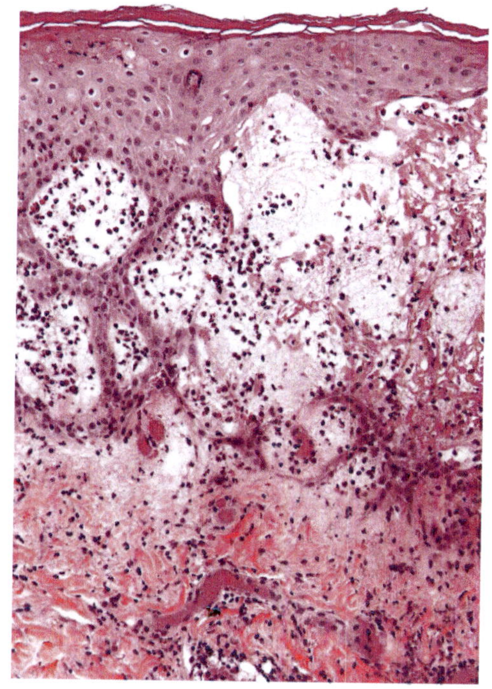

Figure 5.4. *Pemphigoid gestationis, an autoimmune reaction that occurs most commonly during the second and third trimesters of pregnancy.*

Source: By Nephron – Own work, CC BY-SA 3.0, https://commons.wikimedia.org/w/index.php?curid=17847568.

5.4.1. Etiology

The hemidesmosomal proteins bullous pemphigoid 180 (BP 180) and bullous pemphigoid 230 (BP 230), which are found in the placental tissue and dermal basement membrane zone, are involved in the maternal autoimmune process that causes the skin lesions in PG. BP 180 and BP 230, also referred to as BPAG2 and collagen, XVII, are recognized by the mother's immune system as foreign proteins. But it's unclear exactly what sets off the formation of these autoantibodies. The maternal HLA-DRB1*0301 (HLA-DR3) and HLA-DRB1*0401/040X (HLA-DR4) are highly correlated with PG, indicating the critical role that major histocompatibility complex (MHC) class II plays in the disease's pathophysiology. Strong correlations have also been found with the human leukocyte antigens PG3 and PG4.

5.4.2. Epidemiology

The number of pregnancies that have PG varies, ranging from 1 in 2,000 to 60,000, and the majority of cases happen in the second and third trimesters of pregnancy. Compared to primiparous women, multiparous women are more likely to experience the condition, which frequently recurs in subsequent pregnancies. Recurrent PG, on the other hand, usually presents with more severe symptoms at an earlier stage. Additionally, a rare correlation between PG and choriocarcinomas and hydatidiform moles has been documented in certain studies.

5.4.3. Pathophysiology

It is believed that PG arises from the loss of the mother's immunotolerance to the fetus and placenta. Maternal IgG autoantibodies are generated against the bullous pemphigoid protein antigens, BP180 and BP 230, which are expressed in the skin, placental cytotrophoblastic and syncytiotrophoblastic cells, and amniotic membrane epithelial cells, although the exact provocation is unclear. An intolerance to this BP 180 placental antigen may lead to autoimmune reactions, which in turn trigger a local allogeneic response against the fetoplacental unit. The placental basement membrane changes along with this process, which is aided by aberrant expression of placental HLA class II antigens. The immune system then reacts at the skin's dermoepidermal junction, disrupting the basement membrane and resulting in the typical bullous skin lesions.

5.4.4. Histopathology

The results of routine histopathologic studies vary depending on the stage and severity of the disease, but they are useful in ruling out other skin disease processes. Papillary edema and dermal infiltration, comprising lymphocytes, histiocytes, and varying numbers of eosinophils, are typical in the pre-bullous stage. Typically, subepidermal blistering is seen during the bullous stage. However, since these results are not unique to PG, histologic examination is usually insufficient for the diagnosis.

5.4.5. History and Physical

5.4.5.1. Clinical Course of Pemphigoid Gestationis

Clinicians are greatly aided in the diagnosis of pemphigoid gestationis (PG), a rare disease, by having a thorough understanding of the characteristic clinical features of PG and the findings that set it apart from similar skin conditions. Getting a thorough history is crucial since the clinical course of postpartum goiter is characterized by flare-ups and remissions, with flare-ups typically occurring during the parturition and postpartum phases. This includes past and present obstetrical histories. PG usually goes away on its own in one to two months after delivery. However, a sudden rise in antibodies after pregnancy may cause symptoms to continue or even worsen. Moreover, it is well documented that recurrence occurs during any subsequent pregnancy (such as miscarriage and abortion) or, less frequently, during menstrual cycles or the combination of oral contraceptive use. Preterm labor, transient neonatal skin lesions, which typically go away a few weeks after birth, and fetal growth restriction are among the other fetal risks linked to pregnancies with PG. There hasn't been any evidence of an elevated risk of stillbirth or miscarriage, but this pregnancy risk seems to be connected with the severity of the illness. As a result, getting a thorough history aids in directing medical professionals when making differential diagnosis decisions.

5.4.5.2. Clinical Features of Pemphigoid Gestationis

The main clinical symptom is pruritus, which in certain patients may appear before skin manifestations. The clinical characteristics can differ because the lesions go through different stages. The polymorphic eruptions can start as papules, erythematous urticarial plaques, eczematous or erythema multiforme-like lesions, and in more than 65% of cases, these lesions progress to vesicles, tense blisters, and bullae. The patient may experience significant psychological effects from the lesions, which can range in severity. First appearing in the umbilical region, the lesions later spread to the thighs, palms, and soles as well as other areas of the abdominal region. Frequently, the face and mucosal membranes remain unharmed. During the initial phase, the physical examination findings and the distribution of skin lesions are often nonspecific. This can make it challenging for clinicians to differentiate Polymorphic Eruption of Pregnancy (PG) from other pruriginal dermatoses of pregnancy, such as PUPPP. PEP and PG share similar clinical characteristics and can also arise during the third trimester of pregnancy. Direct immunofluorescence is usually used to confirm diagnosis because the differential diagnoses in the pre-bullous stage are difficult to distinguish both symptomatically and histopathologically.

5.4.6. Evaluation

Diagnostic studies, such as histopathology, direct immunofluorescence, and enzyme-linked immunosorbent assay (ELISA), are commonly used to diagnose PG because clinical features alone are nonspecific. On the other hand, skin biopsy specimens stained with direct immunofluorescence (DIF) are thought to be the most sensitive and specific diagnostic test for PG confirmation. IgG autoantibodies at the basement membrane zone and linear C3 deposits are characteristic findings of PG on DIF. Since C3 deposits have been seen in every DIF stain from PG patients, they are thought to be diagnostic of the disease. Interestingly, after a clinical remission, DIF can occasionally stay positive for four years or six months.

To diagnose PG, a number of additional studies can be used in addition to DIF. The results of routine histopathologic studies vary depending on the stage and severity of the disease, but they are useful in ruling out other skin disease processes. Papillary edema and dermal infiltration, comprising lymphocytes, histiocytes, and varying numbers of eosinophils, are typical in the pre-bullous stage. PG patients' immunochemistry tests reveal C4d deposits at the dermal-epidermal junction. Between 30 and 100% of patients with PG have circulating IgG antibodies in their serum, according to indirect immunofluorescence microscopy. ELISA testing uses the presence of BP 180 IgG antibodies in serum specimens to differentiate PG from other pregnancy dermatoses. With an estimated sensitivity and specificity of 95%, ELISA has the potential to replace direct immunofluorescence, which is the industry standard at the moment. The requirements for non-formalin tissue fixation and appropriately equipped laboratory facilities come with a higher cost for both DIF and indirect immunofluorescence, which can be challenging in developing nations.

5.4.7. Treatment/Management

The degree and stage of the skin lesions determine how PG is treated. Relieving itching and preventing the development of new blisters are the primary objectives. Topical high-potency corticosteroids and antihistamines are the cornerstones of treatment. However, patients who do not respond to the first therapy may require additional therapies. To minimize the use of high-dose steroids and avoid potential pregnancy complications, more modern treatment plans have been implemented.

Oral antihistamines and topical corticosteroids have traditionally been the recommended treatments for post-glaucoma (PG), even though the majority of treatment recommendations are based on case studies. This is particularly true when the disease is localized and blistering is minimal. Systemic corticosteroids may be necessary for patients who do not respond to topical treatment or whose condition is severe enough to affect more than 10% of their body surface area. Oral prednisolone 0.5 mg/kg per day is the recommended daily dosage for treatment, with a maximum of 20 mg. Because prednisone and prednisolone have a lower concentration that crosses the placenta than other agents, they are preferred. If doctors should gradually wean patients off of corticosteroid medication. Immunosuppressant drugs like azathioprine, dapsone, or cyclosporine are thought to be effective in controlling disease in nonresponsive patients; however, physicians need to be aware of the possible side effects of these drugs, which include liver impairment, preterm birth, and suppression of bone marrow. Compared to immunosuppressants, intravenous immunoglobulins (IVIG) have a better safety record and have been used more successfully recently, either by themselves or in combination with other agents.

Most recently, biotherapy has made use of dupilumab, a monoclonal antibody that targets the alpha subunit of the interleukin 4 receptor, particularly in refractory and corticosteroid-dependent bullous pemphigoid disease. This appears to be a novel and promising treatment, particularly for women who may not benefit from systemic steroid therapy due to co-morbid conditions like diabetes. Using dupilumab was linked to quick symptom remission and the ability to wean off of high-dose systemic steroid use. Furthermore, when administered before conception, rituximab has supposedly shown promise in preventing recurrent PG. After the final infusion, patients should wait 12 months before getting pregnant again.

5.4.8. Differential Diagnosis

Other conditions that should be considered when evaluating patients for PG include:

- Urticaria.
- Allergic contact dermatitis.
- Bullous pemphigoid.
- Cicatricial pemphigoid.
- Dermatitis herpetiformis.
- Erythema multiforme.
- Impetigo.
- Intrahepatic cholestasis of pregnancy.
- Linear IgA dermatosis.
- Bullous drug eruption.
- Atopic eruption of pregnancy.

5.4.9. Prognosis

For PG, the prognosis is generally favorable. Recurrence of postpartum hemorrhage is more likely in subsequent pregnancies. Mothers who have experienced PG-affected pregnancies are also susceptible to the future onset of other autoimmune diseases, particularly Grave's disease. Neonatal pemphigoid is caused by the transplacental passage of maternal antibodies in about 10% of affected pregnancies. These newborn lesions typically resolve spontaneously.

Preterm labor and intrauterine growth retardation are the two biggest fetal risks. Timely clinical and histopathological diagnosis of pemphigoid gestationis is essential for minimizing and preventing the risk of adverse effects for the fetus. To reduce fetal and maternal complications, it is essential to screen for intrauterine fetal growth restriction during pregnancy and to keep an eye out for any side effects of high-dose steroid treatment. Pregnant women and their unborn children benefit greatly from a multidisciplinary approach to care that includes dermatology, pediatrics, obstetrics, and neonatology during and after the pregnancy, as well as in subsequent pregnancies.

5.4.10. Complications

PG has few complications for both mother and fetus, but the itching it causes can be excruciating. Furthermore, prolonged use of corticosteroids during pregnancy may raise the risk of venous thromboembolism, preeclampsia, premature rupture of the membranes, preterm birth, congenital abnormalities, pyelonephritis, and possibly intrauterine fetal death. It is unclear whether the use of long-term corticosteroids during pregnancy results in small gestational-age babies more frequently or if the underlying condition being treated is the primary cause. Steroid use may be linked to aberrant placentation, which results in fetal growth restriction, according to certain animal studies. There is still much to learn about the precise mechanism and association. Long-term steroid use during pregnancy carries risks and benefits that should be considered when developing a treatment plan. If a mother needs corticosteroid treatment during her pregnancy, more research is necessary to determine whether the children will experience any long-term effects.

5.4.11. Enhancing Healthcare Team Outcomes

PG is an uncommon illness that usually doesn't have a major negative impact on health. However, until the right diagnostic tests are carried out, this condition frequently results in severe maternal distress and presents a diagnostic conundrum. Because the disease typically responds well to treatment with topical steroids and antihistamines, clinicians should start evaluation and treatment as soon as patients present with clinical symptoms. It takes an interprofessional approach to ensure coordinated monitoring, including evaluating abnormal fetal growth and signs of prematurity, between obstetric and dermatologic clinicians and ancillary health professionals. To lessen severe pruritus, pharmacists, and other members of the health team should support the direction of adverse effect treatment and promote medication compliance.

5.5. Prurigo of Pregnancy

Pregnancy-related prurigo, also known as early-onset prurigo or Papular eruption, is the second most prevalent pregnancy-specific dermatosis (1:300 incidences). Three variations exist for this condition. Only localized lesions are characteristic of the milder and more prevalent form of prurigo gestationis (Besnier). Papular dermatitis (Spangler) is the term used to describe the generalized variant. Although they are clinically related to this group, pruritic folliculitis and linear IgM disease of pregnancy are distinguished by their histopathology or IF results (Figure 5.5).

Besnier coined the term prurigo gestationis for the first time in 1904. Back then, atopic dermatitis was referred to as "prurigo." Pregnancy-related eczema, prurigo gestationis, papular dermatitis, and pruritic folliculitis all exhibited significant histopathological and clinical overlap. Thus, atopic eruption of pregnancy (AEP) serves as a summary of this disease complex. A recent prospective study on the pruritic skin diseases mentioned above that show a high prevalence of atopic eczema in all of them could provide one explanation.

Although the cause is unknown, elevated IgE is present in many patients. Normal pregnancy is characterized by a lack of strong T-helper

1 (Th1) cytokine production and maternal cell-mediated immunity to prevent fetal rejection. Consequently, the humoral immune response, which produces T-helper 2 (Th2) cytokines, is the predominant one. Since atopic dermatitis is generally thought to be a Th2-dominant illness, the Th2 shift brought on by pregnancy may contribute to an atopic dermatitis flare-up.

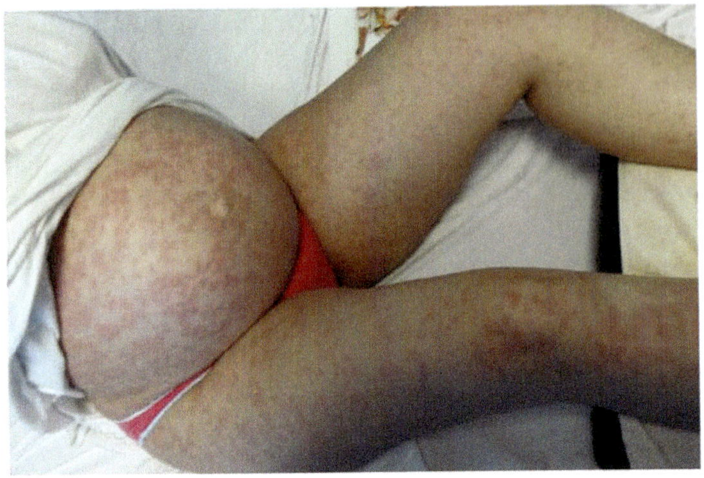

Figure 5.5. *A monomorphic rash consisting of erythematous papules and round oval plaques disseminated on the abdomen and lower limbs, that spares the umbilicus.*

Source: Mehedintu C, Isopescu F, Ionescu O-M, Petca A, Bratila E, Cirstoiu MM, Carp-Veliscu A, Frincu F. Diagnostic Pitfall in Atypical Febrile Presentation in a Patient with a Pregnancy-Specific Dermatosis—Case Report and Literature Review. Medicina. 2022; 58(7):847. https://doi.org/10.3390/medicina58070847.

There have been reports of cholestasis in other patients, indicating a possible overlap with pregnancy-related cholestasis. Given the likelihood of group heterogeneity, several pathways might be pertinent.

Prurigo of pregnancy is linked to twin pregnancies and is typically accompanied by the pregnant woman gaining more weight.

This disease complex occurs earlier in pregnancy compared to other specific skin conditions. It usually begins before the third trimester. The milder form of prurigo gestationis is characterized by small, itchy bumps on the forearms and trunk, mostly on the outside of the arms. Blisters do not form in this variant. The bumps may or may not be associated with hair follicles and are typically 0.5–1.0cm in size, sometimes with a crust in the center. While prurigo gestationis is limited to the forearms and trunk, papular dermatitis can appear all over the body.

The uncommon late-pregnancy dermatitis known as "papular dermatitis" is characterized by a widespread, itchy eruption. Lesions are composed of 3–5 mm soft, reddish-violet to reddish-brown papules, some with a centrally hemorrhagic crust, and occasionally forming large patches. Atopy is typically preexisting. Recent research has linked papular dermatitis to decreased plasma hydrocortisone, a shorter half-life of hydrocortisone, and elevated urine levels of human chorionic gonadotropin (HCG).

Pregnancy's pruritic folliculitis usually appears between weeks four and nine. It goes away two to three weeks after delivery. It's a type of acne brought on by fluctuations in hormones. Legs and the trunk are frequently affected by skin lesions. Pregnancy-related cholestasis and bacterial folliculitis need to be included in the differential diagnosis (Picard et al., 2015).

The results of purigo gestationis and papular dermatitis histopathology are nonspecific. Acanthosis, parakeratosis, and lymphatic perivascular infiltrate are present. Laboratory tests and immunofluorescence are negative.

Pruritic foliculitis histopathology results show a variable number of eosinophils, lymphocytes, mononuclear cells, and intrafollicular neutrophils. Labs and the IMF are not good. Direct IF, which displays a bright linear IgM along the BMZ, is crucial for the diagnosis of linear IgM disease. The pathology lacks specificity.

There is no evidence of fetal or maternal risk and no skin involvement for the newborn. Postpartum, the illness may linger for several weeks or even months. It goes away on its own and may or may not recur in later pregnancies.

In severe cases, oral steroids, topical steroids, and antipruritics are used as treatments. There is no need for intervention because there is no proof of fetal or maternal risk.

5.6. Striae Gravidarum: Risk Factors, Prevention, and Management

Between 55 and 90% of women experience the common and disfiguring gestational change known as striae gravidarum (SG). Atrophic linear scars are the typical appearance of SG, which can be distressing and frequently lower quality of life. The fact that SG is frequently disregarded as a cosmetic issue does not lessen the load on patients. There has been little or no success in the current research on risk factors, prevention, and management of this condition, and/or the results have been inconsistent (Chang et al., 2004).

Stretch marks have historically caused anxiety and distress to expectant mothers. The poet Ovid made references to pregnant women who would self-abort to avoid stretch marks as early as 16 BC. Many remedies for treating stretch marks were documented by the ancient Egyptians, and in the first century, AD, Soranus, and Pliny the Elder recommended unripe olive oil and sea salt, respectively. One of the most frequently suggested remedies is frankincense. Stretch marks have been linked to a wide range of additional therapeutic options, ranging from topical drugs to surgical modalities, which heightens the concern surrounding this condition.

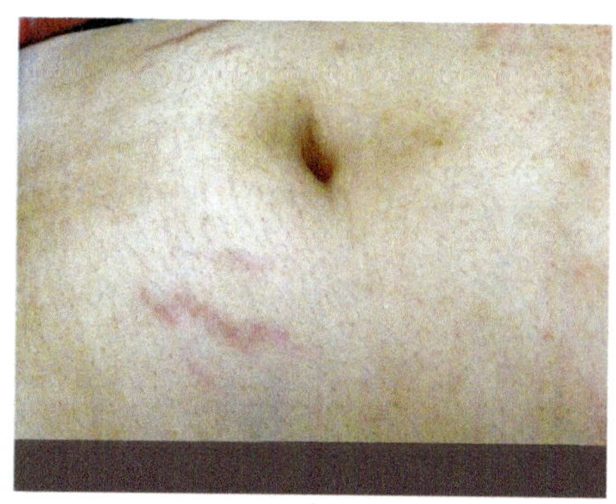

Figure 5.6. *Immature striae (striae rubra) on the abdomen.*

Source: https://www.ncbi.nlm.nih.gov/pmc/articles/PMC5440454/.

SG first appear as flat, pink-to-red bands, also known as immature striae or striae rubra, which later rise and become violet-red, longer, and wider (Figure 5.6) (Figure 5.7). The marks fade and become hypopigmented (striae alba or mature striae) over months to years, showing up parallel to skin tension lines as wrinkled, atrophic, scar-like marks (Figure 5.8). Usually found on the breasts, belly, hips, and thighs, SG can be uncomfortable, itchy, and burning. 90% or more of SG are found in primigravidas. The late second and early third trimesters have historically been reported as the onset period; however, a study has shown that 43% of women experience SG before 24 weeks of pregnancy.

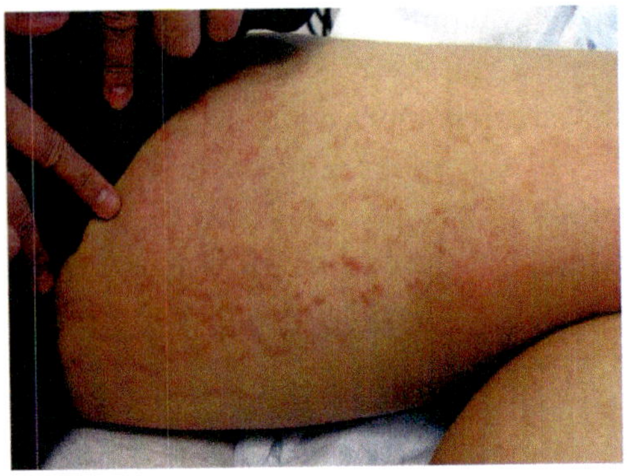

Figure 5.7. *Striae rubra on the thigh.*

Source: https://www.ncbi.nlm.nih.gov/pmc/articles/PMC5440454/.

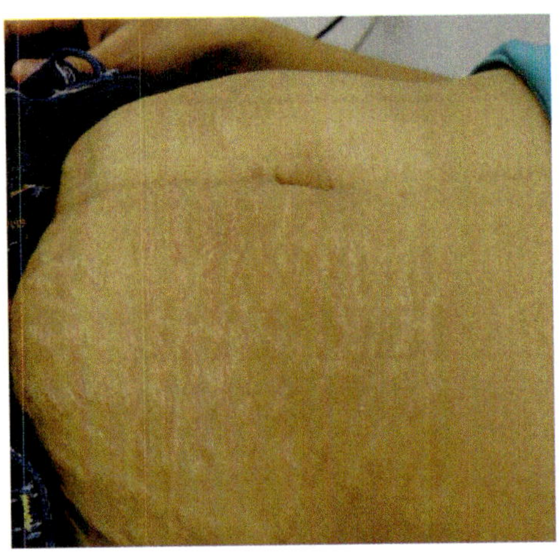

Figure 5.8. *Mature striae (striae alba) on the abdomen.*

Source: https://www.ncbi.nlm.nih.gov/pmc/articles/PMC5440454/.

A combination of genetic, hormonal, and increased mechanical stress on connective tissue plays a role in the etiopathogenesis. It's interesting that research has shown that there is conflicting evidence linking SG to both belly and hip girth stretch and maternal weight gain. This makes skin stretch a contentious trigger. In terms of hormones, striae have been found to have twice as many estrogen receptors as healthy skin, as well as higher levels of androgen and glucocorticoid receptors. It is believed that the unique hormonal environment of pregnancy affects connective tissue, which is prone to SG when stretched. The pathophysiology of SG is ultimately thought to be caused by abnormalities in collagen fibrils, elastic fibers, and other extracellular membrane components (Wang et al., 2015).

In terms of histology, SG resembles striae distensae (SD) and is dependent on the age of the lesion. Active lesions are primarily made of fine elastic fibers in the early stages, but aging lesions show a thinning of the dermis and a decrease in the amount of collagen in the upper dermis. When SG tissue samples are compared to tissue samples from normal skin, the SG biopsy tissue exhibits a disarray, shortening, and thinning of the elastic fiber network. Fibrils are tropoelastin-rich despite their thinness and disarray, which is probably because of their uncoordinated synthesis. The epidermis flattens, with atrophy, loss of rete ridges, and an increase in glycosaminoglycans, as seen by light microscopy. However, each patient has a different lesion development and severity, indicating a variable genetic predisposition.

5.6.1. Risk Factors

Younger age, maternal, and family history of SG, higher pre-pregnancy and pre-delivery weight, and higher birth weight are the most common risk factors for SG. The majority of research revealed a statistically significant correlation between SG and these risk factors, however, Findik et al found no evidence linking mother age or pre-pregnancy weight to risk. The majority of research also showed that a history of striae on the thighs, hips, and breasts was linked to the development of SG; nevertheless, a study involving 299 Caucasian women revealed that while striae on the breasts raised the risk of SG, striae on the thighs reduced that risk. The research conducted by Chang and colleagues found that non-white women had a higher prevalence of SG. Numerous studies regarding socioeconomic status revealed that SG was also linked to unemployment, receiving state medical assistance, and having less education. Confounding variables should be taken into account, though. In some studies, women who developed SG were also more likely to drink more alcohol, drink less water, have lower blood vitamin C levels, and expect a male child. The research included here did not find a correlation between diabetes or glycosylated hemoglobin levels, despite theorizing that both conditions may contribute to the pathophysiology of SG. The size, type, and patient population of the studies all had limitations (Fitzpatrick and Freedberg, 2003; Fitzpatrick, 2008).

5.6.2. Prevention

The effectiveness of preventative measures has been patchy. The strongest evidence supports the use of creams containing *Centella asiatica* extract, particularly Trofolastin cream, in preventing or lessening the severity of SG. The medicinal herb *Centella asiatica* is believed to promote the synthesis of collagen and elastic fibers. Mallol and associates. showed that applying Trofolastin cream, which is applied daily from gestational week 12 until delivery and contains collagen-elastin hydrolysates, α-tocopherol, and *Centella asiatica* extract, significantly decreased the incidence of SG when compared to placebo. Mallol et al. and Hernández García et al. discovered that among women who did develop SG, creams containing *Centella asiatica* significantly decreased the intensity and/or severity of SG. Alonso García et al. additionally showed that the patient group receiving a placebo experienced a significant increase in the severity of prior striae, but the patient group receiving Centella cream did not experience a change in severity.

The use of almond oil, olive oil, or cocoa butter did not effectively reduce the occurrence of SG compared to the placebo group. Although two studies did show a decrease in SG development when almond oil or olive oil was used in conjunction with daily massages, the positive results might be due to the massage itself rather than the oils used.

Two studies have demonstrated that Alphastria cream and Verum cream, both containing hyaluronic acid along with vitamins and fatty acids, were effective in reducing the occurrence of SG. Hyaluronic acid, the key ingredient in both creams, is believed to enhance resistance to mechanical forces and combat atrophy by stimulating fibroblast activity and collagen production. The creams were applied through massage during the second trimester in both studies, raising the question of whether the benefits observed were due to the creams themselves or the act of massage alone.

5.6.3. Management

While many studies have been conducted using topical medications or lasers to treat nongestational SD, very few of these studies specifically addressed the treatment of SG. Early on in SG, rather than after striae have developed and irreversible changes have taken place, treatment should be started. Inadequate evidence limits the use of many homeopathic and alternative therapies, such as fruit and vegetable oils that moisturize the skin.

5.6.3.1. Topical Medications

Clinical research demonstrated that SG could be improved by retinoin cream and a 20%

glycolic acid + 10% ascorbic acid combination. Daily application of tretinoin 0.05% and 0.1% creams for three to seven months produced a consistent improvement in the overall global SG of up to 47% and a decrease in the mean length and width of lesions of up to 20% and 23%, respectively. A research project by Pribanich and colleagues. demonstrated that 0.05% is the lowest effective concentration of tretinoin cream. Although there was no statistically significant difference between the two combinations, the appearance of SG was improved by combining 20% glycolic acid with either 10% ascorbic acid or 0.05% tretinoin. Tretinoin boosted the amount of elastin in the lesions' reticular and papillary dermis, but ascorbic acid and untreated regions did not exhibit the same improvement. In SG lesions, both treatments resulted in an increase in epidermal thickness and a decrease in papillary dermal thickness (Fitzpatrick and Freedberg, 2003; Fitzpatrick, 2008).

Clinical research demonstrated that SG could be improved by retinoin cream and a 20% glycolic acid + 10% ascorbic acid combination. Daily application of tretinoin 0.05% and 0.1% creams for three to seven months produced a consistent improvement in the overall global SG of up to 47% and a decrease in the mean length and width of lesions of up to 20% and 23%, respectively. A research project by Pribanich and colleagues demonstrated that 0.05% is the lowest effective concentration of tretinoin cream. Although there was no statistically significant difference between the two combinations, the appearance of SG was improved by combining 20% glycolic acid with either 10% ascorbic acid or 0.05% tretinoin. Tretinoin boosted the amount of elastin in the lesions' reticular and papillary dermis, but ascorbic acid and untreated regions did not exhibit the same improvement. In SG lesions, both treatments resulted in an increase in epidermal thickness and a decrease in papillary dermal thickness.

5.6.3.2. Laser Treatments

Three months after treatment, a 1540-nm non-ablative fractional laser showed a discernible difference and a statistically significant clinical improvement in SG that ranged from 1 to 24%. Fractional and non-fractional lasers have been used for nongestational SD, with differing degrees of success.

Both ablative carbon dioxide (CO_2) lasers and non-ablative Erbium (Er): Glass lasers have been researched as fractional lasers. There have been reports of lesions improving by an average of 50 to 75% following two to six nonablative Er: Glass treatments. Histologic investigations revealed a rise in collagen synthesis and elastic fibers. Patients tolerated their treatments well, and this laser was generally safe. In an investigation conducted by Lee and colleagues improvements of 50 to 75% were shown with ablative CO_2 lasers, particularly in striae alba. Other research, meanwhile, has produced contradictory findings. Compared to non-ablative lasers, CO_2 lasers can cause more pain and require longer recovery periods.

Non-fractional lasers such as excimer, pulsed dye, copper bromide, neodymium-doped yttrium aluminum garnet (Nd:YAG), and diode have been investigated for the treatment of nongestational SD patients. By causing repigmentation, the excimer 308-nm laser can treat mature striae alba and has been shown to increase pigmentation by up to 75%. Nevertheless, the effects are usually transient, and pigmentation of the surrounding normal skin is an undesirable side effect. While there has been some success using pulsed dye laser to treat striae alba, the effects are primarily textural. It might help striae rubra by lessening erythema. Even though it is intended only for immature striae rubra, the vascular Nd:YAG laser showed remarkable improvement of up to 70% or more. In a small study using copper bromide laser, 13 out of 15 women experienced a complete resolution or modest improvement of striae for up to 2 years. Dark-skinned people with SD were treated with the diode laser, however, this laser was ineffective and 64% of patients experienced undesired hyperpigmentation.

5.6.3.3. Light Treatments

Nongestational SD has been treated with light therapy techniques like intense pulsed light (IPL), ultraviolet (UV), and infrared light. Strokes appear to improve at least somewhat with IPL; however, treatment may become more difficult if erythema and post-inflammatory hyperpigmentation persist. It has been demonstrated that UV light, particularly a mix of UV-B and UV-A, regularly repigments striae alba. However, maintenance therapy is necessary because the results are not long-lasting. In just four treatment sessions, striae alba can improve by 25 to 50% when exposed to infrared light at 800 to 1800 nm. To validate these findings, longer-term research studies with bigger sample numbers are required.

(Fitzpatrick and Freedberg, 2003; Fitzpatrick, 2008).

5.6.3.4. Other Modalities

While tripolar third generation radiofrequency (Tripollar) produced a 25 to 75% improvement at one week following the end of treatment, bipolar radiofrequency showed improvements in both clinical and histologic aspects of SD. Numerous studies have demonstrated the efficacy of modalities like microdermabrasion and microneedling in improving nongestational striae. For striae rubra, microdermabrasion has proven to be particularly beneficial. Abrasive materials are blasted onto a treated area during microdermabrasion, and the area is then vacuumed afterward. A different study discovered that while microdermabrasion combined with sonophoresis improved striae, needling therapy produced a statistically significant and even greater improvement in striae than microdermabrasion. To stimulate the production of new collagen and elastin in the papillary dermis, needling therapy intentionally injures the skin.

5.7. Pruritic Folliculitis of Pregnancy

Pregnancy-related pruritic folliculitis is a skin condition that affects one in three individuals, or approximately 0.2% of cases, during the second or third trimester. It causes an inflamed or infected hair follicle, which leads to a pus-filled bump. Pregnancy-related dermatological conditions include pruritic urticarial papules and plaques, atopic eruption, pemphigoid gestationis, intrahepatic cholestasis, and pustular psoriasis, in addition to pruritic folliculitis. This pregnancy-related pruritic folliculitis is not like the usual kind; instead of primarily affecting the upper back, shoulders, and chest, the pregnancy-related pruritic folliculitis is characterized by inflamed sterile hair follicles involving the trunk. This illness was initially discovered when certain pregnant women displayed folliculitis symptoms that had never been seen before. It was believed that an ingrown hair, bacterial, fungal, or viral infection, or an imbalance in hormones, was the source of the inflammation. However, as of yet, the exact cause is unknown. Usually, these lumps start on the abdomen and move to the thighs and upper body parts.

This condition usually goes away after the baby is delivered and does not harm either the mother or the fetus. The rate of incidence may be higher, but it is hard to tell because of the condition's unclear etiology, misdiagnosis, and range of severity. According to a retrospective study conducted in 2006, pruritic folliculitis of pregnancy is now categorized as atopic eruption of pregnancy (AEP). The study compared pruritic folliculitis of pregnancy with eczema and prurigo of pregnancy, which occurred in 49.7%

and 0.88% of cases, respectively, with eczema being clearly more common. Pregnancy-related pruritic folliculitis resolves spontaneously after delivery or during the postpartum period, in contrast to ordinary pruritic folliculitis, which does not go away on its own. Pregnancy-related pruritic folliculitis does not cause death or have a major negative impact on either the mother or the fetus.

Since the cause of this condition is unknown, there are currently no treatment guidelines available; however, non-pharmacological interventions, like taking warm baths or dressing loosely, are highly recommended for relieving symptoms. Benzoyl peroxide, topical steroids of low to mid potency, or antihistamines can be tried if the itching and discomfort don't go away. Novel therapies, such as ultraviolet phototherapy, have also demonstrated promise in treating case studies of pruritic folliculitis of pregnancy. To fully understand its effectiveness and safety in patients who are pregnant in the second or third trimester, more research is still needed.

5.7.1. History

In 1981, this condition was first noted in six individuals. Various theories were put forth at the time, but no concrete evidence of a cause could be found. These women experienced variable-severity papules that began at different points in the second and third trimesters. Over the course of 15 months, biopsies were taken from these individuals to look at the makeup of these papules. Upon staining the samples with HandE, hematoxylin, and eosin, the researchers discovered a limited number of inflammatory cells, including neutrophils, monocytes, lymphocytes, and eosinophils. Immunofluorescence microscopy was used to examine the expression levels of a protein of interest by binding fluorescent antibodies to it in four of the samples; however, no indications of immunoglobulins, such as IgG, IgM, IgA, or C3, were detected. There have been very few case reports since this condition was first described, indicating the rarity of pruritic folliculitis. This was also shown by a prospective study that was conducted in 1994 by Roger et al. that concluded that one individual out of 3192 pregnant mothers (0.03%) had symptoms sthat were consistent with the diagnosis of pruritic folliculitis (Fitzpatrick and Freedberg, 2003; Fitzpatrick, 2008).

5.7.2. Pathophysiology

In response to infection or damage to the hair follicles, a common inflammatory process of the follicles is called folliculitis. Ingrown hairs, viruses, fungi, or bacteria can all trigger this inflammatory reaction. Pruritic folliculitis of pregnancy, on the other hand, is unique in that it only affects expectant mothers and only manifests in the second or third trimester of pregnancy. The exact process by which pruritic folliculitis of pregnancy arises is unknown. There isn't enough research done at this time to determine the cause of this rare condition. According to some research, an imbalance in hormone levels during pregnancy may be the cause of this condition. Additional studies suggest that immunological alterations, such as the decrease in T helper 1 immune cells and the increase in T helper 2 immune cells that happen especially during pregnancy, maybe the cause of this illness. Nevertheless, there isn't enough data to firmly back up these assertions. While the pathophysiology of pregnancy-related pruritic folliculitis remains unclear, there has been no discernible correlation between the condition and harm to the mother or unborn child. Furthermore, this illness goes away after pregnancy and has no effect on the baby's growth or the mother's recuperation following delivery.

5.7.2.1. Suspected Risk Factors

There are currently no studies into the etiology behind pruritic folliculitis specifically in pregnancy; however, suspected risk factors include:

- Dry skin.
- Genetics affecting hormone production.
- Poor personal hygiene.
- Family history of pruritus in pregnancy.
- Family history of eczema, hay fever, or asthma.
- Pruritus while taking contraceptive pills before pregnancy.

5.7.3. Signs and Symptoms

During the second or third trimester of pregnancy, pruritic folliculitis of pregnancy can cause redness of the skin, small red bumps surrounding a hair follicle, and red, pus-filled bumps that usually start on the abdomen and spread to the chest, upper back, shoulders, arms, and thighs. Usually mildly pruritic or asymptomatic, these symptoms can linger anywhere from a week to several months. However, within a month of delivery, symptoms typically go away on their own.

5.7.4. Diagnosis

The diagnosis of pruritic folliculitis of pregnancy is made based on microscopic testing that reveals the absence of bacteria, microorganisms, or other conditions that could cause itchy skin, as well as clinical features such as redness of the skin with small red bumps surrounding a hair follicle and histopathologic features such as immune cells within the pus. Patients must undergo a biopsy to be diagnosed with pruritic folliculitis of pregnancy. This procedure involves removing tissue samples to determine whether the lesions on the patient's skin match the physical characteristics of pruritic folliculitis. Obstetric cholestasis, a condition that affects the liver during pregnancy, must be ruled out in addition to other skin diseases linked to pregnancy.

Eczema, prurigo, and pruritic folliculitis are three conditions that coexist quite a bit during pregnancy. They are placed in a class known as atopic eruption of pregnancy as a result. Atopic eruption of pregnancy is a class of skin condition that manifests much earlier than other pregnancy-related skin conditions.

5.7.5. Management/Treatment

Since the etiology and clinical manifestations of pruritic folliculitis of pregnancy are still being investigated, there are currently no official treatment guidelines. Nevertheless, the aim of treatment is to alleviate symptoms without endangering the mother or fetus. Before employing pharmaceutical agents to treat symptoms, nonpharmacological interventions are advised.

The first line of treatment for pruritic folliculitis in pregnancy should be non-pharmacological since it manifests in the later stages of pregnancy and goes away on its own after delivery. The main goal of these interventions is to incorporate lifestyle modifications, such as dressing in looser clothing, applying emollients, taking warm baths, avoiding harsh soaps, and practicing proper personal hygiene.

First-generation antihistamines and topical corticosteroids with low to medium potencies may be taken into consideration if itching symptoms are still present, as they may enhance the appearance of skin lesions. They might not, however, offer total relief. First generation H1 receptor blockers like diphenhydramine or chlorpheniramine, 10% topical benzoyl peroxide, 1% topical hydrocortisone, and a brief course of systemic corticosteroids like prednisone are commonly used to treat pruritic folliculitis of pregnancy. In one case study, narrowband ultraviolet B phototherapy was also investigated as a novel treatment option for pruritic folliculitis during pregnancy. It will take more research leading to clinical trials before we can fully comprehend the safety and effectiveness of this non-traditional treatment option.

According to a thorough review of the literature on skin diseases in pregnancy conducted between 1990 and 2005 using the Medline and Cochrane databases, pruritic folliculitis during pregnancy is a condition that will resolve after giving birth and does not pose any risks to the mother or fetus.

According to a 2007 American Family Physician article, topical corticosteroids, topical benzoyl peroxide, or ultraviolet B light therapy can all be used to treat pruritic folliculitis of pregnancy. There has been no evidence of any negative effects on pregnancy risks associated with this condition (Fitzpatrick and Freedberg, 2003; Fitzpatrick, 2008).

A Closer Look

A Case of Pruritic Urticarial Papules and Plaques of Pregnancy

PUPPP, or pruritic urticarial papules and plaques of pregnancy, is a red papule-colored erythema resembling urticaria that primarily affects pregnant women in the latter stages of their first pregnancy on the abdomen. Although there is a 1/200 frequency of occurrence and a good response to topical steroids and oral antihistamines, the pathophysiology of PUPPP is still unknown.

Case Presentation

At 38 weeks and 5 days into her second pregnancy, a 28-year-old woman with a history of normal deliveries observed the target lesions on both forearms. She went to the antenatal clinic three days after the erythema started, and there, she received 100 mg of hydrocortisone sodium phosphate for two days. Despite this, the erythema with severe pruritus spread throughout her body. Seven days after the erythema first appeared, she consulted our department. She had an edematous eczema on her abdomen, mostly around the stretch marks, and her body temperature was 37.6°C.

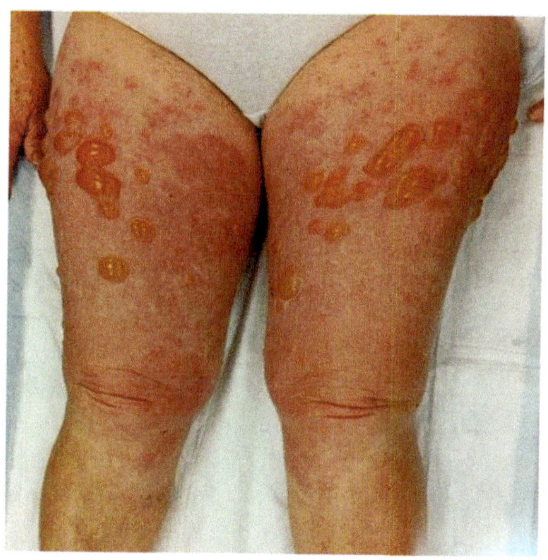

Example: *Clinical presentation of bullous pemphigoid showing tense bullae with a clear content overlying wheal-and-flare plaques on lower limbs.*

https://karger.com/cde/article/13/1/18/69090/A-Case-of-Pruritic-Urticarial-Papules-and-Plaques.

Source: Schettini N, Corazza M, Schenetti C, Pacetti L, Borghi A. Urticaria: A Narrative Overview of Differential Diagnosis. Biomedicines. 2023; 11(4):1096. https://doi.org/10.3390/biomedicines11041096.

Additionally, there were sporadic erythematous target lesions on the extremities; however, the mucosa remained unaffected. She didn't have a history of allergies, infections, illnesses, or oral medications. The following laboratory results were recorded: CRP was 0.38 mg/dL; WBC was 13.46 × 10^3/μL; band cells were 0.5%; segmented cells were 73.5%; monocytes were 2 points5%; lymphocytes were 14%; eosinophils were 8.5%; D-dimer was 12 points09 μg/mL; non-specific IgE was 174 IU/mL; C3, 151 mg/dL; C4, 29.3 mg/dL; CH50 was 50.4 U/mL; urine protein was 30 mg/dL; urine blood was negative. Electrolyte levels and liver and renal function were both normal. Postinfection patterns included measles, rubella, varicella zoster virus, herpes simplex virus, and autoantibodies showed no evidence of an autoimmune disease. For her full-term pregnancy, the patient underwent an induced delivery, and the following day, she gave birth without incident. Without medical intervention, the erythema cleared up right away after delivery.

Serum were collected 7 days before and 7 days after delivery and stored at –80°C before use. Two weeks after delivery, patch, and prick tests were performed using her serums and the results were negative. The serum IgG levels against dominant bacteria and fungus on human skin were as follows: *Staphylococcus aureus* A, 9.76 and 13.8 mg/L; *S. aureus* B, 26.6 and 40.9 mg/L; enterotoxin TSST, 30.2 and 47.0 mg/L; enterotoxin C, 9.35 and 16.0 mg/L; Malassezia, 2.98 and 5.30 mg/L; and Candida, 61.6 and 80.6 mg/L, before, and after delivery, respectively. We also measured cytokine concentration in the serum: IFN-γ, TNF-α, TNF-β, IL-1β, IL-2, IL-4, IL-5, IL-6, IL-8, IL-9, IL-10, IL-12p70, IL-17A, IL-17F, IL-22, IL-33, GM-CSF, and TSLP by flow cytometric analyses using AimPlex (COSMO BIO Co., Ltd., Tokyo, Japan). Th2 cytokines including IL-33 were elevated before delivery. On the other hand, inflammatory markers such as IL-12, TNF-α, and IFN-γ were unchanged before and after deliver

Discussion

PUPPP is unquestionably a skin eruption phenomenon that started after the first pregnancy and subsided right away after delivery. The target lesions on the extremities in this instance were the initial phenotype. An autoimmune condition, a drug eruption, or a viral or bacterial infection could cause the target lesion. Given the lack of evidence of infection, we hypothesized that an immunological or allergic response related to pregnancy may be the cause of the unusual occurrence.

Initially, we conducted patch and prick tests using the patient's serum obtained both before and after delivery, speculating that the mother's blood during pregnancy contains some antigenic substances, including fetal components. The outcomes were all unfavorable. Second, different antibody titers were measured against external factors such as fungi and bacteria that reside on the skin. Consequently, the serum after delivery had higher IgG antibody titers against S. aureus, enterotoxin, Malassezia, and Candida than it did before delivery. The findings showed that the immune system's defense against bacteria and fungi that live on the skin would be strengthened when an eruption occurred; this is partly because the pathogen can more easily infiltrate the eczematous abdominal skin that becomes longer during pregnancy. Finally, before, and after delivery, different serum cytokine levels were assessed. To contract the uterus, the concentration of IL-8 is raised towards the end of pregnancy. It is well known that during pregnancy, the Th2 system outperforms the Th1 system in terms of fetal tolerance. Indeed, there was an increase in Th2 cytokines, such as IL-33 and IL-9, in this instance, most likely from Th2 and ILC2 cells. However, the severe eczematous and enlarged lesions encouraged the production of IL-33 from epithelial cells, which is what forms the placenta during pregnancy. IL-9 stimulates the activation of intracellular targets and the survival of various mast cells, B cells, T cells, and structural cells. It is primarily produced by memory B cells and Th9. IL-9 is often undetectable or slightly elevated during a typical pregnancy, however, in this instance, IL-9 was elevated. In PUPPP, IL-9 may amplify the Th2 immune response.

In conclusion, because of the abdominal hyperextension that occurs during pregnancy, it will be simple to develop eczema and to let certain antigens into the skin. The pathophysiology of PUPPP may involve the immune mechanism of an upregulated Th2 cytokine profile, including IL-9 and IL-33, as well as the response against bacteria and fungi that reside on the skin.

Summary

- The dermatoses of pregnancy represent a unique, heterogeneous group of pathologic skin disturbances, caused by the gravid state.
- The first specific dermatosis of pregnancy reported was pemphigoid gestationis, which Milton described in 1872 under the name herpes gestationis.
- Pruritic urticarial papules and plaques of pregnancy (PUPPP) is a chronic hives-like rash that strikes some women during pregnancy.
- Skin distension (stretching) is thought to be a possible trigger for PUPPP as it most commonly affects primigravida (women in their first pregnancy), those with large fundal measurements (distance from the pubic bone to the top of the uterus) and/or those who are carrying large babies or multiples.
- Impetigo herpetiformis (IH) is a rare dermatosis of pregnancy that can be life-threatening. It is currently considered as a form of generalized pustular psoriasis despite the previous opinion that illustrated it to be a separate entity.
- An important aspect of impetigo herpetiformis is the complications that might accompany IH or occur as a result of it endangering the life of mother and fetus.
- Pemphigoid gestationis (PG), formerly herpes gestationis, is a rare, self-limiting, autoimmune subepidermal bullous dermatosis of pregnancy.
- Prurigo of pregnancy also referred to as "early onset prurigo of pregnancy," or "Papular eruption of pregnancy" is the second most common of the pregnancy-specific dermatosis (1:300 incidences).
- Striae gravidarum (SG) is a common, disfiguring, gestational change that affects between 55% and 90% of women. SG presents as atrophic linear scars and can cause distress, often leading to a decrease in quality of life.
- Pruritic folliculitis of pregnancy is a skin condition that occurs in one in 3000 people, about 0.2% of cases, who are in their second to third trimester of pregnancy where the hair follicle becomes inflamed or infected, resulting in a pus-filled bump.

References

1. Abdel-Latif, A. M., & Elbendary, A. (2008). Treatment of striae distensae with microdermabrasion: A clinical and molecular study. *Journal of the Egyptian Women's Dermatologic Society, 5*, 24–30.
2. Al-Dhalimi, M. A., & Abo Nasyria, A. A. (2013). A comparative study of the effectiveness of intense pulsed light wavelengths (650 nm vs 590 nm) in the treatment of striae distensae. *Journal of Cosmetic and Laser Therapy, 15*, 120–125.
3. Aldahan, A. S., Shah, V. V., Mlacker, S., Samarkandy, S., Alsaidan, M., & Nouri, K. (2016). Laser and light treatments for striae distensae: A comprehensive review of the literature. *American Journal of Clinical Dermatology, 17*, 239–256.
4. Andrulonis, R., & Ferris, L. K. (2012). Treatment of severe psoriasis with ustekinumab during pregnancy. *Journal of Drugs in Dermatology (JDD), 11*(10), 1240–1241.
5. Ash, K., Lord, J., Zukowski, M., & McDaniel, D. H. (1998). Comparison of topical therapy for

striae alba (20% glycolic acid/0.05% tretinoin versus 20% glycolic acid/10% L-ascorbic acid). *Dermatologic Surgery, 24*, 849–856.

6. Atwal, G. S., Manku, L. K., Griffiths, C. E., & Polson, D. W. (2006). Striae gravidarum in primiparae. *British Journal of Dermatology, 155*, 965–969.
7. Bak, H., Kim, B. J., Lee, W. J., Bang, J. S., Lee, S. Y., & Choi, J. H. (2009). Treatment of striae distensae with fractional photothermolysis. *Dermatologic Surgery, 35*, 1215–1220.
8. Buchanan, K., Fletcher, H. M., & Reid, M. (2010). Prevention of striae gravidarum with cocoa butter cream. *International Journal of Gynecology & Obstetrics, 108*, 65–68.
9. Chang, A. L., Agredano, Y. Z., & Kimball, A. B. (2004). Risk factors associated with striae gravidarum. *Journal of the American Academy of Dermatology, 51*, 881–888.
10. Cho, S. B., Lee, S. J., Lee, J. E., Kang, J. M., Kim, Y. K., & Oh, S. H. (2010). Treatment of striae alba using the 10,600-nm carbon dioxide fractional laser. *Journal of Cosmetic and Laser Therapy, 12*, 118–119.
11. Cordeiro, R. C., Zecchin, K. G., & de Moraes, A. M. (2010). Expression of estrogen, androgen, and glucocorticoid receptors in recent striae distensae. *International Journal of Dermatology, 49*, 30–32.
12. Davey, C. M. (1972). Factors associated with the occurrence of striae gravidarum. *Journal of Obstetrics and Gynaecology of the British Commonwealth, 79*, 1113–1114.
13. de Angelis, F., Kolesnikova, L., Renato, F., & Liguori, G. (2011). Fractional nonablative 1540-nm laser treatment of striae distensae in Fitzpatrick skin types II to IV: Clinical and histological results. *Aesthetic Surgery Journal, 31*, 411–419.
14. de Buman, M., Walther, M., & de Weck, R. (1987). Effectiveness of Alphastria cream in the prevention of pregnancy stretch marks (striae distensae). Results of a double-blind study. *Gynäkologische Rundschau, 27*, 79–84.
15. Di Lernia, V., Bonci, A., Cattania, M., & Bisighini, G. (2001). Striae distensae (rubrae) in monozygotic twins. *Pediatric Dermatology, 18*, 261–262.
16. Elsaie, M. L., Baumann, L. S., & Elsaaiee, L. T. (2009). Striae distensae (stretch marks) and different modalities of therapy: An update. *Dermatologic Surgery, 35*, 563–573.
17. Ersoy, E., Ersoy, A. O., Yasar Celik, E., Tokmak, A., Ozler, S., & Tasci, Y. (2016). Is it possible to prevent striae gravidarum? *Journal of the Chinese Medical Association, 79*, 272–275.
18. Findik, R. B., Hascelik, N. K., Akin, K. O., Unluer, A. N., & Karakaya, J. (2011). Striae gravidarum, vitamin C and other related factors. *International Journal of Vitamin and Nutrition Research, 81*, 43–48.
19. Fitzpatrick, T. B., & Freedberg, I. M. (2003). *Fitzpatrick's Dermatology in Clinical Medicine* (6th ed.). New York, NY: McGraw-Hill Professional.
20. Fitzpatrick, T. B., & Wolff, K. (2008). *Fitzpatrick's Dermatology in General Medicine*. New York, NY: McGraw-Hill Medical.
21. García Hernández, J. Á., Madera González, D., Padilla Castillo, M., & Figueras, F. T. (2013). Use of a specific anti-stretch mark cream for preventing or reducing the severity of striae gravidarum: Randomized, double-blind, controlled trial. *International Journal of Cosmetic Science, 35*, 233–237.

22. Ghasemi, A., Gorouhi, F., Rashighi-Firoozabadi, M., Jafarian, S., & Firooz, A. (2007). Striae gravidarum: Associated factors. *Journal of the European Academy of Dermatology and Venereology, 21*, 743–746.

23. Goldberg, D. J., Sarradet, D., & Hussain, M. (2003). 308-nm Excimer laser treatment of mature hypopigmented striae. *Dermatologic Surgery, 29*, 596–598.

24. Goldman, A., Rossato, F., & Prati, C. (2008). Stretch marks: Treatment using the 1,064-nm Nd:YAG laser. *Dermatologic Surgery, 34*, 686–691.

25. J-Orh, R., Titapant, V., Chuenwattana, P., & Tontisirin, P. (2008). Prevalence and associated factors for striae gravidarum. *Journal of the Medical Association of Thailand, 91*, 445–451.

26. Kang, S., Kim, K. J., Griffiths, C. E., Wong, T. Y., Talwar, H. S., & Fisher, G. J. (1996). Topical tretinoin (retinoic acid) improves early stretch marks. *Archives of Dermatology, 132*, 519–526.

27. Kasielska-Trojan, A., Sobczak, M., & Antoszewski, B. (2015). Risk factors of striae gravidarum. *International Journal of Cosmetic Science, 37*, 236–240.

28. Korgavkar, K., & Wang, F. (2015). Stretch marks during pregnancy: A review of topical prevention. *British Journal of Dermatology, 172*, 606–615.

29. Lee, S. E., Kim, J. H., Lee, S. J., Lee, J. E., Kang, J. M., & Kim, Y. K. (2010). Treatment of striae distensae using an ablative 10,600-nm carbon dioxide fractional laser: A retrospective review of 27 participants. *Dermatologic Surgery, 36*, 1683–1690.

30. Longo, L., Postiglione, M. G., Marangoni, O., & Melato, M. (2003). Two-year follow-up results of copper bromide laser treatment of striae. *Journal of Clinical Laser Medicine & Surgery, 21*, 157–160.

31. Lurie, S., Matas, Z., Fux, A., Golan, A., & Sadan, O. (2011). Association of serum relaxin with striae gravidarum in pregnant women. *Archives of Gynecology and Obstetrics, 283*, 219–222.

32. Madlon-Kay, D. J. (1993). Striae gravidarum: Folklore and fact. *Archives of Family Medicine, 2*, 507–511.

33. Malekzad, F., Shakoei, S., Ayatollahi, A., & Hejazi, S. (2014). The safety and efficacy of the 1540nm non-ablative fractional XD probe of star lux 500 device in the treatment of striae alba: Before-after study. *Journal of Lasers in Medical Sciences, 5*, 194–198.

34. Mallol, J., Belda, M. A., Costa, D., Noval, A., & Sola, M. (1991). Prophylaxis of striae gravidarum with a topical formulation: A double-blind trial. *International Journal of Cosmetic Science, 13*, 51–57.

35. Manuskiatti, W., Boonthaweeyuwat, E., & Varothai, S. (2009). Treatment of striae distensae with a TriPollar radiofrequency device: A pilot study. *Journal of Dermatologic Treatment, 20*, 359–364.

36. McDaniel, D. H., Ash, K., & Zukowski, M. (1996). Treatment of stretch marks with the 585-nm flashlamp-pumped pulsed dye laser. *Dermatologic Surgery, 22*, 332–337.

37. Montesi, G., Calvieri, S., Balzani, A., & Gold, M. H. (2007). Bipolar radiofrequency in the treatment of dermatologic imperfections: Clinicopathological and immunohistochemical aspects. *Journal of Drugs in Dermatology, 6*, 890–896.

38. Murphy, K. W., Dunphy, B., & O'herlihy, C. (1992). Increased maternal age protects against striae gravidarum. *Journal of Obstetrics and Gynaecology, 12*, 297–300.

39. Nassar, A., Ghomey, S., El Gohary, Y., & El-Desoky, F. (2016). Treatment of striae distensae with needling therapy versus microdermabrasion with sonophoresis. *Journal of Cosmetic and Laser Therapy, 18*, 330–334.

40. Osman, H., Rubeiz, N., Tamim, H., & Nassar, A. H. (2007). Risk factors for the development of striae gravidarum. *American Journal of Obstetrics and Gynecology, 196*, 62.e1–62.e5.

41. Osman, H., Usta, I. M., Rubeiz, N., Abu-Rustum, R., Charara, I., & Nassar, A. H. (2008). Cocoa butter lotion for prevention of striae gravidarum: A double-blind, randomised and placebo-controlled trial. *BJOG: An International Journal of Obstetrics and Gynaecology, 115*, 1138–1142.

42. Picard, D., Sellier, S., Houivet, E., Marpeau, L., Fournet, P., & Thobois, B. (2015). Incidence and risk factors for striae gravidarum. *Journal of the American Academy of Dermatology, 73*, 699–700.

43. Pinkus, H., Keech, M. K., & Mehregan, A. H. (1966). Histopathology of striae distensae, with special reference to striae and wound healing in the Marfan syndrome. *Journal of Investigative Dermatology, 46*, 283–292.

44. Poidevin, L. O. (1959). Striae gravidarum: Their relation to adrenal cortical hyperfunction. *The Lancet, 2*, 436–439.

45. Pribanich, S., Simpson, F. G., Held, B., Yarbrough, C. L., & White, S. N. (1994). Low-dose tretinoin does not improve striae distensae: A double-blind, placebo-controlled study. *Cutis, 54*, 121–124.

46. Rangel, O., Arias, I., García, E., & Lopez-Padilla, S. (2001). Topical tretinoin 0.1% for pregnancy-related abdominal striae: An open-label, multicenter, prospective study. *Advances in Therapy, 18*, 181–186.

47. Rathore, S. P., Gupta, S., & Gupta, V. (2011). Pattern and prevalence of physiological cutaneous changes in pregnancy: A study of 2000 antenatal women. *Indian Journal of Dermatology, Venereology and Leprology, 77*, 402.

48. Sadick, N. S., Magro, C., & Hoenig, A. (2007). Prospective clinical and histological study to evaluate the efficacy and safety of a targeted high-intensity narrow band UVB/UVA1 therapy for striae alba. *Journal of Cosmetic and Laser Therapy, 9*, 79–83.

49. Sheu, H. M., Yu, H. S., & Chang, C. H. (1991). Mast cell degranulation and elastolysis in the early stage of striae distensae. *Journal of Cutaneous Pathology, 18*, 410–416.

50. Soltanipoor, F., Delaram, M., Taavoni, S., & Haghani, H. (2012). The effect of olive oil on prevention of striae gravidarum: A randomized controlled clinical trial. *Complementary Therapies in Medicine, 20*, 263–266.

51. Soltanipour, F., Delaram, M., Taavoni, S., & Haghani, H. (2014). The effect of olive oil and the Saj® cream in prevention of striae gravidarum: A randomized controlled clinical trial. *Complementary Therapies in Medicine, 22*, 220–225.

52. Taavoni, S., Soltanipour, F., Haghani, H., Ansarian, H., & Kheirkhah, M. (2011). Effects of olive oil on striae gravidarum in the second trimester of pregnancy. *Complementary Therapies in Clinical Practice, 17*, 167–169.

53. Tay, Y. K., Kwok, C., & Tan, E. (2006). Non-ablative 1,450-nm diode laser treatment of striae distensae. *Lasers in Surgery and Medicine, 38*, 196–199.

54. Thomas, R. G., & Liston, W. A. (2004). Clinical associations of striae gravidarum. *Journal of Obstetrics and Gynaecology, 24*, 270–271.

55. Timur Taşhan, S., & Kafkasli, A. (2012). The effect of bitter almond oil and massaging on striae gravidarum in primiparous women. *Journal of Clinical Nursing, 21*, 1570–1576.

56. Trelles, M. A., Levy, J. L., & Ghersetich, I. (2008). Effects achieved on stretch marks by a nonfractional broadband infrared light system treatment. *Aesthetic Plastic Surgery, 32*, 523–530.

57. Tretti Clementoni, M., & Lavagno, R. (2015). A novel 1565 nm non-ablative fractional device for stretch marks: A preliminary report. *Journal of Cosmetic and Laser Therapy, 17*, 148–155.

58. Wang, F., Calderone, K., Smith, N. R., Do, T. T., Helfrich, Y. R., & Johnson, T. R. (2015). Marked disruption and aberrant regulation of elastic fibers in early striae gravidarum. *British Journal of Dermatology, 173*, 1420–1430.

59. Watson, R. E., Parry, E. J., Humphries, J. D., Jones, C. J., Polson, D. W., & Kielty, C. M. (1998). Fibrillin microfibrils are reduced in skin exhibiting striae distensae. *British Journal of Dermatology, 138*, 931–937.

60. Wierrani, F., Kozak, W., Schramm, W., & Grünberger, W. (1992). Attempt of preventive treatment of striae gravidarum using preventive massage ointment administration. *Wiener Klinische Wochenschrift, 104*, 42–44.

61. Yamaguchi, K., Suganuma, N., & Ohashi, K. (2012). Quality of life evaluation in Japanese pregnant women with striae gravidarum: A cross-sectional study. *BMC Research Notes, 5*, 450.

Chapter

SKIN CANCER

6

Contents

Introduction

Cancers that originate in the skin are known as skin cancers. They result from the growth of aberrant cells that can infiltrate or spread to different areas of the body. The most common type of cancer in humans to be diagnosed is skin cancer. Melanoma, squamous-cell skin cancer (SCC), and basal-cell skin cancer (BCC) are the three primary forms of skin cancer. Nonmelanoma skin cancer (NMSC) is the term used to describe the first two types of skin cancer as well as several less common types. Although basal-cell cancer is unlikely to spread to distant locations or cause death, it can cause damage to the surrounding tissue and grows slowly. It frequently manifests as a painless elevated patch of skin that may be shiny and have tiny blood vessels running across it, or it may look like a raised ulcerated area of skin. The spread of squamous-cell skin cancer is higher. It may develop into an ulcer, but it typically manifests as a hard lump with a scaly top. Aggressive melanomas are the most common. A mole that has changed in size, shape, or color, has uneven edges, is multicolored, itchy, or bleeds are among the warning signs.

In more than 90% of cases, sun exposure results in UV radiation exposure. There is an increased risk of all three primary forms of skin cancer with this exposure. A thinner ozone layer has contributed to an increase in exposure. Another typical source of UV radiation is tanning beds. Childhood exposure is especially dangerous for basal-cell carcinomas and melanomas. All exposure matters more for squamous-cell skin cancers, regardless of when it happens. 20 to 30% of melanomas start off as moles. Individuals with paler skin tones and those with compromised immune systems due to medication side effects or HIV/AIDS are more susceptible. Biological diagnosis is essential (Cakir et al., 2012).

It seems that using sunscreen and reducing UV radiation exposure are good ways to prevent squamous-cell skin cancer and melanoma. If sunscreen reduces the risk of basal-cell cancer is unclear. Skin cancer that is not melanoma is often curable. The most common form of treatment is surgery to remove the tumor; less frequently, radiation therapy or topical drugs like fluorouracil are used. A combination of surgery, chemotherapy, radiation therapy, and targeted therapy may be used to treat melanoma. Palliative care can help people whose disease has spread to other parts of their body and improve their quality of life. With over 86% of patients in the UK and over 90% in the US surviving for more than five years, melanoma has one of the highest survival rates of all cancers.

At least 40% of cancer cases worldwide are skin cancer, making it the most prevalent type of cancer. Nonmelanoma skin cancer is the most prevalent kind, affecting at least 2–3 million individuals annually. However, since accurate statistics are not maintained, this is only an estimate. About 80% of nonmelanoma skin cancers are basal-cell tumors, while 20% are squamous-cell tumors. Skin cancers of the basal and squamous cells seldom cause death. Less than 0.1% of cancer-related deaths in the US were caused by them. Melanoma affected 232,000 individuals worldwide in 2012, and it was the cause of 55,000 deaths. The highest rates of melanoma worldwide are found in white people living in Australia, New Zealand, and South Africa. In the past 20 to 40 years, there has been an increase in the prevalence of the three main types of skin cancer, particularly in areas where White people predominate.

Orientation and Directional Terms

Term	Definition	Illustration
Squamous cell carcinoma (SCC)	Squamous cell carcinoma (SCC) of the skin is the second most common form of skin cancer, characterized by abnormal, accelerated growth of squamous cells.	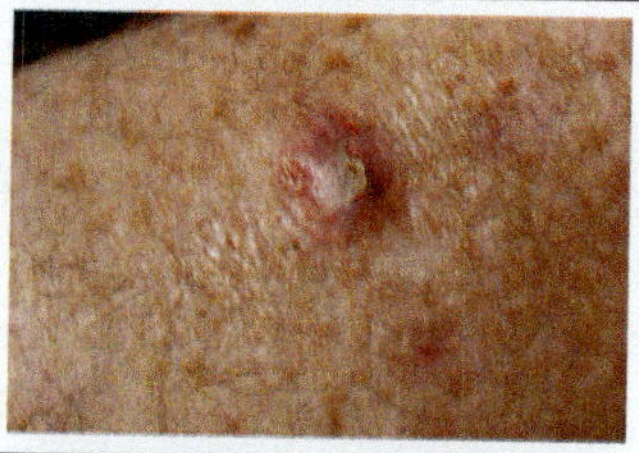
Palliative care	Palliative care is a type of medical care that helps people with serious illnesses improve their quality of life. It can be used at any age, regardless of the stage of the disease, and can be given alongside other treatments.	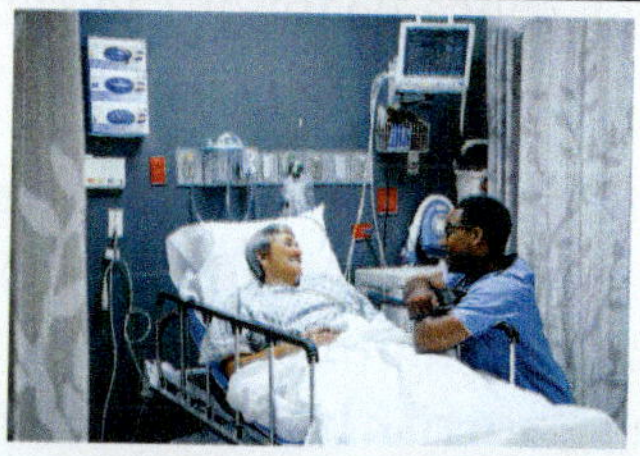
Immune system	The immune system is a network of biological systems that protects an organism from diseases. It detects and responds to a wide variety of pathogens, from viruses to parasitic worms, as well as cancer cells and objects such as wood splinters, distinguishing them from the organism's own healthy tissue.	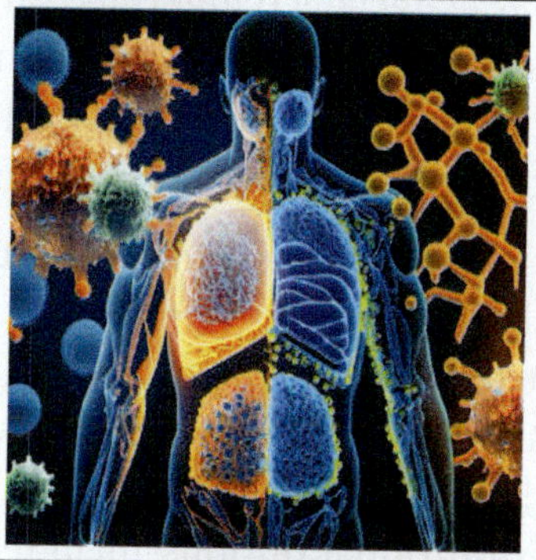
Cryosurgery	Cryosurgery is the use of extreme cold in surgery to destroy abnormal or diseased tissue; thus, it is the surgical application of cryoablation. Cryosurgery has been historically used to treat a number of diseases and disorders, especially a variety of benign and malignant skin conditions.	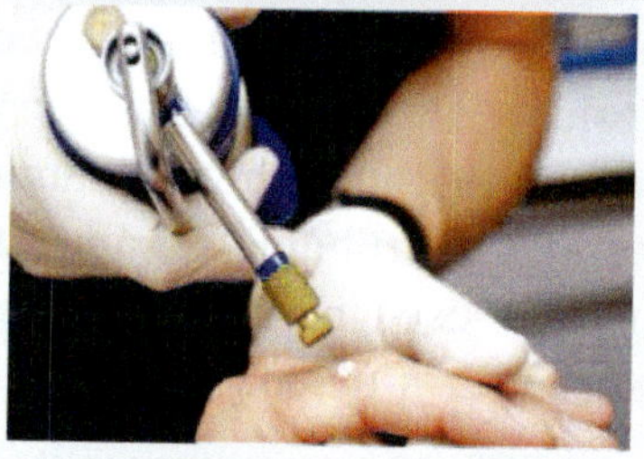
Chemotherapy	Chemotherapy is the type of cancer treatment that uses one or more anti-cancer drugs in a standard regimen. Chemotherapy may be given with a curative intent, or it may aim only to prolong life or to reduce symptoms.	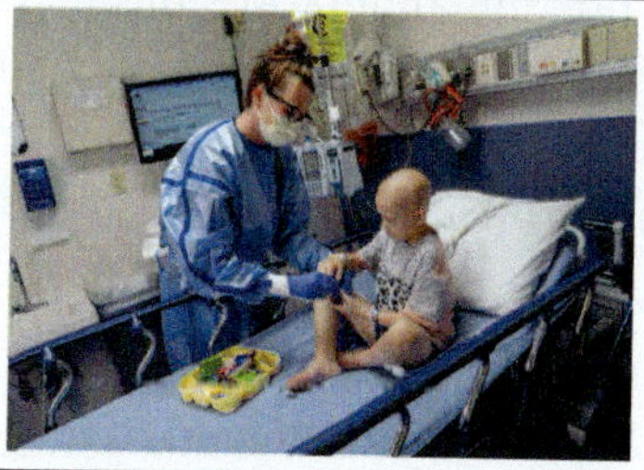

6.1. Basal-Cell Carcinoma

The most prevalent kind of skin cancer is called basal-cell carcinoma (BCC), sometimes referred to as rodent ulcer, basalioma, or basal-cell cancer. It frequently manifests as a raised, painless patch of skin that may be shiny and covered in tiny blood vessels. It could also show up as an ulcerated raised area. Although basal-cell cancer is unlikely to spread to distant locations or cause death, it can cause damage to the surrounding tissue and grows slowly.

UV light exposure, lighter skin tones, radiation therapy, prolonged exposure to arsenic, and compromised immune system performance are risk factors. Childhood UV light exposure is especially dangerous. An additional popular source of UV radiation is tanning beds. The diagnosis is often made based on a skin examination and tissue biopsy confirmation.

The impact of sunscreen on the risk of basal-cell cancer is still unknown. Surgery is usually used as a form of treatment. If the cancer is small, it may be treated with simple excision; if not, Mohs surgery is usually advised. Additional options include the use of imiquimod, a topical immune-activating drug, electrodesiccation, and curettage, cryosurgery, topical chemotherapy, photodynamic therapy, and laser surgery. Chemotherapy or targeted therapy may be used in the rare instances where distant spread has taken place.

At least 32% of cancer cases worldwide are basal-cell cancers. About 80% of skin cancers that are not melanoma are basal-cell cancers. In the US, approximately 25% of white women and 35% of white men will experience BCC at some point in their lives (Figure 6.1).

The basal cells that make up the epidermal bottom layer are the source of the name "basal-cell carcinoma." It is believed to originate from the trichoblasts, which are folliculo-sebaceous-apocrine germinative cells (it should be noted that trichoblastic carcinoma is a term occasionally used to refer to a rare type of aggressive skin cancer that can closely resemble basal cell carcinoma as well as a benign trichoblastoma) (Figure 6.2).

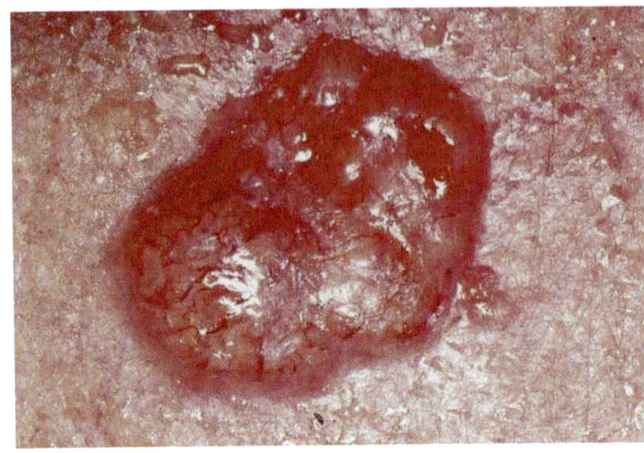

Figure 6.1. *Basal cell carcinoma on a patient's back.*

Source: https://en.wikipedia.org/wiki/Basal-cell_carcinoma#/media/File:Basal_cell_carcinoma.jpg.

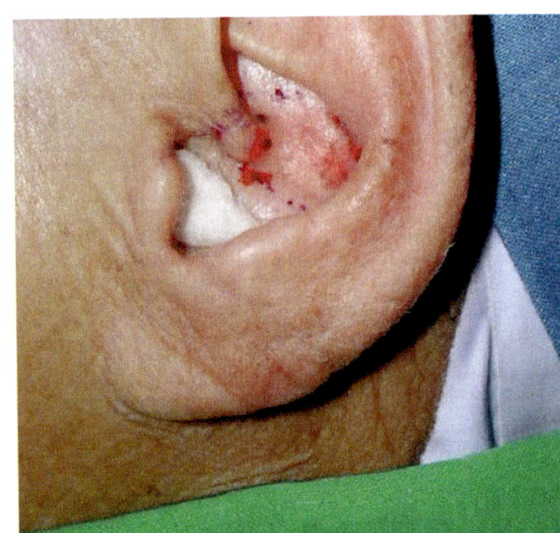

Figure 6.2. *Ulcerated basal cell carcinoma of the ear concha.*

Source: https://www.researchgate.net/figure/a-Basal-cell-carcinoma-on-the-left-ear-concha-b-Skin-defect-after-wide-excision-of_fig5_281820910

6.1.1. Signs and Symptoms

People who have basal-cell carcinoma usually have a pearly, shiny skin nodule when they first appear. On the other hand, superficial basal-cell carcinoma may appear as an eczema-like red patch. It can be challenging to diagnose infiltrative or morpheaform basal-cell carcinomas without tactile feeling and a skin biopsy because they can appear as skin thickening or scar tissue. Visually, basal-cell cancer can be hard to distinguish from actinic elastosis, acne scar, and inflammation from recent cryodestruction.

6.1.2. Pathophysiology

Because of the way the cancer cells appear under a microscope, basal-cell carcinoma gets its name from the basal cells that make up the epidermal bottom layer. However, not every case of basal-cell carcinoma starts from within the basal layer. Trichoblasts, which are folliculo-sebaceous-apocrine germinative cells, are thought to be the source of basal-cell carcinomas. The term "trichoblastic carcinoma" refers to a rare and potentially aggressive cancer that may resemble a benign trichoblastoma and is believed to originate from trichoblasts (differential diagnosis can be challenging). Lesions identified as "trichoblastic carcinoma" may actually be basal-cell carcinoma, according to certain theories (Figure 6.3).

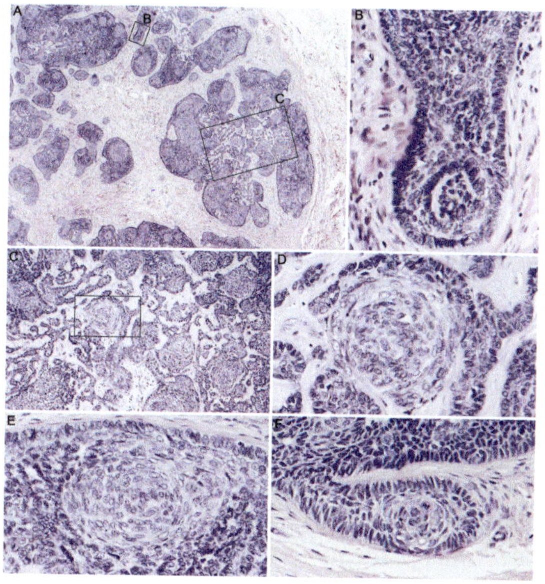

Figure 6.3. *Microphotograph of trichoblastomas.*

Source: By Article authors: John P. Sundberg, Timothy M. Stearns., Joongho Joh., Mary Proctor, Arvind Ingle, Kathleen A. Silva, Soheil S. Dadras, A. Bennett Jenson, Shin-je Ghim – (2014). "Immune Status, Strain Background, and Anatomic Site of Inoculation Affect Mouse Papillomavirus (MmuPV1) Induction of Exophytic Papillomas or Endophytic Trichoblastomas." PLoS ONE 9 (12): e113582. DOI:10.1371/journal.pone.0113582. ISSN 1932-6203."Figure 2- available via license: Creative Commons Attribution 4.0 International," CC BY 4.0, https://commons.wikimedia.org/w/index.php?curid=83279730.

One type of DNA damage caused by overexposure to the sun is the formation of thymine dimers. Most UV-induced damage is eliminated by DNA repair, but not all crosslinks are removed. Therefore, DNA damage accumulates over time and results in mutations. In addition to causing mutagenesis, prolonged exposure to sunlight weakens the immune system in the area, which may lead to less immune surveillance for nascent tumor cells.

Actinic keratosis, seborrheic keratosis, and squamous cell carcinoma are among the skin lesions that frequently coexist with basal-cell carcinomas. A small percentage of cases also result in basal-cell nevus syndrome, also known as Gorlin Syndrome, which is characterized by rib abnormalities, calcification of the falx cerebri (the brain's central line), palmar or plantar pits, and keratocystic odontogenic tumors of the jaw. A mutation in the PTCH1 tumor suppressor gene, which is found on chromosome 9q22.3, is the cause of this syndrome because it inhibits the hedgehog signaling pathway. Basal-cell carcinoma is also caused by a mutation in the SMO gene, which is also on the hedgehog pathway.

6.1.3. Diagnosis

Histopathologic analyses of a skin biopsy are used to diagnose basal-cell carcinomas. A shave biopsy performed under local anesthesia is the most popular technique. Though some variants, like intradermal naevus, sebaceomas, fibrous papules, early acne scars, and hypertrophic scarring, can be difficult to differentiate from benign lesions, the majority of nodular basal-cell cancers can be diagnosed clinically. When there is a high level of clinical suspicion, exfoliative cytology methods can confirm the diagnosis of basal cell carcinoma with high sensitivity and specificity. However, their utility in other situations is unclear. Basal-cell carcinoma cells are typically well differentiated and resemble epidermal basal cells in appearance. BerEP4 immunohistochemistry has a high sensitivity and specificity in identifying only BCC cells; it can be used in cases of uncertainty.

6.1.3.1. Main Classes

Basal-cell carcinoma can broadly be divided into three groups, based on the growth patterns.

- A superficial proliferation of neoplastic basal cells is the hallmark of superficial basal-cell carcinoma, also known as *in-situ* basal-cell carcinoma. Topic chemotherapy with drugs like imiquimod or fluorouracil can usually be used to treat this tumor; however, surgery is a better option to guarantee total removal and ensure that no more aggressive subtype of the tumor exists that was not sampled during the initial biopsy.
- Given its propensity to infiltrate deeper layers of the skin, infiltrative basal-cell carcinoma—which includes morpheaform and micronodular basal-cell carcinoma—is more challenging to treat with conservative techniques.
- Nodular basal-cell carcinoma includes most of the remaining categories of basal-cell cancer. It is not unusual to encounter heterogeneous morphologic features within the same tumor.

6.1.3.2. Nodular Basal-Cell Carcinoma

50% of cases of basal-cell carcinoma (BCC) are nodular BCC, also referred to as classic BCC. It usually appears on the parts of the head and neck that are exposed to the sun. Histopathology reveals basaloid cell aggregates with distinct borders, a peripheral cell palisading, and one or more typical clefts. These clefts result from mucin shrinking during tissue fixation and staining. Mucin and central necrosis with granular, eosinophilic features may also be present. A cystic structure is determined by the large mucin aggregates. There could also be calcification, particularly in lesions that have been there for a while. Usually, not very noticeable, mitotic activity can have a high rate in more aggressive lesions. As a subtype of NBCC, adenoidal BCC is distinguished by basaloid cells that have reticulated structures and extend into the dermis.

6.1.4. BCC Risk Factors

It is well known that some hereditary disorders predispose to an early onset of BCCs in terms of genetic risk factors for the disease. One of the most prevalent autosomal dominant genodermatoses, Gorlin syndrome (GS), also called basal cell nevus syndrome, is characterized by the development of multiple BCCs. Its disease incidence in the general population ranges from 1:56,000 to 1:164,000. Multiple germline mutations affecting the patched 1 (PTCH1) gene on chromosome 9q22.3–q316 are the cause of GS. The sonic hedgehog ligand's dysregulation is known to play a significant role in the carcinogenesis of numerous tumors, including BCC. The PTCH1 gene encodes the receptor for this ligand. Diseases of the bones, skin, eyes, and nervous system are linked to GS, and there is also a higher chance of developing BCC. Bazex syndrome and Xeroderma Pigmentosum are two more hereditary conditions that predispose people to BCC.

There is evidence linking melanocortin-1 receptor (MC1R) gene polymorphisms to the risk of BCC. A membrane G coupled protein involved in the synthesis of melanin is called MC1R. There are approximately 80 or more distinct alleles that have been linked to variations in red hair color (RHC). In addition to having red hair, RHC variants also cause fair skin, freckles, and a poor reaction to UV rays when tanning. Patients with solar keratosis, pronounced elastosis, and non-melanoma skin cancer (NMSC) are more likely to have certain MC1R variants. Moreover, single nucleotide polymorphisms affecting the TYR and ASIP genes, which control melanin hormone, have been linked to an increased risk of developing BCC. In fact, TYR gene mutations may result in ocular albinism, a genetic disorder linked to a higher risk of NMSCs. Research has indicated that there is a genetic predisposition to multiple BCCs. Specifically, polymorphisms in the glutathione S-transferase (GST) and cytochrome (CYP) supergene families, which are essential for metabolic and detoxification processes in cells, have been linked to the number of BCCs.(Ramachandran et al., 1999).

The genetic mechanisms behind sporadic basal cell carcinomas (BCCs) in the general population remain poorly understood. A recent study using whole exome sequencing on 293 BCC cases identified the most commonly mutated genes and pathways involved in BCC development. Both sporadic and hereditary BCCs often feature genetic alterations in the Hedgehog (Hh) signaling pathway. In fact, approximately 85% of sporadic BCCs contain mutations in Hh pathway genes such as PTCH1, SMO, SUFU, and TP53, with many of these alterations involving specific UV-induced mutations at certain DNA sites. Somatic mutations in the PTCH1 gene are found in the majority of BCC cases, while a subset of patients (10–20%) have activating mutations in the SMO gene, which is normally suppressed by PTCH1. A small percentage of cases also exhibit mutations in the PTCH2 gene, a homolog of PTCH1, and SUFU, another gene in the Hh pathway. Some BCCs may not show genetic alterations in the Hh pathway, but they show increased expression of GLI1 and GLI2, transcription factors downstream of the Hh pathway, suggesting potential dysregulation of other molecules that activate this signaling cascade. (Figure 6.4).

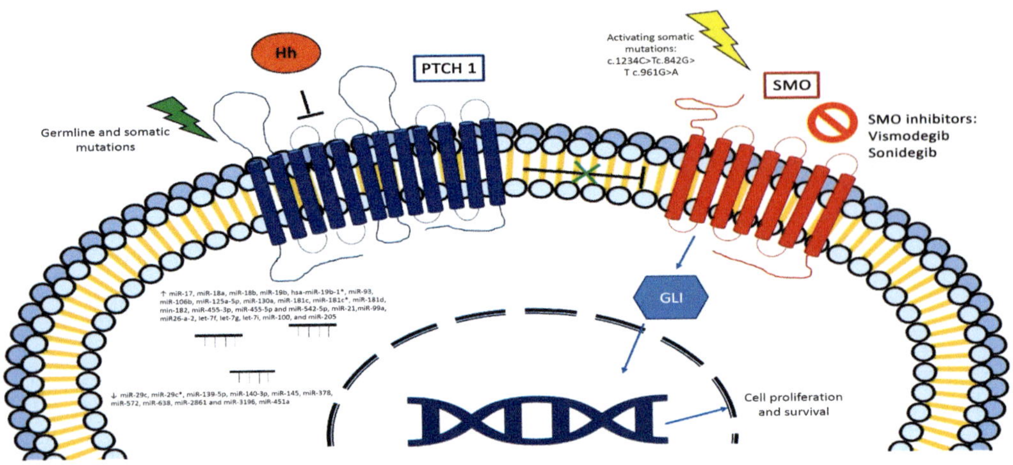

Figure 6.4. *Main molecular pathways involved in basal cell carcinoma.*

Source: *Dika E, Scarfì F, Ferracin M, Broseghini E, Marcelli E, Bortolani B, Campione E, Riefolo M, Ricci C, Lambertini M. Basal Cell Carcinoma: A Comprehensive Review. International Journal of Molecular Sciences. 2020; 21(15):5572. https://doi.org/10.3390/ijms21155572.*

BCCs typically have somatic inactivating mutations in the TP53 gene, with a frequency ranging from 40% to 65%. Many cancer types, including BCC, are known to have an early onset associated with P53, and P53's LOH appears to be mutually exclusive with PTCH1.

Moreover, the TP53-encoded p53 protein is involved in the senescence of keratinocytes; thus, its loss of function may promote the growth of BCCs in this situation. There are occasionally claims that other pathways, like the MYCN/FBXW7 pathway and the Hippo-YAP pathway, are involved in the genesis of BCC. In rare cases, BCC is associated with additional mutations in the protein kinase C (PKC) family, the phosphatidylinositol 3-kinase (PI3K)/AKT pathway, and the epidermal growth factor receptor (EGFR) pathway (Riobo et al., 2006).

6.1.5. Prevention

Basal-cell carcinoma, a common skin cancer, typically affects fair-skinned individuals with a family history of the disease. Sunlight is a significant factor in about two-thirds of cases, leading doctors to recommend sunscreen with at least SPF 30 for protection. However, a Cochrane review on the effectiveness of sunscreen in preventing basal-cell carcinoma and cutaneous squamous cell carcinoma found insufficient evidence to support its use for preventing these types of skin cancer. The review noted that the certainty of these results was low and future evidence could change this conclusion. Additionally, one-third of cases occur in areas not typically exposed to sun, indicating that the causes of these cancers may be more complex than just UV exposure.

A chemotherapeutic agent like imiquimod or 5-fluorouracil can be used to stop skin cancer from developing. People with a history of multiple skin cancers, significant sun damage, or early stages of cancer (solar keratosis) are typically advised to get it. To further reduce the risk of skin cancer, it is frequently repeated every two to three years.

6.1.6. Treatment

The following methods are employed in the treatment of BCC:

6.1.6.1. Standard Surgical Excision

The most effective treatment for basal-cell carcinoma is believed to be surgery to remove the affected area and surrounding skin. A known increased recurrence rate of basal-cell carcinomas of the face, particularly in the vicinity of the nose, eyelids, and facial structures, is a drawback of standard surgical excision. Comparing the efficacy of surgical excision versus Mohs micrographic surgery for BCC of the eye is not well-researched or methodical.

For lower lip excisions due to basal cell carcinoma, a keystone flap can be used to cover the wound. Creating a flap beneath the defect and pulling it superiorly to cover the wound results in a keystone flap. If the skin is loose enough to cover the defect and the flap receives enough blood flow, this procedure can be carried out.

6.1.6.2. Mohs Surgery

Mohs surgery should be taken into consideration for many new (primary) and all recurrent forms of basal cell carcinoma following prior surgery, particularly those affecting the head, neck, hands, feet, genitalia, and anterior legs (shins).

Developed by Frederic E., Mohs surgery, also known as Mohs micrographic surgery, is an outpatient procedure. In the 1930s, Mohs performed surgery to remove a tumor, which was then promptly examined under a microscope. This type of pathology processing is known as CCPDMA, and it entails examining the entire surgical margin, including the deep and edge portions. Every time a tissue is removed during surgery, the tissue is checked for cancer cells while the patient waits. The results of that examination determine whether or not to remove more tissue. In addition, squamous-cell carcinoma, melanoma, dermatofibrosarcoma protuberans, Merkel cell carcinoma, microcystic adnexal carcinoma, and several other skin cancers are treated with Mohs surgery; these cases typically have greater cure rates than those of other surgical and non-surgical treatments.

The Mohs surgeon performing the procedure and personally reviewing the Mohs pathology slides is a crucial component of Mohs surgery. The majority of routine excisions performed in an office setting are sent to an outside laboratory to be processed using the common bread loafing technique. Because each tissue slice is only 6 micrometers thick, only 3 to 4 serial slices are obtained per section, and only 3 to 4 sections are obtained per specimen, it is likely that less than 5% of the surgical margin is examined using this method.

6.1.6.3. Cryosurgery

Cryosurgery is an established method used to treat various skin cancers. When performed accurately using a temperature probe and cryotherapy instruments, it can have a high cure rate. However, there are drawbacks such as lack of margin control, tissue necrosis, potential for over or under treating the tumor, and a lengthy recovery period. While there is enough data to support cryosurgery as a viable treatment for basal cell carcinoma (BCC), there is a lack of studies comparing it to other methods like Mohs surgery, excision, or electrodesiccation and curettage, making it difficult to determine its effectiveness in comparison. Additionally, the impact of curetting lesions before cryosurgery on treatment efficacy is unknown. Despite the existence of textbooks on the subject, only a few physicians continue to use cryosurgery on certain patients.

6.1.6.4. Electrodesiccation and Curettage

The process of electrodesiccation and curettage (EDC, also referred to as curettage and cautery, or just curettage) involves scraping away the soft cancer with a round knife, or curette. Electric current is then used to burn the skin. This further softens the skin, making it possible for the next curettage layer to be cut more deeply with the knife. With a safety margin of curettage of normal skin surrounding the visible tumor, the cycle is repeated. The free skin margin treated is typically 4 to 6 mm, and this cycle is repeated three to five times. The size and type of the tumor, in addition to the user, have a significant impact on the cure rate. It can be challenging to completely eradicate infiltrative or morpheaform BCCs using EDC. Typically, the trunk (torso) and other unimportant cosmetic areas are treated with this technique. Some medical professionals think that older patients over 70 can have their faces treated with EDC. However, such an objective criterion cannot be supported as life expectancy rises. Depending on how aggressive the EDC is and how much free margin is treated, the cure rate can change. Some support curettage only, using the same cure rate and without electrodesiccation.

6.1.6.5. Chemotherapy

Local therapy using the chemotherapy drug 5-fluorouracil is effective in treating certain superficial cancers. With this treatment, a significant amount of inflammation is to be expected. After the invasive portion of the cancer is removed, chemotherapy is frequently used to eradicate any remaining superficial basal-cell carcinoma following Mohs surgery. The FDA has approved 5-fluorouracil.

If the remaining superficial tumor is removed surgically alone, significant, and challenging-to-repair surgical defects may arise. To ensure that the surgical wound has sufficiently healed, immunotherapy, and chemotherapy are frequently started one month or longer after surgery. These experimental methods are not considered standard practice.

Although sonidegib and vismodegib are approved medications for the specific treatment of BCC, they are costly and not suitable for use in pregnant patients. Traditionally used as an anti-fungal drug, ittraconazole has also recently drawn interest for its possible application in the management of BCC, particularly those that are incurable. Itraconazole, which has anti-Hedgehog pathway activity, has been clinically shown to have some efficacy for primary and recurrent BCC, either by itself or in combination with vismodegib/sonidegib. One case report of effectiveness in metastatic BCC exists.

6.1.6.6. Immunotherapy

This method destroys cancer cells by stimulating the immune system. To treat skin cancer, immune system improvement must reach the cancerous cells.

Topical treatment with 5% Imiquimod cream (IMQ) applied five times a week for six weeks has been shown to reduce, if not completely eradicate, basal-cell carcinoma (BCC) cases. The FDA has approved imiquimod, and the European Medicines Agency has approved topical IMQ for the treatment of small superficial basal-cell carcinoma. There have been reports of imiquimod being used off-label for invasive basal-cell carcinoma. Before surgery, imiquimod may be used to shrink the size of the carcinoma.

Before undergoing Mohs surgery to remove the cancer's superficial component, some people recommend using imiquimod. Studies indicate that Euphorbia peplus, a common garden weed, may be used as a treatment. This is being developed by the Australian biopharmaceutical company Peplin as a topical treatment for BCC.

6.1.6.7. Radiation

Radiation therapy can be administered as brachytherapy, which primarily consists of internal radiotherapy, or as external beam radiation. While radiotherapy is typically administered to elderly patients who are not surgical candidates, it is also used in situations where reconstructing the nose after surgery would be difficult or disfiguring (particularly on the tip of the nose and the nostril rims). External radiation therapy can require as few as five visits or as many as 25. Generally speaking, the more therapy visits planned, the fewer complications or harm to the surrounding normal tissue that supports the tumor. Additionally, radiotherapy may be helpful if surgical excision is not completed or if the postoperative pathology report indicates a high risk of recurrence, such as when nerve involvement has been shown. The cure rate for small tumors can reach 95%, while for large tumors it can drop to 80%. Epidermal radioisotope therapy, such as the Rhenium-SCT with 188Re, is a variant of external brachytherapy. It is applied in compliance with the standard brachytherapy indications, with a focus on complex localizations or structures (such as the earlobe) and the genitalia.

Surgery is typically used to treat recurrent tumors following radiation therapy rather than radiation. Additional radiation therapy will harm healthy tissue even more, and the tumor may become resistant to additional radiation. Treatment with radiation therapy may not be appropriate for nevoid basal-cell carcinoma syndrome. According to a 2008 study, radiation therapy is suitable for both primary and recurrent bladder cancers, but not for BCCs that have returned after receiving prior radiation therapy.

6.1.6.8. Photodynamic Therapy

Photodynamic therapy (PDT) is a new treatment method for basal-cell carcinoma, where photosensitizers are applied to the affected area and activated by light to destroy target cells. The EU has approved methyl aminolevulinate as a photosensitizer for this therapy since 2001. This treatment is also used for other types of skin cancer. A study from 2008 found that PDT is effective for treating primary superficial basal-cell carcinomas and reasonable for primary low-risk nodular basal-cell carcinomas, but less effective for high-risk lesions.

6.1.7. Prognosis

If the right treatment is applied to early primary basal-cell cancers, the prognosis is excellent. Cancers that recur are more difficult to treat and have a higher chance of doing so despite treatment. While it rarely spreads, basal-cell carcinoma grows locally by invading and destroying nearby tissues. When cancer affects important structures like nerves, it may cause loss of function, sensation, or, in rare cases, even death. Most cases can be successfully treated before they result in significant complications. For the aforementioned treatment options, the recurrence rate varies from 50% to one% or less.

6.1.8. Epidemiology

A very common type of skin cancer is basal-cell cancer. It is far more prevalent in fair-skinned people with a family history of basal-cell carcinoma, and its incidence rises at higher altitudes and closer to the equator. It is extremely prevalent in older adults (above 80 years of age). About 800,000 new cases are reported each year in the US alone. Basal-cell carcinomas can occur in up to 30% of white individuals over their lifetime. Basal-cell carcinoma, which accounts for up to one-third of all cancer diagnoses in Canada, is the most common type of skin cancer, affecting one in seven people in their lifetime.

Approximately 3 out of 10 Caucasian individuals in the US will experience basal-cell carcinoma at some point in their lives. About 70% of skin cancers that are not melanoma are caused by this tumor. Skin on the head or neck is affected by basal-cell carcinoma in 80% of cases.

On sun-exposed skin, the majority of sporadic BCC occurs in small numbers in individuals over 50, though younger people can also be impacted. Early onset of multiple basal-cell carcinomas may be a sign of nevoid basal-cell carcinoma syndrome, sometimes referred to as Gorlin syndrome.

6.2. Cutaneous Squamous-Cell Carcinoma

Along with basal-cell carcinoma and melanoma, cutaneous squamous-cell carcinoma (cSCC) is one of the three main forms of skin cancer. It is also referred to as squamous-cell carcinoma of the skin or squamous-cell skin cancer.

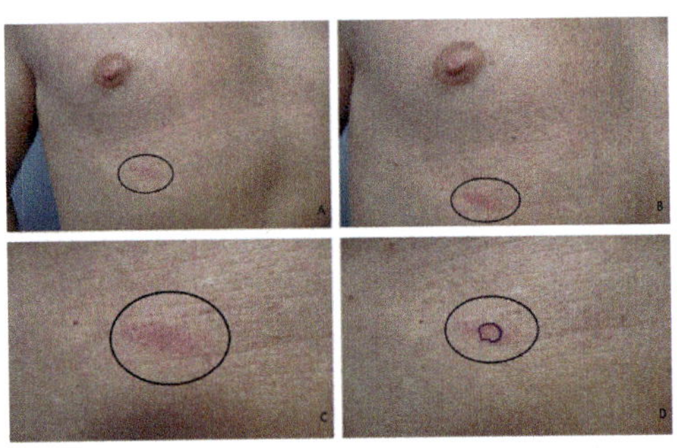

Figure 6.5. *Morphologic features of a cutaneous basal cell carcinoma in situ.*

Distant (A) and closer (B, C, and D) views of a cutaneous basal cell carcinoma in situ presenting as an asymptomatic, red, triangular-shaped 5 x 4 x 4 cm plaque (black oval) on the right upper abdomen of a 43-year-old Fitzpatrick skin type 1 Caucasian male. The biopsy site is designated by the purple oval (D).

Source: Cohen P R (September 23, 2022) Cutaneous Basal Cell Carcinoma In Situ: A Case Series. Cureus 14(9): e29479. doi:10.7759/cureus.29479.

Further, cSCC can appear as an ulcer, but it usually manifests as a hard lump with a scaly surface. Development and onset frequently take place over a few months. When it comes to metastasis, cSCC is more likely to spread than basal cell carcinoma. Bowen's disease is the name given to the pre-invasive or in situ form of cSCC that is limited to the epidermis, the outermost layer of skin (Figure 6.5).

One of the primary risk factors for cSCC is prolonged exposure to ultraviolet radiation from the sun over a person's lifetime. Other risk factors include previous scars, chronic wounds, actinic keratosis, light skin that is prone to sunburn, Bowen's disease, exposure to arsenic, radiation therapy, smoking, weak immune system function, previous basal cell carcinoma, and HPV infection. The risk from UV radiation is related to the total amount of exposure rather than exposure in early life. Tanning beds are now recognized as a significant source of UV radiation. Certain genetic conditions, like xeroderma pigmentosum and specific types of epidermolysis bullosa, can also increase the chances of developing cSCC. The cancer originates from squamous cells in the upper layers of the skin. Diagnosis usually involves a skin examination and confirmation through a skin biopsy.

Studies conducted *in vitro* and *in vivo* suggest that the progression of colorectal cancer cells (cSCC) is significantly influenced by the upregulation of FGFR2, a member of the fibroblast growth factor receptor immunoglobin family. TPL2 gene mutations cause FGFR2 to be overexpressed, which in turn triggers the mTORC1 and AKT pathways in primary and metastatic cSCC cell lines. *In vitro* studies on cSCC have demonstrated a reduction in cell migration and proliferation upon the use of a pan FGFR inhibitor (Figure 6.6).

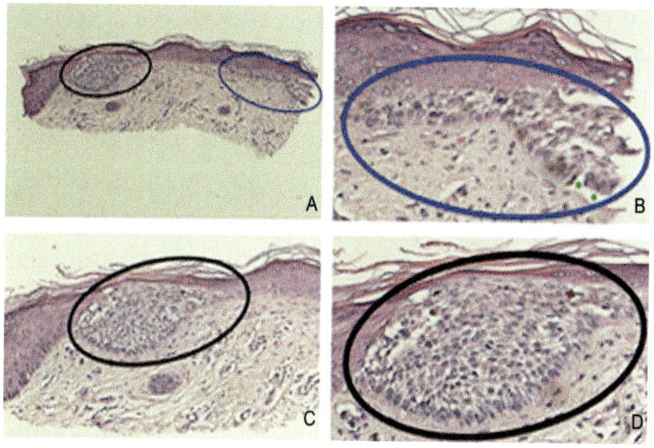

Figure 6.6. *Pathologic features of a basal cell carcinoma in situ of the skin.*

Distant (A) and closer (B, C, and D) views of microscopic findings of a cutaneous basal cell carcinoma in situ.

Source: Cohen P R (September 23, 2022) Cutaneous Basal Cell Carcinoma In Situ: A Case Series. Cureus 14(9): e29479. doi:10.7759/cureus.29479.

Using sunscreen and reducing UV radiation exposure are two preventive measures against cSCC. The usual course of treatment is surgical removal, which can involve Mohs surgery for more extensive cases or simple excision for less severe ones. Radiation therapy and cryotherapy are further options. In cases where there is distant metastasis, biologic therapy or chemotherapy may be used.

In 2015, around 2.2 million individuals worldwide were living with cutaneous squamous cell carcinoma (cSCC), accounting for roughly 20% of all skin cancer cases. In the United States, about 12% of males and 7% of females will be diagnosed with cSCC at some point in their lives. The prognosis for cSCC is generally positive when the cancer has not spread, but if it metastasizes, the five-year survival rate drops to approximately 34%. In 2015, there were approximately 52,000 global deaths due to cSCC. The average age of diagnosis is around 66 years old. After successful treatment of an initial cSCC lesion, there is a high risk of developing additional lesions.

6.2.1. Signs and Symptoms

Skin SCC usually develops from an actinic keratosis and starts off as a small nodule that sloughs and becomes necrotic in the center. Eventually, the nodule grows into an ulcer. Keratinocytes have the capacity to develop into cancer and cause cutaneous squamous-cell carcinoma if they start to grow out of control.

- The lesion caused by cSCC is often asymptomatic.
- Ulcer or reddish skin plaque that is slow-growing.
- Intermittent bleeding from the tumor, especially on the lip.
- The clinical appearance is highly variable.
- Usually, the tumor presents as an ulcerated lesion with hard, raised edges.
- The tumor may be in the form of a hard plaque or a papule, often with an opalescent quality, with tiny blood vessels.
- The tumor can lie below the level of the surrounding skin and eventually ulcerates and invades the underlying tissue.
- The tumor commonly presents on sun-exposed areas (e.g., back of the hand, scalp, lip, and superior surface of pinna).
- On the lip, the tumor forms a small ulcer, which fails to heal and bleeds intermittently.
- Evidence of chronic skin photodamage, as in multiple actinic keratoses (solar keratoses).
- The tumor grows relatively slowly.

6.2.1.1. Spread

Squamous-cell carcinoma (SCC) carries a greater risk of spreading to other parts of the body compared to basal-cell carcinoma (BCC).

Clinically, there is a greater chance of metastasis in patients receiving solid organ transplants who are immunosuppressed, have scarring, or appear on the lower lips, ears, or mucosa. Additionally, SCC with diameters greater than 2 cm, growth into the fat layer and along nerves, lymphovascular invasion present, histologically poorly differentiated cell architecture, or thickness greater than 6 mm are more likely to metastasize. (Cohen, 2022).

6.2.2. Causes

The second most common type of skin cancer, after basal-cell carcinoma but more common than melanoma, is cutaneous squamous cell carcinoma. It typically happens in sun-exposed areas. Skin SCC is associated with immunosuppression and sunlight exposure, with prolonged sun exposure being the main environmental risk factor. Although the risk of metastasis is higher than with basal-cell carcinoma, it is still low and can occur more than 10 years after the first detectable signs of squamous-cell carcinoma. There is a significant chance of distant metastasis and local recurrence in squamous-cell cancers of the lip and ears. A recent study has also demonstrated that the development of normal keratinocytes into squamous-cell carcinoma may be facilitated by the deletion or severe down-regulation of a gene called Tpl2 (tumor progression locus 2).

About 20% of non-melanoma skin cancers are cSCCs, and the head and neck region is home to 80–90% of cSCCs with the potential to spread.

Additionally, there is a higher chance of cutaneous squamous-cell carcinoma with tobacco use. Most cases of cSCC are found on exposed skin and are frequently brought on by UV exposure. cSCC typically affects areas of the body like the face, ears, neck, hands, or arms that are frequently exposed to the sun. The main symptom is a growing bump with flat, reddish patches and possibly a rough, scaly surface. In contrast to basal-cell carcinoma, colorectal cancer (cSCC) has a greater chance of metastasis and has the potential to spread to the local lymph nodes.

Erythroplasia of Queyrat (SCC in situ of the glans or prepuce in males, M:or the vulva in females.) may be induced by human papilloma virus. It is reported to occur in the corneoscleral limbus. Erythroplasia of Queyrat may also occur on the anal mucosa or the oral mucosa.

Genetically, cSCC tumors have high frequencies of p53 and NOTCH mutations along with less frequent changes in histone acetyltransferase EP300, DNA-repair deubiquitinase USP28, a subunit of the SWI/SNF chromatin remodeling complex PBRM1, and NF-κB signaling regulator CHUK.

6.2.2.1. Immunosuppression

Due to the use of chronic immunosuppressive medication, people who have received solid organ transplants are significantly more likely to develop squamous cell carcinoma. All skin cancers are more likely to develop when taking these drugs, but the effect is most pronounced for colorectal cancer (cSCC), where hazard ratios as high as 250 have been reported, compared to 40 for basal cell carcinoma. After transplantation, the incidence of cSCC development rises with time. Recipients of heart and lung transplants are most vulnerable to developing cSCC because these patients require more potent immunosuppressive drugs.

Regardless of location, cutaneous squamous-cell carcinomas are typically far more aggressive in those receiving immunotherapy or suffering from lymphoproliferative diseases like leukemia.

cSCC risk, as well as the risk of non-melanoma skin cancers in general, is dependent on the immunosuppressive medication regimen selected. The risk is lowest with mTOR inhibitors like sirolimus and everolimus and highest with calcineurin inhibitors like cyclosporine and tacrolimus. The risk profile of the antimetabolites mycophenolic acid and azathioprine is in the middle.

6.2.3. Risk Factors

Environmental, immunological, and genetic factors are among the many components of the multifactorial etiology of cSCC. Cumulative ultraviolet radiation (UVR) exposure, which includes sun exposure and tanning devices, is the main environmental factor. Considering the correlation between cumulative sun exposure (including exposure from both work and play), cSCC is more common in men than in women and affects the elderly population (80% of cases occur in those over 60). Fair skin tone is another significant risk factor. The risk of BCC is increased by intermittent and intense sun exposure, whereas the risk of cSCC is primarily linked to cumulative lifetime sun exposure. Using tanning beds increases the risk of colorectal cancer (cSCC), especially if one does so before the age of 25. Additionally, individuals who have received ultraviolet A (PUVA) and psoralen therapy for skin conditions may also be more vulnerable. Additional risk factors include immunosuppression, smoking, and infection with beta-human papilloma virus (HPV) subtypes.

Increased incidence of colorectal cancer (cSCC) has been noted in recipients of organ transplants, individuals infected with HIV, and patients undergoing hematopoietic stem cell transplantation. The length of immunosuppression may have an impact on the carcinogenesis of cSCC. Extensive cSCC can arise spontaneously, from an underlying in situ cSCC (AK or Bowen's disease, BD), or in conjunction with persistent photoexposure or inflammation of certain skin regions. Chronic cutaneous inflammation, as in the case of burns, scars, ulcers, sinus tracts, or chronic wounds, appears to be a factor in the development of cSCC. The development of cSCC is more likely with pharmacological treatments involving BRAF inhibitor monotherapy (e.g., vemurafenib, dabrafenib, or encorafenib) than with combined BRAF/mitogen-activated protein kinase (MEK) inhibitors. It has also been documented that voriconazole and vismodegib, an inhibitor of the Hedgehog pathway, cause the development of cSCC. Debate has surrounded the use of photosensitizing thiazide antihypertensives and the development of cSCC. Despite the fact that Gandini et al. found no correlation between this treatment and cSCC; however, Tang et al.'s meta-analysis did describe a potential relationship. Moreover, a prior history of cSCC increases the risk of developing further skin cancers, such as melanoma and other NMSCs. Flohil and associates. demonstrated that the percentage of cSCC patients who went on to develop melanoma, BCC, or cSCC was, respectively, 13.3%, 15.9%, and 0% (0.3%–0.6%). According to a recent study, patients with NMSC had a relative risk (RR) of 6.2 for melanoma when compared to controls. Patients who had NMSC before the age of 40 had an even higher RR for melanoma (RR 25.1). Lastly, a few genetic disorders, including albinism, xeroderma pigmentosum, Lynch syndrome/Muir-Torre syndrome, Fanconi anemia, recessive dystrophic epidermolysis bullosa, and xeroderma pigmentosum, may make cSCC development more likely.

6.2.4. Clinical Features

The anatomical site and subtype have an impact on the highly variable clinical characteristics of cSCC.

6.2.4.1. Bowen's Disease (BD)

A red, scaly plaque with distinct boundaries is the primary characteristic of BD, also referred to as in situ cSCC. It is most commonly found on skin that has been exposed to the sun on the head, neck, and extremities. It is possible for up to 5% of in situ cSCC to develop into invasive cSCC. On the penis, erythroplasia of Queyrat is a specific type of in situ cSCC. The characteristic lesion is velvety and erythematous (Figure 6.7).

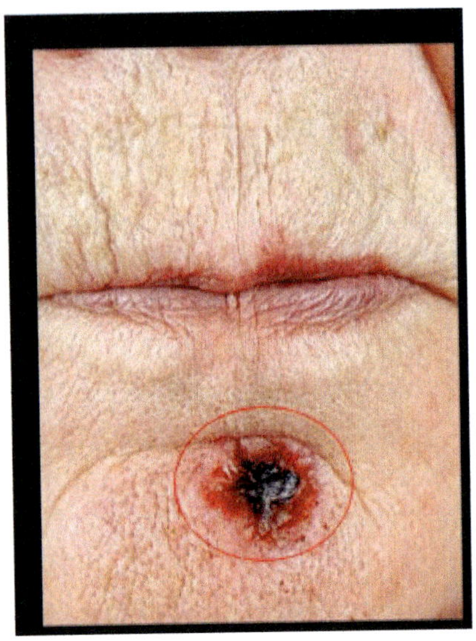

Figure 6.7. *Ulcerated squamous cell carcinoma on the chin.*

Source: Fania L, Didona D, Di Pietro FR, Verkhovskaia S, Morese R, Paolino G, Donati M, Ricci F, Coco V, Ricci F, Candi E, Abeni D, Dellambra E. Cutaneous Squamous Cell Carcinoma: From Pathophysiology to Novel Therapeutic Approaches. Biomedicines. 2021 Feb 9;9(2):171. doi: 10.3390/biomedicines9020171. PMID: 33572373; PMCID: PMC7916193.

6.2.4.2. Keratoacanthoma (KA)

It is also possible to think of KA as a subtype of cSCC. It is more commonly found in male Caucasian individuals in their 60s. Moreover, immunodeficiency, ultraviolet (UV) irradiation, HPV exposure, and abnormalities in DNA repair are linked to KA. In addition, trauma, scarring, and laser resurfacing can all result in KA. Additionally, patients with inherited syndromes like Witten-Zak and Muir-Torre syndrome have been reported to develop multiple KA. Its primary clinical characteristic is a spontaneous regression following a period of rapid expansion.

6.2.4.3. Invasive cSCC

Most cases of invasive cSCC are found on skin that is frequently exposed to the sun and typically appear as a persistent sore or wound that doesn't heal. Around 55% of cSCC cases are located on the head and neck, while the hands and forearms are affected in about 18% of cases. Other areas such as the legs, back, and upper extremities are involved in smaller percentages. However, cSCC can occur on any part of the body, including the lips, anus, and genitals. The clinical presentation of cSCC varies depending on how differentiated the lesion is. Well-differentiated cSCC often appears as scaly nodules or patches, while poorly differentiated cSCC typically presents as soft, ulcerated, or bleeding lesions. Marjolin's ulcer is a specific type of cSCC that develops on burn wounds, usually on the lower extremities, and can be associated with lymph node and distant metastases. HPV-related cSCC usually presents as a new or growing wart in the genital or periungual areas, with patients often reporting a history of stubborn warts.(Esther et al., 1999).

Common primary or advanced cSCC can be distinguished based on the extension. Common primary cSCCs are nonmetastatic cSCCs that are easily surgically removed; based on the likelihood of recurrence, they can be further classified as high-risk or low-risk cSCCs. Numerous clinical and pathological variables, such as lesion location and size, poorly defined borders, and a rapidly growing tumor, are considered high-risk factors. Additional information about high-risk variables is provided in Table 6.1.

Table 6.1. *Clinical and Pathological Risk Factors*

Clinical Risk Factors for Recurrence	
Size and location of lesion *	≥20 mm on area L ≥10 mm on area M ≥6 mm on area H
Undefined borders	
Recurrent lesion	
SOTRs **	
Previous radiotherapy or site of chronic inflammation	
Rapidly growing lesion	
Neurological symptoms	
Pathological risk factors for recurrence	
Not clearly differentiated lesion	
Adenoid, adenosquamous, or desmoplastic subtypes	
Clark level ≥IV	
Modified Breslow thickness ≥4 mm	
Perineural and/or vascular involvement	

* Area H: high risk of recurrence mask areas of face, ears, genitalia, hands, and feet; area M: middle risk of recurrence, cheeks, forehead, neck, and scalp; area L: low risk of recurrence, trunk, and extremities. ** SOTRs, solid organ transplant recipients.

Source: Fania L, Didona D, Di Pietro FR, Verkhovskaia S, Morese R, Paolino G, Donati M, Ricci F, Coco V, Ricci F, Candi E, Abeni D, Dellambra E. Cutaneous Squamous Cell Carcinoma: From Pathophysiology to Novel Therapeutic Approaches. Biomedicines. 2021 Feb 9;9(2):171. doi: 10.3390/biomedicines9020171. PMID: 33572373; PMCID: PMC7916193.

6.2.5. Diagnosis

A skin biopsy of the tissue or tissues suspected to be impacted by SCC is used to confirm the diagnosis. The biopsy's depth affects how squamous-cell cancer looks pathologically. For this reason, a biopsy that includes the basilar epithelium and subcutaneous tissue must be performed to make an accurate diagnosis. A skin biopsy may not yield sufficient information for a diagnosis. Inadequate biopsy results could be interpreted as follicularly involved actinic keratosis. The true cancer may become visible with a deeper biopsy that reaches the dermis or subcutaneous tissue. Although ideal, an excision biopsy is typically impractical. It is preferable to do an incisional or punch biopsy. The least desirable biopsy is a shave biopsy, particularly if only the superficial layer is obtained.

6.2.5.1. Histological Characteristics

Histopathologically, hyperkeratosis, and parakeratosis will be visible in the epidermis of patients with cSCC in situ (Bowen's disease). Acanthosis will also be evident, causing the rete ridges to thicken and elongate. Overly keratinocyte cells, which are frequently extremely atypical and may even have a more peculiar appearance than invasive cSCC, will result from these alterations. The entire thickness of the epidermis is affected by the atypia, and the keratinocytes exhibit pleomorphism, intense mitotic activity, and noticeably enlarged nuclei. Additionally, they will exhibit a loss of polarity and maturity, which will make the epidermis appear disorganized or blown by the wind.

There are two different kinds of multinucleated cells that can be observed: a dyskeratotic cell that is engulfed in the cytoplasm of a keratinocyte, and a multinucleated giant cell. Upper epidermis cells can occasionally vacuolate, revealing a copious amount of strongly eosinophilic cytoplasm. The upper dermis may have a mild to moderate lymphohistiocytic infiltrate.

6.2.5.2. In Situ Disease

Since Bowen's disease does not invade through the basement membrane, it is essentially the same as cSCC in situ and can be used interchangeably. It is categorized as precancerous or cSCC in situ (technically cancerous but non-invasive) depending on the source. Atypical squamous cells proliferate throughout the entire thickness of the epidermis in cSCC in situ, also known as Bowen's disease. The whole tumor does not spread into the dermis; rather, it remains contained within the epidermis. Under a microscope, the cells are frequently incredibly atypical and may even appear more peculiar than the cells of some invasive squamous-cell carcinomas. A specific kind of Bowen's disease called erythroplasia of Queyrat can develop on the vulva in females and the glans or prepuce in males. It mostly affects males over 40 who are not circumcised.

6.2.5.3. Invasive Disease

In cases of invasive cSCC, cancer cells penetrate the basement membrane. Detecting this infiltration can be challenging during the initial stages, but signs like full thickness epidermal atypia and involvement of hair follicles can aid in diagnosis. Advanced stages of invasion are marked by the development of abnormal tumor cell clusters in the dermis, typically accompanied by inflammation.

6.2.6. Prevention

While timely diagnosis and appropriate treatment are essential for bettering the prognosis of colorectal cancer (cSCC), prevention is also essential for lowering the disease's incidence. Reducing UV exposure—both occupational and recreational—is the most crucial preventive measure. In fact, as opposed to BCC, the risk of cSCC is primarily associated with lifetime sun exposure rather than sporadic or intense sun exposure. Moreover, it is well known that exposure to UV light, particularly in childhood and adolescence, raises the risk of colorectal cancer. Numerous studies have looked into the connection between lifetime UV exposure and cSCC. Average annual UV exposure was found to have a strong positive Sun exposure above a threshold of 70,000 cumulative hours of exposure over the course of a lifetime statistically significantly increased the risk of cSCC. Additionally, it was noted that working outside significantly raised the risk of developing cSCC (OR 1.6 for more than 54,000 cumulative hours of exposure for a lifetime). In fact, it is commonly known that occupational UV exposure is a critical risk factor for colorectal cancer (cSCC), whereas nonoccupational UV exposure has not been shown to be substantially associated with the development of cSCC. It is important to note that while UV exposure doses were evaluated in these studies, the biological effects of UV exposure on skin were not. It is true that extrinsic factors like UV protection as well as intrinsic factors like age, sex, and

Fitzpatrick skin types alter the effects of UV radiation.

It has been demonstrated in experimental and prospective studies that using sunscreen on a regular basis lowers the incidence of cSCC. Green et al. found that daily use of sunscreen decreased the incidence of squamous-cell tumors. Additionally, it has been discovered that sunscreens can lessen the depletion of Langerhans cells and prevent UV-induced immune suppression of contact hypersensitivity in mice.

Patients with a clinical history of multiple cSCC, multiple AKs, or diffuse field cancerization should be evaluated for preventive treatments. In high-risk patients (such as psoriatic patients who had previously received PUVA treatment, patients with xeroderma pigmentosum (XP), and solid organ transplant recipients (SOTRs), a preventive with oral retinoids, such as acitretin and isotretinoin, was evaluated in prospective studies, demonstrating a significant reduction of development of cSCC. It was found that 25 mg/d of oral aromatic retinoid decreased risk by approximately one-fourth in a nested cohort study on psoriatic patients treated with PUVA. This advantage, though, was only present during the retinoid intake period. In a controlled prospective study that lasted three years, Kraemer et al. observed that among XP patients taking isotretinoin (2 mg per kilogram of body weight), there was an average 63% reduction in skin cancers. On the other hand, compared to the frequency during treatment, the tumor frequency increased up to 19 times (mean value = 8.5 times) after the drug was stopped. In a double-blind, placebo-controlled trial as well as a prospective study conducted over a five-year period, it was found that actretin effectively decreased the incidence of chronic stem cell carcinoma in recipients of renal allografts. A prospective, open, randomized crossover trial on recipients of renal allografts corroborated these findings, demonstrating the efficacy of acitretin in preventing cSCC in patients with a prior history of NMSC. However, Chen, and colleagues revealed that the primary limiting factor is tolerability, as per a recent systematic review. Additionally, it was discovered that a nicotinamide supplement taken on a regular basis for a year decreased the rate of new cSCC by 30%, but only while the supplement was being taken.

A systematic review and meta-analyses revealed that NSAIDs consumption was also linked to a lower risk of cSCC, with the greatest risk reduction seen in COXIB users who were currently taking the medication (Torti et al., 2011).

6.2.7. Management

The majority of cutaneous squamous-cell carcinomas are typically removed through surgical procedures, with some cases also being treated with topical medication. Surgical excision with a clear margin of healthy tissue is a common approach, while radiotherapy in the form of external beam or brachytherapy can also be utilized. However, there is limited evidence available to compare the efficacy of various treatments for non-metastatic cSCC.

Mohs surgery is commonly used; in addition to being the preferred course of treatment for squamous-cell carcinoma of the skin, doctors have also used it to treat squamous-cell carcinoma of the mouth, throat, and neck. If there isn't a doctor with Mohs training, a pathologist can use an equivalent approach to the CCPDMA standards. Following surgery, radiation therapy is frequently administered to patients with high-risk cancer. For the treatment of cSCC, radiation or radiotherapy can also be used independently. Brachytherapy is a non-invasive treatment that can be used to treat sensitive but challenging areas, such as the genitalia or earlobes, without causing pain. One instance of this type of treatment is high-dose brachytherapy Rhenium-SCT, which utilizes rhenium-188's ability to emit beta radiation. A compound that is applied to a thin protective foil directly over the lesion encloses the radiation source. In this manner, the radiation source can be used in difficult-to-reach areas while reducing radiation exposure to healthy tissue.

Following cancer removal, patients with limited skin laxity require closure of the skin through the use of a split-thickness skin graft. A donor site is carefully selected, and the necessary amount of skin is extracted to ensure proper healing. The procedure involves removing only the epidermis and a portion of the dermis from the donor site, allowing it to heal effectively. Skin harvesting can be done using a mechanical dermatome or a Humby knife.

Certain skin squamous-cell carcinomas can be treated with electrodessication and curettage (EDC). If the patient is not immunosuppressed and the cSCC is known to be non-aggressive, EDC can be carried out with a good to adequate cure rate.

Excision, topical 5-fluorouracil or imiquimod, cryotherapy, photodynamic therapy with 5-aminolevulinic acid, and cryotherapy are available treatments for cSCC in situ (Bowen's disease). Evidence from a meta-analysis suggested that PDT produces better cosmetic results and is more effective than cryotherapy. Evidence comparing the efficacy of all available treatment options is generally lacking.

High-risk squamous-cell carcinoma is characterized by its large size, poor differentiation, rapid growth, and occurrence around the eye, ear, or nose. It calls for more aggressive, multidisciplinary treatment.

Nodal spread:

- Surgical block dissection if palpable nodes or in cases of Marjolin's ulcers but the benefit of prophylactic block lymph node dissection with Marjolin's ulcers is not proven.
- Radiotherapy.
- Adjuvant therapy may be considered in those with high-risk cSCC even in the absence of evidence for local metastasis. Imiquimod (Aldara) has been used with success for squamous-cell carcinoma in situ of the skin and the penis, but the morbidity and discomfort of the treatment is severe. An advantage is the cosmetic result: after treatment, the skin resembles normal skin without the usual scarring and morbidity associated with standard excision. Imiquimod is not FDA-approved for any squamous-cell carcinoma.

Squamous cell carcinomas typically have a high chance of local recurrence, with up to 50% of cases occurring. Following treatment, routine skin examinations with a dermatologist are advised.

6.2.8. Prognosis

Squamous cell carcinoma's long-term prognosis depends on several variables, including the patient's age, associated diseases, location, severity, and type of carcinoma, as well as treatments that are currently available. With a metastasis rate of 1.9–5.2% and a mortality rate of 1.5–3.4%, the long-term prognosis is typically favorable.

The lungs, brain, bone, and other skin locations are the most frequently affected organs when it does spread to other organs. Immunosuppressed individuals (those with organ transplants, HIV infection, or chronic lymphocytic leukemia) have a significantly higher risk of developing cSCC and experiencing metastases from squamous-cell carcinoma than the general population.

According to one study, squamous-cell carcinoma of the penis has a much higher death rate—roughly 23%—than some other forms of the disease. However, this relatively high death rate could be linked to patients delaying genital exams until their symptoms are incapacitating or refusing to have their genitalia operated on, which could leave scars.

6.2.9. Epidemiology

Globally, the prevalence of cutaneous squamous-cell carcinoma is still on the rise. Numerous theories have been put forth to explain this, including the aging of the population, an increase in the prevalence of immunocompromised individuals, and the rising use of tanning beds.

According to a recent study, there were between 180,000 and 400,000 instances of cSCC in the US in 2013. Geographical location, age, gender, race, and genetics are all risk factors for cSCC. The incidence of colorectal cancer (cSCC) rises with age, with people 75 years of age or older having a 5–10 times higher chance of getting the disease than people under the age of 55. The incidence of cSCC in males is 3:1 higher than in females. Additionally at risk are people with fair skin, red, blonde, or light-colored eyes.

Although squamous-cell carcinoma of the skin can occur anywhere on the body, it most commonly affects areas of the body that are exposed to sunlight, such as the arms, legs, and face. Patients who have received solid organ transplants (heart, lung, liver, pancreas, etc.) are also more likely to develop aggressive, high-risk cSCC. A few uncommon congenital illnesses can also increase the risk of cutaneous cancer. Exposure to arsenic from industrial sources or well water can dramatically raise the risk of cSCC in some areas of the world (Fania et al., 2021).

6.3. Melanoma

Melanoma, the most deadly kind of skin cancer, arises from melanocytes, which are cells that produce melanin. Though it rarely happens in the mouth, intestines, or eye (uveal melanoma), it usually affects the skin. Melanomas typically develop on the legs in women and the back in men. Malignant melanoma is a term commonly used to describe melanoma. The medical community advises against using the term "malignant melanoma" as it is redundant and emphasizes that there is no such thing as a "benign melanoma."

About 25% of melanomas develop from moles. Changes in a mole that can indicate melanoma include an increase—especially rapid increase—in size, irregular edges, change in color, itchiness, or skin breakdown.

UV exposure is the main factor contributing to melanoma in people whose skin pigment melanin levels are low. The sun or other sources, like tanning equipment, could be the source of the UV light. People who have a lot of moles, a family history of the condition, and weakened immune systems are more vulnerable. Additional rare genetic conditions that raise the risk include xeroderma pigmentosum. The process of diagnosing involves taking a biopsy and analyzing any skin lesion that exhibits indications of being malignant (Lens and Dawes., 2004).

Melanoma may be avoided by avoiding UV radiation and by wearing sunscreen when the sun is brightly shining. Surgery is usually used to remove the melanoma and any potentially affected surrounding tissue when it borders the area. It may be necessary to test the lymph nodes in the vicinity of patients with somewhat larger cancers for metastasis. If metastases have not formed, the majority of patients are cured. Immunotherapy, biological therapy, radiation therapy, or chemotherapy may increase survival for those whose melanoma has spread. In the US, the five-year survival rates after receiving treatment are as follows: 25% for patients with distant spread, 65% for those whose disease has spread to lymph nodes, and 99% for those with localized disease. The thickness, rate of cell division, and state of the overlying skin breakdown all influence the chance of melanoma returning or spreading (Figure 6.8).

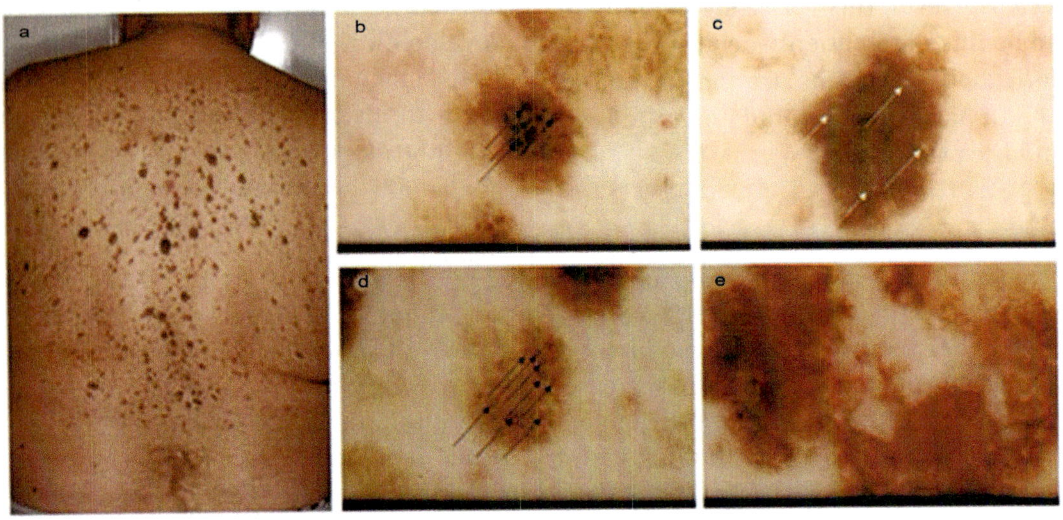

Figure 6.8. *Melanoma among several seborrheic keratoses (SK) on the back. This 67-year-old male patient was diagnosed with a melanoma on his back (in situ melanoma, pTis) near the shoulders and many SK lesions (**a**). Non-polarized dermoscopic images of SKs (**b–d**) and melanoma (**e**). SKs (**b–d**) show a dull surface, including fingerprint and cerebriform patterns, milia-like cyst (yellow arrows) and comedo-like opening (black arrows). Melanoma (**e**) contains an irregular pigment network and blue-white veil with multiple colors. The case of this patient also emphasizes the importance of full body examinations.*

Source: Bozsányi S, Farkas K, Bánvölgyi A, Lőrincz K, Fésűs L, Anker P, Zakariás S, Jobbágy A, Lihacova I, Lihachev A, et al. Quantitative Multispectral Imaging Differentiates Melanoma from Seborrheic Keratosis. Diagnostics. 2021; 11(8):1315. https://doi.org/10.3390/diagnostics11081315.

The most deadly kind of skin cancer is melanoma. In 2012, it happened for the first time in 232,000 people worldwide. 59,800 people died from active disease in 2015, out of 3.1 million cases. Globally, the highest rates of melanoma are found in Australia and New Zealand. While it is less common in Asia, Africa, and Latin America, high rates are also found in Northern Europe and North America. Men are approximately 1 in 6 times more likely than women to get melanoma in the US. Since the 1960s, malignant melanoma has increased in frequency in regions primarily inhabited by people of European descent.

6.3.1. Signs and Symptoms

Changes in the color or form of pre-existing moles, or the appearance of a new lump anywhere on the skin in the case of nodular melanoma, are early indicators of melanoma. The mole may itch, ulcerate, or bleed in later stages.

Early signs of melanoma are summarized by the mnemonic "ABCDEEFG":

- **A**symmetry.
- **B**orders (irregular with edges and corners).
- **C**olor (variegated).
- **D**iameter (greater than 6 mm (0.24 in), about the size of a pencil eraser).
- **E**volving over time.

This classification does not apply to nodular melanoma, which has its own classifications:

- Elevated above the skin surface.
- Firm to the touch.
- Growing.

Fatigue, nausea, vomiting, and loss of appetite are examples of non-specific paraneoplastic symptoms that can be brought on by metastatic melanoma. Less than 25% of melanomas diagnosed at an early stage go on to spread; however, metastatic disease is a possibility. Patients with metastatic melanoma are especially likely to develop brain metastases. Additionally, it may spread to distant lymph nodes, the liver, bones, or the abdomen.

6.3.2. Causes

The most common cause of melanomas is UV light exposure-induced DNA damage. Genes also have an impact. Additionally, skin areas with minimal sun exposure (such as the mouth, soles of feet, palms of hands, and genital areas) are susceptible to melanoma. Melanoma risk is elevated in those with dysplastic nevus syndrome, also referred to as familial atypical multiple mole melanoma. More than 50 moles suggest a higher chance of developing melanoma. A compromised immune system facilitates the growth of cancer by impairing the body's capacity to combat cancerous cells.

6.3.2.1. UV Radiation

The risk of developing melanoma is increased by exposure to UV radiation from tanning beds. The International Agency for Research on Cancer has classified tanning beds as "carcinogenic to humans" and has found that individuals who start using these devices before the age of 30 are 75% more likely to develop melanoma.

There seems to be a higher risk for those who work in airplanes, which is thought to be related to increased UV exposure.

UVB rays, which have wavelengths between 315 and 280 nm and are emitted by the sun, are directly absorbed by skin cell DNA. which causes cyclobutane pyrimidine dimers, a form of direct DNA damage. Two adjacent pyrimidine bases in a DNA strand can join to form thymine, cytosine, or cytosine-thymine dimers. UVA light is visible at longer wavelengths than UVB (between 400 and 315 nm). It can also be directly absorbed by skin cells' DNA, albeit with efficiencies of only 1/100 to 1/1000 of UVB.

UVA and UVB radiation exposure is a major factor in the development of melanoma. Melanoma is causally linked to sporadic extreme sun exposure that causes sunburn on human body parts; this intermittent sun exposure appears to be the reason why melanoma is more common on men's backs and women's legs. Rather than being strongly influenced by indoor versus outdoor occupations, the risk appears to be strongly influenced by socioeconomic conditions; professional and administrative workers are more likely to experience it than unskilled workers. Tumor suppressor gene mutations or complete loss are additional factors. With their intensely penetrating UVA rays, sunbed use has been connected to the emergence of skin cancers, including melanoma.

Factors that may contribute to an increased risk of melanoma include the amount and length of time spent in the sun, the age when sun exposure occurs, and the level of skin pigmentation. Melanoma rates are highest in regions where migrants from Northern Europe have settled, such as Australia, due to the intense sunlight that their skin is not accustomed to. Studies have shown that exposure to sunlight during childhood is a more significant risk factor for melanoma than exposure in adulthood, particularly in migrant populations in Australia.

The chance that subsequent sunburns will progress to melanoma increases if there are several severe sunburns because of the cumulative damage. Living near the equator increases exposure to UV radiation. The main sources of UV radiation that raise the risk for melanoma are tanning beds and UV-high sunlight.

6.3.2.2. Genetics

There are several uncommon mutations that significantly raise the risk of melanoma and frequently run in families. Numerous genes raise the odds. Certain more common genes, like the red hair-causing MC1R gene, have a relatively lower elevated risk of melanoma than certain rare genes, which have a relatively high risk. The mutations can be found by genetic testing.

The gene CDKN2A is affected by one class of mutations. This gene has an alternative reading frame mutation that causes p53, a transcription factor involved in apoptosis and 50% of human cancers, to become unstable. A different mutation in the same gene causes CDK4, a cyclin-dependent kinase that stimulates cell division, to become nonfunctional. Melanoma susceptibility is also increased by mutations that cause xeroderma pigmentosum (XP), a skin condition. These mutations, which are dispersed throughout the genome, impair a cell's capacity to repair DNA. Both the XP and CDKN2A mutations are highly penetrant, meaning that a carrier has a high probability of expressing the phenotype. The chromosome arms 1p, 9p, and 12q contain loci for familial melanoma, which is a genetically heterogeneous condition. The pathogenesis (disease development) of melanoma has been linked to multiple genetic events. The low-molecular weight protein inhibitor of cyclin-dependent protein kinases (CDKs), p16INK4a, is encoded by the multiple tumor suppressor 1 (CDKN2A/MTS1) gene and has been found to be located in the p21 region of the human chromosome. A family history of melanoma and 50 or more combined moles are typical characteristics of FAMMM. It is mostly linked to CDKN2A mutations and is transmitted autosomally dominantly. Pancreatic cancer risk is 38 times higher in those with FAMMM associated with CDKN2A mutations.

Although they are more prevalent in the population, some mutations carry a lower risk. Melanoma risk is two to four times higher in individuals with MC1R gene mutations compared to those with two wild-type (normal, unaffected type) copies. Every redhead has a mutated copy of MC1R, which is a highly common mutation. Younger women are more susceptible to complications when there is a mutation in the MDM2 SNP309 gene.

Individuals with fair or red hair, those with numerous atypical or dysplastic nevi, and those who were born with large congenital melanocytic nevi are more vulnerable.

A person's risk of developing melanoma is significantly increased if they have a family history of the disease, as melanoma-prone families have multiple gene mutations. Individuals who have previously experienced one melanoma are more likely to experience a second primary tumor. Less melanin in the skin indicates less protection from UV rays, which is why fair skin is the result.

6.3.3. Pathophysiology

Melanocytes that grow uncontrollably initiate the initial phase of melanoma. Between the epidermis, which is the skin's outermost layer, and the dermis, which is the skin's innermost layer, are melanocytes. When the tumor is less than 1 mm thick and spreads to the level of the basal epidermis, it is referred to as the radial growth phase in the early stages of the disease. This early-stage melanoma is unlikely to spread to other parts of the body because the cancer cells have not yet entered the blood vessels deeper within the skin. Surgery can typically remove the melanoma entirely if it is discovered at this stage. Cell behavior drastically changes when the tumor cells begin to migrate in a different direction, up, and into the epidermis and papillary dermis (Figure 6.9).

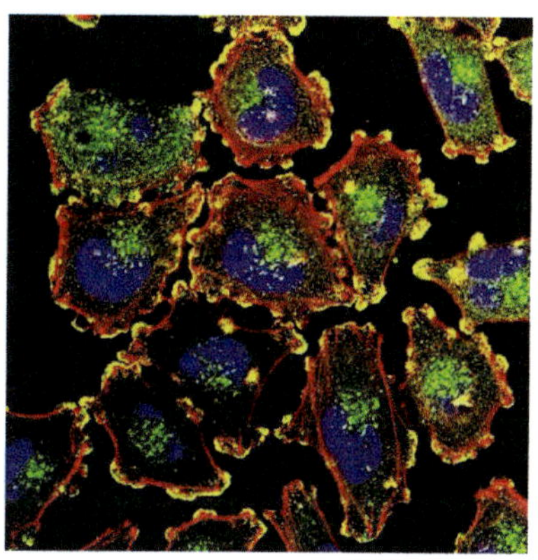

Figure 6.9. *Molecular basis for melanoma cell motility: actin-rich podosomes (yellow), along with cell nuclei (blue), actin (red), and an actin regulator (green).*

Source: https://en.wikipedia.org/wiki/Melanoma#/media/File:Metastatic_Melanoma_Cells_Nci-vol-9872-300.jpg.

The invasive radial growth phase, in which individual cells begin to acquire invasive potential, is the next stage of evolution. Melanoma has the potential to spread from this point forward. The lesion's Breslow's depth is typically less than 1 mm (0.04 in), and the Clark level is typically 2. The vertical growth phase (VGP) following is invasive melanoma. The tumor becomes able to grow into the surrounding tissue and can spread around the body through blood or lymph vessels. The tumor thickness is usually more than 1 mm (0.04 in), and the tumor involves the deeper parts of the dermis.

During the VGP, the host triggers an immune response against the tumor, which is determined by the presence and activity of TILs, or tumor infiltrating lymphocytes. Regression is the last stage of development, where these cells occasionally totally eradicate the original tumor. Sometimes only the metastatic tumor is found after the primary tumor has been totally destroyed. Activating mutations affecting the B-Raf protein's structure are present in about 40% of human melanomas. These mutations cause constitutive signaling via the Raf to MAP kinase pathway.

DNA damage is a common cause of most cancers. Thymine dimers are mostly caused by UVA light. At 1/10, 1/10, and 1/3rd the frequencies of UVA-induced thymine dimers, respectively, oxidized pyrimidines, oxidized purine 8-oxoguanine (a mutagenic DNA alteration), and single-strand breaks are the main DNA damage caused by reactive oxygen species, which are also produced by UVA.

Cyclobutane pyrimidine dimer (CPD) photoproducts can cause mutations during DNA replication or repair if they are not repaired. This is because they produce incorrect translesion synthesis. The most common mutations resulting from incorrect synthesis beyond CPDs are transitions from cytosine to thymine (C>T) or CC>TT. Since they are the most specific mutation brought on by UV light and are typically found in skin that has been exposed to the sun but are rarely found in internal organs, these mutations are known as UV fingerprint mutations. Chromosome translocations, deletions, and insertions can also result from mistakes made in the DNA repair of UV photoproducts or from incorrect synthesis proceeding beyond these photoproducts.

25 melanomas had their entire genomes sequenced. Each melanoma genome contained, on average, 80,000 mutated bases (mostly C>T transitions) and roughly 100 structural rearrangements. This exceeds the approximately 70 mutations that occur between parents and children in a single generation. Approximately 6,000 protein-coding genes contained missense, nonsense, or splice site mutations among the 25 melanomas. Additionally, more than 100 melanoma transcriptomes have been sequenced and examined. Melanoma expresses nearly 70% of all human protein-coding genes. About 200 genes exhibit a more distinct expression pattern in melanoma than in other cancer types, while the majority of these genes are also expressed in other normal and cancerous tissues. Some genes that are specific to melanoma include tyrosinase, MLANA, and PMEL.

When UV radiation damages a cell's DNA, it usually results in thymine dimerization, which, if left unrepaired, can lead to gene mutations. The tumor type with the most mutations is cutaneous melanoma due to this potent mutagenic factor. These mutations are passed on to new cell generations during cell division. A tumor may form if the mutations affect tumor suppressor or protooncogene genes, which can cause the rate of mitosis in the cells carrying the mutation to become uncontrollable. Studies on skin cancer in mice tend to confirm a role for activating transcription factor-2 in the progression of cancer; data from patients suggest that aberrant levels of activating transcription factor in the nucleus of melanoma cells are associated with increased metastatic activity of melanoma cells.

6.3.3.1. Gene Mutations

Extensive investigations, like The Cancer Genome Atlas, have identified recurrent somatic changes that are probably responsible for the onset and progression of cutaneous melanoma. Four subtypes have been identified by the Cancer Genome Atlas study: triple wild-type, NF1 mutant, RAS mutant, and BRAF mutant.

The 600th codon of BRAF is where the most common mutation (50% of cases) is found. Normally involved in cell growth, BRAF is made constitutively active by this particular mutation, which makes it independent of normal physiological regulation and promotes tumor growth. 30% of TCGA cases have recurrent mutations in the RAS genes (NRAS, HRAS, and KRAS), and oncogenic activity is triggered by mutations in the 61st or 12th codons. Mutations resulting in loss of function frequently impact tumor suppressor genes, including NF1, TP53, and CDKN2A. Other oncogenic changes include kinase fusions involving BRAF, RAF1, ALK, RET, ROS1, NTRK1, NTRK3, and MET. It is noteworthy that kinase fusions and mutations involving BRAF, RAS, and NF1 are remarkably mutually exclusive, occurring in distinct patient subsets. Therefore, determination of mutation status can enhance patient matching and guide the use of particular inhibitors in targeted therapy. Copy-number amplification occurs in 3–7% of mutated versions of BRAF and NRAS.

6.3.3.2. Metastasis

The study demonstrated that melanoma cells with high pigmentation had a Young's modulus of approximately 4.93, compared to 0.98 in non-pigmented cells. In a different experiment, the researchers discovered that the elasticity of melanoma cells plays a crucial role in the metastasis and growth of the cancer: non-pigmented tumors grew more rapidly and were larger than pigmented ones. They demonstrated that melanoma tumors contain both pigmented and non-pigmented cells, allowing for the possibility of both drug resistance and metastasis.

6.3.4. Diagnosis

The most common way to suspect melanoma is to look at or visually inspect the area in question. Generally, irregularly shaped or colored moles are considered candidates. It is advised to become knowledgeable about melanomas, to routinely check moles for changes (in size, shape, color, itching, or bleeding), and to seek medical advice from a qualified professional when a candidate is identified to detect melanomas and improve survival rates. Examining suspicious skin lesions in person yields more accurate results than looking at pictures of them. When utilized by qualified professionals, dermoscopy is a more useful tool than the human eye alone for identifying malignant lesions. In the diagnosis of cutaneous melanoma, reflectance confocal microscopy may be more sensitive and specific than dermoscopy; however, further research is required to validate this finding (Dinnes et al., 2018).

Nonetheless, a large number of melanomas manifest as lesions with a diameter of less than 6 mm, and all melanomas are malignant when they initially resemble tiny dots. All moles are usually examined by doctors, even those with a diameter of less than 6 mm. False alarms may result from seborrheic keratosis, which may satisfy some or all of the ABCD criteria. Dermatoscopy and examination are usually sufficient for doctors to differentiate between melanoma and seborrheic keratosis.

Some argue that evolving should be used in place of enlarging because changing and evolving moles are concerning. On the other hand, some practitioners favor elevation. A melanoma can be identified with elevation; however, elevation alone does not rule out melanoma diagnosis. In the US, the majority of melanomas are found before they grow larger. They might have advanced into the more dangerous invasive stage by the time elevation becomes apparent.

6.3.4.1. Ugly Duckling

Using the ugly duckling sign is one technique. Common lesion characteristics are correlated. When a lesion doesn't match the typical traits, it's called an ugly duckling, and a professional examination is needed. The Little Red Riding Hood symbol indicates that people with light-colored hair and fair skin may have amelanotic melanomas, which can be challenging to diagnose. Examining such individuals requires extra caution because they may have severely dysplastic nevi and multiple melanomas. Because many melanomas in these people resemble nonmelanomas or are thought to be wolves in sheep's clothing, dermatoscopes are necessary for the detection of ugly ducklings. These fair-skinned people frequently have amelanotic or light-pigmented melanomas, which do not exhibit noticeable color variations and changes. Their borders are frequently blurry, making it difficult to identify them visually without a dermatoscope.

Melanotic melanomas and melanomas arising in fair-skinned individuals are extremely difficult to diagnose because they break the ugly duckling sign, don't exhibit many of the ABCD rule's characteristics, and are difficult to differentiate from dermatofibromas, lentigines, acne scarring, or insect bites.

6.3.4.2. Biopsy

After a visual and dermatoscopic examination, the doctor may choose to biopsy a suspicious mole for further evaluation. A skin biopsy, typically done under local anesthesia, can help confirm a diagnosis and determine the severity of the condition. Elliptical excisional biopsies are often used to remove tumors, followed by histological analysis and Breslow scoring. Incisional biopsies, like punch biopsies, are generally not recommended for suspected melanomas due to the risk of sampling error or local implantation leading to inaccurate tumor thickness estimates. Despite concerns, there is no evidence to suggest that biopsies increase the risk of metastatic disease.

Following up with high-risk patients frequently involves total body photography, which is taking pictures of every inch of the body. The method's effectiveness has been questioned because it cannot detect macroscopic changes, despite reports that it allows for early detection and is cost-effective (using any digital camera). Combining the two methods seems to yield very high detection rates. The diagnosis method should be used in addition to dermoscopic imaging, not as a substitute for it.

6.3.5. Prevention

There is no evidence to support or refute adult population screening for melanoma.

6.3.5.1. Ultraviolet Radiation

Protection can be obtained by minimizing exposure to UV radiation sources (the sun and sunbeds), adhering to sun safety precautions, and donning sun protective gear (long-sleeved shirts, long pants, and wide-brimmed hats).

Although it was originally thought that tanning under artificial light could help prevent skin cancer, melanomas can actually become more common as a result of this practice.

UV nail lamps, a common and widespread source of UV radiation that could be avoided, are used in nail salons to dry nail polish. Even though there is little chance of getting skin cancer from using a UV nail lamp, it is still advised to put on fingerless gloves and/or sunscreen with an SPF of 30 or higher before using one.

The body uses UV light to create vitamin D, so it's important to strike a balance between getting enough sunlight to maintain healthy levels and lowering the risk of melanoma. Fair-skinned people can get a sunburn in about 30 minutes, which is also how long it takes the body to produce its daily supply of vitamin D. Sunlight exposure does not have to come from the sun all at once.

6.3.5.2. Sunscreen

It seems that using sunscreen helps avoid melanoma. Sunscreens with an SPF of 50 or higher were advised to be used on exposed areas in the past because these older sunscreens were better at blocking UVA rays. Even at lower SPFs, zinc oxide, titanium dioxide, and avobenzone—three of the more recent sunscreen ingredients—effectively block UVA and UVB rays. Sunscreen also guards against another type of skin cancer called squamous cell carcinoma. Concerns have been raised that sunscreen might create a false sense of security against sun damage.

6.3.5.3. Medications

There is preliminary evidence, according to a 2005 review, that fibrate medication and statins can lower the risk of melanoma. However, a 2006 review found no evidence of any advantages.

6.3.6. Treatment

Utilizing a skin biopsy, the clinical diagnosis is confirmed. Usually, a larger excision of the tumor or scar occurs next. A sentinel lymph node biopsy may be done, depending on the stage. Sentinel lymph node biopsy trial results are controversial, and as of 2015, there was conflicting evidence regarding the procedure's benefits. Advanced malignant melanoma is treated using a multidisciplinary strategy.

6.3.6.1. Surgery

Although the tumor may be removed by excisional biopsies, additional surgery is frequently required to lower the chance of recurrence. It is customary to perform a full surgical excision with sufficient surgical margins, assess for detectable metastatic disease, and follow up over the short and long terms. This is frequently accomplished by a wide local excision (WLE) with margins of 1–2 cm (0.4–0.8 in). Narrower surgical margins are typically used to treat lentigo malignas and melanoma-*in-situ*, measuring 0.2–0.5 cm (0.1–0.2 in). For standard excision of melanoma-*in-situ*, many surgeons recommend a margin of 0–5 cm (0.2 in). However, in margin-controlled surgery (also known as Mohs surgery or the double-bladed technique with margin control), a margin of 0.2 cm (0.1 in) may be acceptable. Wide excision is performed to lower the chances of tumor regrowth at the initial location. This is a frequent issue seen with melanoma treatment. Research has been conducted to determine the optimal margins for excision, with a shift towards less aggressive treatment over the past few decades. A meta-analysis in 2009 of various randomized controlled trials showed only a slight survival advantage for wide excision of primary skin melanomas, but the results did not reach statistical significance.

Mohs surgery has shown cure rates ranging from 77% to 98.0% for melanoma-*in-situ*. The effectiveness of CCPDMA and "double scalpel" peripheral margin controlled surgery is on par with Mohs surgery for this type of melanoma.

Melanomas typically spread to nearby lymph nodes before spreading to other areas of the body. While surgically removing lymph nodes (lymphadenectomy) was previously attempted to improve survival rates, it often led to complications without providing an overall survival benefit. A newer technique called sentinel lymph node biopsy has been developed to reduce complications associated with lymph node surgery and still determine if the nodes are affected by the tumor.

When treating cutaneous melanoma, a biopsy of sentinel lymph nodes is a commonly performed procedure.

It is not necessary to perform sentinel lymph node biopsy or other diagnostic tests for early, thin melanoma, such as melanoma in situ, T1a melanoma, or T1b melanoma ≤ 0.5mm. These individuals have a high 5-year survival rate of 97% and are unlikely to have cancer spread to their lymph nodes or elsewhere. Therefore, these tests are considered unnecessary for them. Additionally, baseline blood tests and radiographic studies should not be done solely based on the identification of this type of melanoma due to their high false-positive rates. Gene expression profiling may be used as a supplementary test for uncertain or small lesions to potentially address false positives.

Sentinel lymph node biopsy is a common procedure, particularly for T1b/T2+ tumors, mucosal tumors, ocular melanoma, and tumors of the limbs. The process involves lymphoscintigraphy, where a radioactive tracer is injected at the tumor site to locate the sentinel node(s). Blue tracer dye is also used for added precision, and surgery is then conducted to biopsy the identified node(s). Hematoxylin and eosin and immunoperoxidase staining are typically sufficient to determine if the node is involved. Polymerase chain reaction (PCR) tests are sometimes used on nodes, mainly for clinical trial eligibility, revealing that some patients with negative sentinel lymph nodes may contain a small number of positive cells. Alternatively, fine-needle aspiration biopsy is often used to test masses.

A radical lymph node dissection is frequently carried out if a lymph node is positive, depending on the degree of lymph node spread. Adjuvant therapy will be considered for the patient if the disease is fully resected. Excisional skin biopsy is the preferred method of management. Here, a sufficient (but tiny, typically 1 or 2 mm) ellipse of surrounding skin and tissue is removed along with the suspected lesion. A narrow surgical margin (1 mm) is the preferred choice for the initial biopsy to prevent disruption of the local lymphatic drainage. The skin's subcutaneous, dermal, and epidermal layers should all be included in the biopsy. This makes it possible for the histopathologist to use a microscope to assess the melanoma's thickness. Breslow's thickness, which is expressed in millimeters, describes this. In cases where lentigo maligna is suspected or where the lesion is located in surgically challenging areas (such as the face, toes, fingers, or eyelids), a small punch biopsy in representative areas will provide sufficient information without interfering with the final staging or depth determination.

The final surgical margin (0.5 cm, 1.0 cm, or 2 cm) should never be included in the initial biopsy under any circumstances because a misdiagnosis could lead to excessive scarring and procedure-related morbidity. A significant initial excision can interfere with subsequent lymphangiogram-directed lymph node dissection and disturb the local lymphatic drainage. When a patient declines a more invasive excisional biopsy due to logistical or personal reasons, a small punch biopsy can be used at any time. Small punch biopsies usually leave no visible scars and are very non-invasive. They also heal quickly.

6.3.6.2. Add on Treatment

Following surgery, the use of adjuvant treatment can help lower the chances of recurrence, particularly in high-risk melanoma cases. Practices differ across countries, with immune checkpoint inhibitor therapy being the most frequently utilized adjuvant treatment for up to one year following surgery.

During the early 2000s, it was common practice to administer high-dose interferon treatment for up to a year to patients at high risk of cancer recurrence. This treatment, known for its severe side effects, was believed to potentially improve the patient's prognosis. However, a 2013 meta-analysis suggested that interferon alpha could increase disease-free and overall survival rates in patients with AJCC TNM stage II-III cutaneous melanoma. A 2011 meta-analysis indicated that while interferon treatment may delay the recurrence of melanoma, it only improved survival rates by 3% after 5 years. The unpleasant side effects of interferon treatment also significantly impact the patient's quality of life. In the European Union, the use of interferon is typically limited to clinical trial settings.

6.3.6.3. Chemotherapy

Since its approval by the FDA in 1975, chemotherapy drugs like Dacarbazine have been a key part of treating metastatic melanoma. However, its effectiveness in terms of increasing survival rates has not been confirmed in randomized controlled trials. With the introduction of immune checkpoint inhibitors, Dacarbazine, and its oral form, Temozolomide, are now considered as possible treatment choices in later stages of therapy.

Isolated limb infusion (ILI) has been shown to be a minimally invasive and well-tolerated technique for administering regional chemotherapy to patients with sarcoma and locally advanced cutaneous malignancies.

6.3.6.4. Targeted Therapy

Melanoma cells harbor mutations that enable their continuous growth and survival within the body. Small-molecule targeted therapies function by impeding the activity of the genes involved in pathways crucial for tumor proliferation and survival. The primary treatments for melanoma include inhibitors targeting BRAF, C-Kit, and NRAS. These inhibitors work by suppressing the downstream pathways associated with cell proliferation and tumor development resulting from particular gene mutations. Individuals who test positive for the specific mutation can receive treatment with small-molecule targeted inhibitors. BRAF inhibitors like vemurafenib and dabrafenib, along with MEK inhibitor trametinib, are the most effective approved treatments for BRAF-positive melanoma. Tumors may acquire resistance to therapy over time, potentially rendering it ineffective. Nonetheless, combining BRAF and MEK inhibitors may produce a rapid and enduring response to melanoma therapy.

Several therapies outlive conventional chemotherapy in terms of improving survival. In patients with BRAF-positive melanoma, biochemotherapy—chemotherapy utilizing the cytokines IL-2 and IFN-α—in conjunction with BRAF inhibitors increased survival. In comparison to chemotherapy, biochemotherapy was more toxic and did not increase overall survival when used alone. Polychemotherapy, the combination of several chemotherapy agents, did not increase survival compared to monochemotherapy. Progression-free survival (PFS) periods are comparatively short as a result of targeted therapies. The 3-year PFS and 5-year PFS of dabrafenib and trametinib therapy, respectively, are 23% and 13%.

In February 2024, the US FDA approved Lifileucel (Amtagvi), an autologous T-cell immunotherapy derived from tumors, for medical use.

6.3.6.5. Immunotherapy

Immunotherapy works by boosting the body's natural defenses against cancer cells to activate the patient's immune system against the tumor. Currently, adoptive cell transfer, immune checkpoint inhibitors, and cytokines are the three main treatment categories used in immunotherapy for melanoma. Patients with metastatic melanoma are most frequently treated with these options, which greatly increase overall survival. These procedures are frequently expensive, though. For instance, pembrolizumab, an immune checkpoint inhibitor, costs between $10,000 and $12,000 USD for a single dose given every three weeks.

For melanoma, cytokine treatments such as IL-2 and IFN-a are utilized. The first novel medication to be licensed for the treatment of metastatic melanoma in 20 years was IL-2 (proleukin). For a tiny proportion of melanoma patients, IL-2 may provide the chance of total and permanent remission from their illness. The complete response rate of intralesional IL-2 for in-transit metastases is high, ranging from 40 to 100%. Likewise, IFN-a's use as a stand-alone therapy has been limited due to its high toxicity and only moderate survival benefits.

Anti-CTLA-4 monoclonal antibodies (ipilimumab and tremelimumab), toll-like receptor (TLR) agonists, CD40 agonists, anti-PD-1 (pembrolizumab, pidilizumab, and nivolumab), and PD-L1 antibodies are examples of immune checkpoint inhibitors. Research indicates that anti-PD-1 antibodies have less systemic toxicity and are more effective than anti-CTLA4 antibodies. The five-year progression-free survival rate for pembrolizumab-based immunotherapy is 21%. When multiple therapies are used in combination, overall survival and progression-free survival are higher than when the individual immunotherapy medications are used alone.

The use of adoptive cell transfer for treatment is still being studied. Adoptive cell transfer, which is currently used to reduce complications from graft-versus-host disease, is the application of pre-stimulated, modified T cells or dendritic cells.

6.3.6.6. Lentigo Maligna

Most surgeons still perform standard excisions. Regretfully, the rate of recurrence is incredibly high—up to 50%. This is because the lesions are located on the face, which frequently requires the surgeon to use a narrow surgical margin, and the visible surgical margin is not well defined. Due to the standard bread-loafing technique of fixed tissue histology's limitations and the narrow surgical margin used, there is a high rate of false negative errors and frequent recurrences. Perimeter margins, or margin control, are required to get rid of false negative errors. Distances from sections should approach 0 point 1 mm if bread loafing is used to ensure that the procedure approaches total margin control. Despite being the most commonly used treatment, a meta-analysis of the literature in 2014 revealed that there were no randomized controlled trials of surgical interventions to treat lentigo maligna or melanoma *in-situ*.

One author reported cure rates for Mohs surgery as low as 77% and as high as 95%. Another method, known as the "double scalpel" peripheral margin controlled excision, is similar to the Mohs method in controlling margins but requires a pathologist with expertise in managing the vertical margins and staining methods on thin peripheral sections.

Imiquimod (Aldara) topical cream, an immune-boosting medication, has been used as an experimental treatment for melanocytic nevi and melanoma-*in-situ* (lentigo maligna). A combination of surgical excision of the cancer and three months of postoperative Aldara cream treatment are being used by some derma-surgeons. Although some research has recommended topical tazarotene as an adjuvant, there is not enough data available at this time to support this recommendation. It may even worsen topical inflammation, which could impair patient compliance.

6.3.6.7. Radiation

Radiation therapy is frequently utilized following surgical removal for patients with advanced melanoma in the local or regional area, or for those with distant metastases that cannot be removed. Kilovoltage X-ray beams are commonly employed in these treatments, delivering the highest radiation dose near the skin's surface. While it may decrease the likelihood of local recurrence, it does not extend survival. The use of radioimmunotherapy for metastatic melanoma is currently being researched. Radiotherapy plays a part in easing the symptoms of metastatic melanoma.

6.3.7. Prognosis

Factors that affect prognosis include:

- tumor thickness in millimeters (Breslow's depth),
- depth related to skin structures (Clark level),
- type of melanoma,
- presence of ulceration,
- presence of lymphatic/perineural invasion,
- presence of tumor-infiltrating lymphocytes (if present, the prognosis is better),
- location of the lesion, and
- presence of satellite lesions.

The prognosis of some melanoma types is poorer than others, but this is explained by their thickness. At the time of staging, less invasive melanomas with lymph node metastases have a better prognosis than deep melanomas without regional metastases. Unless they are at the site of a wide local excision (as opposed to a staged excision or punch/shave excision), local recurrences typically behave similarly to a primary because they tend to indicate lymphatic invasion.

One of the most crucial variables when melanomas have spread to the lymph nodes is the number of malignant nodes. A node's level of malignancy is also significant; micrometastases, where the cancer is only microscopic, have a better prognosis than macrometastases. Micrometastases can sometimes only be found with specialized staining, and the prognosis is better if malignancy is only found with the infrequently used polymerase chain reaction (PCR) test. The prognosis is much worse for macrometastases where the malignancy is clinically evident (in certain cases, the cancer completely replaces a node). The prognosis is even worse if the nodes are matted or if there is extracapsular extension. Apart from these variables, the assessment of the prognosis of malignant melanoma may also be supported by the expression levels and copy number variations of several relevant genes.

The most fatal form of skin cancer is stage IV melanoma, which has spread and has a 22.5% five-year survival rate. It is usually accepted that cancer is incurable when distant metastases are present. The survival rate after five years is less than 10%. 6–12 months is the median survival time. Palliative care is given with the goal of extending life and improving quality of life. Depending on how aggressively the treatment is administered, patients with metastatic melanoma may live for several months or even years in certain situations. The prognosis for skin and lung metastases is better. A worse prognosis is linked to liver, bone, and brain metastases. When there is metastasis and the primary tumor's location is unknown, survival is improved.

Even though mucosal melanoma (such as rectal melanoma) and melanoma of the soft parts, such as ocular melanoma, tend to metastasize more readily, there is not enough conclusive evidence to properly stage these cases and provide a prognosis. Regression may improve survival, but it is impossible to determine the initial size of a melanoma after it has regressed, and as a result, the original tumor is frequently worse than what a pathology report may suggest.

Approximately 200 genes have been identified as prognostic markers in melanoma. Some of these genes are considered unfavorable, as high expression levels are linked to poorer survival outcomes, while others are considered favorable, with high expression associated with longer survival times. Examples of unfavorable genes include MCM6 and TIMELESS, while an example of a favorable gene is WIPI1. An increased neutrophil-to-lymphocyte ratio is associated with worse outcomes.

A Closer Look

How do Dermatologists Treat Skin Cancer?

One of the most prevalent forms of cancer in the world, skin cancer is diagnosed in an increasing number of people each day. Experts in identifying, treating, and even preventing it before it begins are dermatologists.

Dermatologists are the superheroes taking a stand against skin cancer, using their expertise, precision, and compassion to combat this disease.

Depending on the type and stage of the disease, dermatologists have a wide range of treatment options when diagnosing skin cancer. It could be removed surgically, treated with creams or light therapy, frozen with cryotherapy, zapped with radiation, or treated with a specialized procedure known as Mohs micrographic surgery.

It goes beyond simply treating skin cancer, though. Dermatologists also instruct patients on preventative measures to avoid developing the condition in the first place. They remind us to regularly check our skin for any changes and discuss the importance of wearing sunscreen, hats, and sunglasses when it's sunny outside. By disseminating this information, they aid in the early detection of skin cancer, which is essential for recovery.

Dermatologists are similar to skin health protectors. In addition to treating skin cancer, they also provide skin safety and health education. With their assistance, skin cancer is highly preventable.

Diagnosing Skin Cancer

Dermatologists are skilled at detecting signs of potential skin issues. By using a dermatoscope, they can closely examine moles and spots for any abnormalities. This tool allows them to see even the smallest details of the skin, making it easier to identify anything that appears concerning. If they come across something suspicious, they will conduct a biopsy by taking a small sample of the area to examine under a microscope and determine if it is cancerous. It is akin to solving a puzzle to safeguard one's health!

Types of Skin Cancer

There are various types of skin cancer, including basal cell carcinoma (BCC), squamous cell carcinoma (SCC), and melanoma. Each type has its own distinctive appearance. BCC typically appears as a shiny bump or a spot that matches the color of the skin. SCC may present as a rough patch or a persistent sore. Melanoma, the most severe type, can manifest in irregular shapes and colors.

Now, let's talk about how dermatologists treat these types of skin cancer:

Surgical Excision: Dermatologists often use surgery to remove skin cancers that haven't spread.

They cut out the cancer along with a bit of healthy skin around it to make sure it's all gone.

Mohs Micrographic Surgery: This special surgery is used when the cancer isn't easy to see or is in a sensitive area, like your face. Dermatologists inspect small skin samples under a microscope to verify the cancer is gone.

Cryotherapy: This treatment freezes and destroys cancer cells. It's often used for cancers that are just on the surface of the skin.

Radiation Therapy: If surgery isn't an option, dermatologists might suggest radiation to target the cancer cells with strong energy rays.

Topical Treatments: For early skin cancers or spots that might become cancerous, dermatologists can prescribe creams that help your body fight off the abnormal cells.

Photodynamic Therapy (PDT): This treatment uses a special light and a medicine to kill the cancer cells while keeping the healthy skin safe.

Immunotherapy: Dermatologists can boost your body's own defenses to fight cancer with medicines that help your immune system recognize and attack the cancer cells.

Follow-up and Surveillance

Dermatologists emphasize the significance of continuing with routine examinations following treatment to ensure overall health. They will monitor for any indications of recurrence of the cancer or the appearance of new lesions. By regularly checking your skin and keeping yourself informed, you can take charge of the health of your skin.

Now, let's talk about preventing skin cancer:

1. *Sun Protection:* It's important to shield yourself from the sun's harmful rays. Try to stay in the shade, especially between 10 in the morning and 4 in the afternoon. Wear protective gear like hats, sunglasses, and lightweight clothes that cover your skin.
2. *Sunscreen:* Remember to apply sunscreen with SPF 30 or higher on your skin, especially areas at risk of sun exposure. Reapply it every two hours or more often if you're swimming or sweating.
3. *Avoid Tanning Beds:* Steer clear of indoor tanning beds, which can increase your risk of skin cancer, including the dangerous melanoma.
4. *Regular Skin Checks:* Evaluate your skin monthly to monitor any changes in moles, freckles, or other spots. Let your dermatologist know right away if you notice anything strange.
5. *Professional Skin Exams:* Schedule regular appointments with a dermatologist, especially if you've had a lot of sun exposure, have a family history of skin cancer, or have a bunch of moles.
6. *Know Your Skin:* Learn about the ABCDEs of melanoma: Asymmetry, irregular Borders, varied Colors, Diameters larger than 6mm, and Evolution, meaning changes in size, shape, or color.

Summary

- Skin cancers are cancers that arise from the skin. They are due to the development of abnormal cells that have the ability to invade or spread to other parts of the body. Skin cancer is the most commonly diagnosed form of cancer in humans.
- Basal-cell carcinoma (BCC), also known as basal-cell cancer, basalioma or rodent ulcer, is the most common type of skin cancer. It often appears as a painless raised area of skin, which may be shiny with small blood vessels running over it.
- Basal-cell carcinoma is named after the basal cells that form the lowest layer of the epidermis. It is thought to develop from the folliculo–sebaceous–apocrine germinative cells called trichoblasts (of note, trichoblastic carcinoma is a term sometimes used to refer to a rare type of aggressive skin cancer that may resemble a benign trichoblastoma, and can also closely resemble basal cell carcinoma).
- Cutaneous squamous-cell carcinoma (cSCC), also known as squamous-cell carcinoma of the skin or squamous-cell skin cancer, is one of the three principal types of skin cancer, alongside basal-cell carcinoma and melanoma. cSCC typically presents as a hard lump with a scaly surface, though it may also present as an ulcer.
- SCC of the skin begins as a small nodule and as it enlarges the center becomes necrotic and sloughs and the nodule turns into an ulcer, and generally are developed from an actinic keratosis.
- Melanoma is the most dangerous type of skin cancer; it develops from the melanin-producing cells known as melanocytes. It typically occurs in the skin, but may rarely occur in the mouth, intestines, or eye (uveal melanoma).
- Early signs of melanoma are changes to the shape or color of existing moles or, in the case of nodular melanoma, the appearance of a new lump anywhere on the skin. At
- Radiation therapy is often used after surgical resection for patients with locally or regionally advanced melanoma or for patients with un-resectable distant metastases.

References

1. Bonilla, X., Parmentier, L., King, B., Bezrukov, F., Kaya, G., Zoete, V., Seplyarskiy, V. B., Sharpe, H. J., McKee, T., Letourneau, A., et al. (2016). Genomic analysis identifies new drivers and progression pathways in skin basal cell carcinoma. *Nature Genetics, 48*, 398–406. https://doi.org/10.1038/ng.3525.
2. Brose, M. S., Volpe, P., Feldman, M., et al. (2002). BRAF and RAS mutations in human lung cancer and melanoma. *Cancer Research, 62*, 6997–7000.
3. Cakir, B. Ö., Adamson, P., & Cingi, C. (2012). Epidemiology and economic burden of nonmelanoma skin cancer. *Facial Plastic Surgery Clinics of North America, 20*(4), 419–422.
4. Chen, K., Craig, J. C., & Shumack, S. (2005). Oral retinoids for the prevention of skin cancers in solid organ transplant recipients: A systematic review of randomized controlled trials. *British Journal of Dermatology, 152*, 518–523. https://doi.org/10.1111/j.1365-2133.2005.06347.x.
5. Cohen, P. R. (2022). Cutaneous basal cell carcinoma *in situ*: A case series. *Cureus, 14*(9), e29479. https://doi.org/10.7759/cureus.29479.

6. De Zwaan, S. E., & Haass, N. K. (2009). Genetics of basal cell carcinoma: Basal cell carcinoma genetics. *Australasian Journal of Dermatology, 51*, 81–92. https://doi.org/10.1111/j.1440-0960.2009.00579.x.

7. Dinnes, J., Deeks, J. J., Grainge, M. J., Chuchu, N., Ferrante di Ruffano, L., Matin, R. N., et al. (2018). Visual inspection for diagnosing cutaneous melanoma in adults. *The Cochrane Database of Systematic Reviews, 2018*(12), CD013194. https://doi.org/10.1002/14651858.CD013194.

8. Dong, J., Phelps, R. G., Qiao, R., Yao, S., Benard, O., Ronai, Z., & Aaronson, S. A. (2003). BRAF oncogenic mutations correlate with progression rather than initiation of human melanoma. *Cancer Research, 63*, 3883–3885.

9. Esther, R. J., Lamps, L., & Schwartz, H. S. (1999). Marjolin ulcers: Secondary carcinomas in chronic wounds. *Journal of the Southern Orthopaedic Association, 8*, 181–187.

10. Fania, L., Didona, D., Di Pietro, F. R., Verkhovskaia, S., Morese, R., Paolino, G., Donati, M., Ricci, F., Coco, V., Ricci, F., Candi, E., Abeni, D., & Dellambra, E. (2021). Cutaneous squamous cell carcinoma: From pathophysiology to novel therapeutic approaches. *Biomedicines, 9*(2), 171. https://doi.org/10.3390/biomedicines9020171.

11. Greene, M., & Fraumeni, J. (1979). The hereditary variant of familial melanoma. In W. Clark, L. Goldman, & M. Mastrangelo (Eds.), *Human Malignant Melanoma* (pp. 139–166). New York, NY: Grune and Stratton.

12. Henrikson, N. B., Morrison, C. C., Blasi, P. R., Nguyen, M., Shibuya, K. C., & Patnode, C. D. (2018). Behavioral counseling for skin cancer prevention: Evidence report and systematic review for the US Preventive Services Task Force. *JAMA, 319*, 1143–1157. https://doi.org/10.1001/jama.2017.21630.

13. King, R., Weilbaecher, K. N., McGill, G., Cooley, E., Mihm, M., & Fisher, D. E. (1999). Microphthalmia transcription factor: A sensitive and specific melanocyte marker for melanoma diagnosis. *American Journal of Pathology, 155*, 731–738.

14. Lens, M. B., & Dawes, M. (2004). Global perspectives of contemporary epidemiological trends of cutaneous malignant melanoma. *British Journal of Dermatology, 150*, 179–185.

15. Muranushi, C., Olsen, C. M., Pandeya, N., & Green, A. C. (2015). Aspirin and nonsteroidal anti-inflammatory drugs can prevent cutaneous squamous cell carcinoma: A systematic review and meta-analysis. *Journal of Investigative Dermatology, 135*, 975–983. https://doi.org/10.1038/jid.2014.531.

16. Nijsten, T. E., & Stern, R. S. (2003). Oral retinoid use reduces cutaneous squamous cell carcinoma risk in patients with psoriasis treated with psoralen-UVA: A nested cohort study. *Journal of the American Academy of Dermatology, 49*, 644–650. https://doi.org/10.1067/S0190-9622(03)01587-1.

17. Ramachandran, S., Lear, J. T., Ramsay, H., Smith, A. G., Bowers, B., Hutchinson, P. E., Jones, P. W., Fryer, A. A., & Strange, R. C. (1999). Presentation with multiple cutaneous basal cell carcinomas: Association of glutathione S-transferase and cytochrome P450 genotypes with clinical phenotype. *Cancer Epidemiology, Biomarkers & Prevention, 8*, 61–67.

18. Reifenberger, J., Wolter, M., Knobbe, C. B., Köhler, B., Schönicke, A., Scharwächter, C., Kumar, K., Blaschke, B., Ruzicka, T., & Reifenberger, G. (2005). Somatic mutations in the PTCH, SMOH, SUFUH, and TP53 genes in sporadic basal cell carcinomas. *British Journal of Dermatology, 152*, 43–51. https://doi.org/10.1111/j.1365-2133.2005.06353.x.

19. Riobo, N. A., Lu, K., Ai, X., Haines, G. M., & Emerson, C. P. (2006). Phosphoinositide 3-kinase and Akt are essential for Sonic Hedgehog signaling. *Proceedings of the National Academy of Sciences, 103*, 4505–4510. https://doi.org/10.1073/pnas.0504337103.

20. Scherer, D., Bermejo, J. L., Rudnai, P., Gurzau, E., Koppova, K., Hemminki, K., & Kumar, R. (2007). MC1R variants associated susceptibility to basal cell carcinoma of skin: Interaction with host factors and XRCC3 polymorphism. *International Journal of Cancer, 122*, 1787–1793. https://doi.org/10.1002/ijc.23257.

21. Soufir, N., Avril, M. F., Chompret, A., et al. (1998). Prevalence of p16 and CDK4 germline mutations in 48 melanoma-prone families in France. *Human Molecular Genetics, 7*, 209–216.

22. Torti, D. C., Christensen, B. C., Storm, C. A., Fortuny, J., Perry, A. E., Zens, M. S., Stukel, T., Spencer, S. K., Nelson, H. H., & Karagas, M. R. (2011). Analgesic and nonsteroidal anti-inflammatory use in relation to nonmelanoma skin cancer: A population-based case-control study. *Journal of the American Academy of Dermatology, 65*, 304–312. https://doi.org/10.1016/j.jaad.2010.05.042.

23. Watt, T. C., Inskip, P. D., Stratton, K., Smith, S. A., Kry, S. F., Sigurdson, A. J., Stovall, M., Leisenring, W., Robison, L. L., & Mertens, A. C. (2012). Radiation-related risk of basal cell carcinoma: A report from the Childhood Cancer Survivor Study. *Journal of the National Cancer Institute, 104*, 1240–1250. https://doi.org/10.1093/jnci/djs298.

Chapter 7

PEDIATRIC DERMATOLOGY

Contents

Introduction

About one-third of all consultations in the context of outpatient pediatric and dermatological services are related to childhood dermatological issues. Parents who have children with skin disorders may experience anxiety. General practitioners should be knowledgeable about the most common skin conditions, as they might not always be able to get a pediatric dermatologist consultation right away.

Orientation and Directional Terms

Term	Definition	Illustration
Hemangiomas	Hemangiomas are common growths of blood vessels found on your skin. These growths can appear anywhere on your body, especially on your face, chest and back, as red or purple lumps. Hemangiomas are usually harmless and tend to resolve on their own.	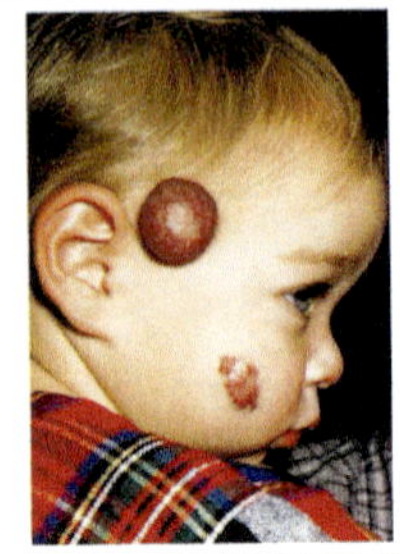
Propranolol	Propranolol is a medication of the beta blocker class. It is used to treat high blood pressure, a number of types of irregular heart rate, thyrotoxicosis, capillary hemangiomas, performance anxiety, and essential tremors, as well to prevent migraine headaches, and to prevent further heart problems in those with angina or previous heart attacks.	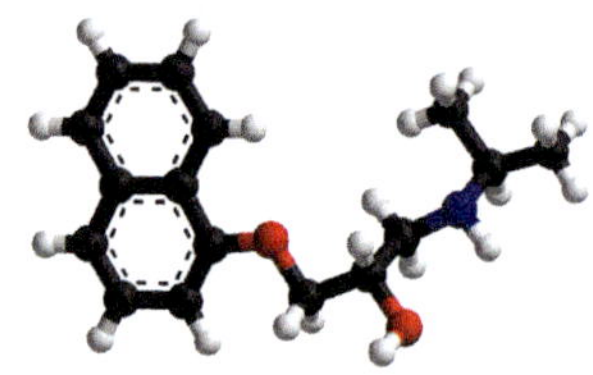
Benign tumor	A benign tumor is a mass of cells that does not invade neighboring tissue or metastasize. Compared to malignant tumors, benign tumors generally have a slower growth rate.	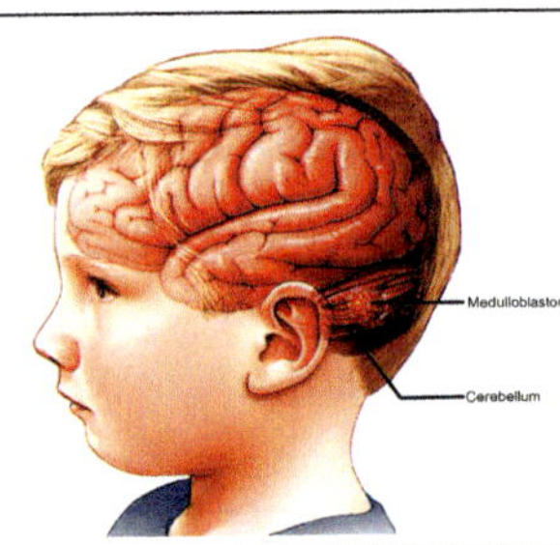
Echocardiography	Echocardiography, also known as cardiac ultrasound, is a non-invasive medical imaging technique that uses ultrasound to produce a picture of the heart. The image is called an echocardiogram, cardiac echo, or simply an echo.	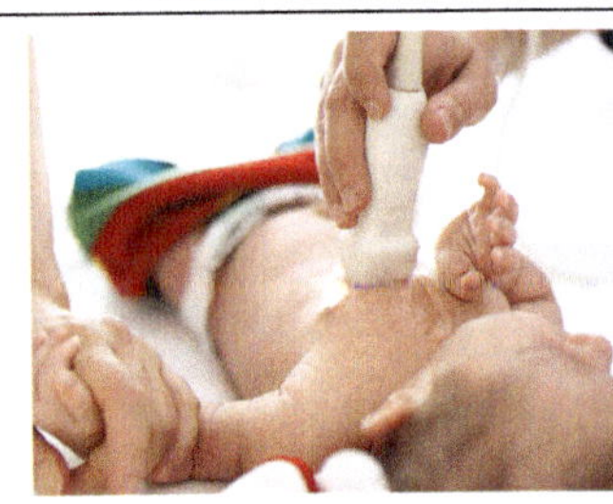
Prednisolone	Prednisolone is a medicine used to treat a wide range of health problems including allergies, blood disorders, skin diseases, inflammation, infections and certain cancers and to prevent organ rejection after a transplant. It helps by reducing swelling (inflammation) and can also calm down your immune system.	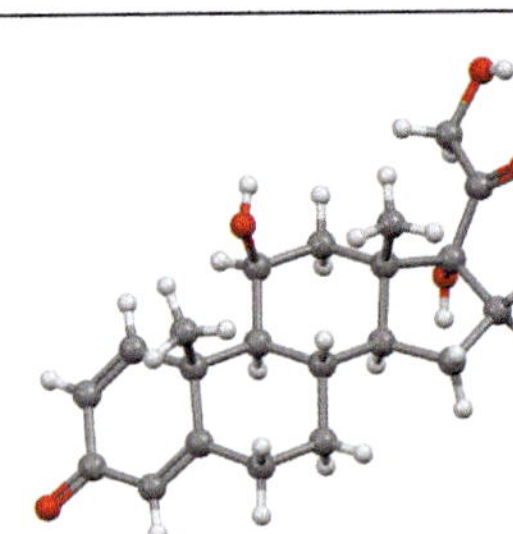

7.1. Infantile Hemangiomas

An infantile hemangioma (IH), also known as a strawberry mark, is a harmless vascular tumor that commonly affects infants. It may also be referred to as capillary hemangioma, strawberry hemangioma, strawberry birthmark, or strawberry nevus. The lesion appears as a raised red or blue mark on the skin and usually develops within the first four weeks of life, reaching its peak size around five months before gradually shrinking and eventually disappearing over the span of a few years. In some cases, residual skin changes may remain even after the hemangioma has faded (Darrow et al., 2015) (Figure 7.1).

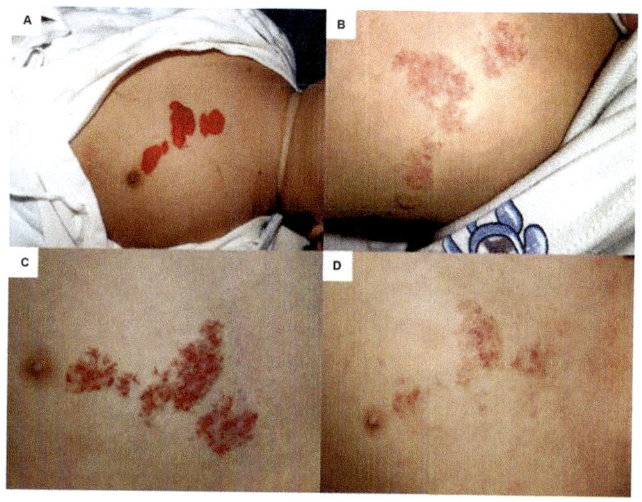

Figure 7.1. *The infantile hemangioma in patient 1 at different periods. (A) Proliferating infantile hemangioma before oral propranolol therapy. (B) Involuted infantile hemangioma when the patient was admitted for pneumonia at the age of 13 months. (C) Infantile hemangioma worsened after nearly 1 day of oral procaterol therapy. (D) Involuted hemangioma after 1 month of oral propranolol therapy and one laser therapy.*

Source: Chen Q, Zhang Y, Sun C, Liu L, Luo X, Wang H and Ni S (2022) Case report: Deterioration of infantile hemangioma related to oral or nebulized administration of β2-AR agonist: Three cases reports. Front. Oncol. 12:1000099. doi: 10.3389/fonc.2022.1000099.

It's unclear why they occur in the first place. About 10% of the time, it seems that they run in families. A few cases have been linked to additional anomalies like PHACE syndrome. In most cases, the diagnosis is made based on the appearance and symptoms. Medical imaging may occasionally help with the diagnosis.

Apart from close observation, no treatment is usually required in these cases. Hemangiomas can grow quickly, then halt and fade gradually; the greatest improvement usually happens by the time a person reaches the age of 35. Although the appearance of this birthmark may be concerning, doctors usually advise letting it go until it goes away on its own, unless it is obstructing the nose or vision. However, in some circumstances, problems may arise, and it is advised to use medications like propranolol or steroids. On rare occasions, laser therapy or surgery may be used. This benign tumor is frequently found in babies, with a prevalence of 5–10% in all births. It is more common in females, white babies, premature infants, and those with low birth weight. These growths can appear on any part of the body, but 83% are typically found on the head or neck region (Chen et al, 2022) (Figure 7.2).

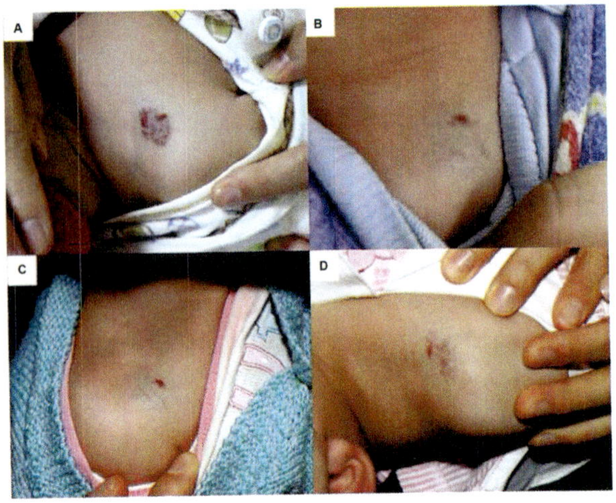

Figure 7.2. *The infantile hemangioma in patient 2 at different periods. (A) Proliferating infantile hemangioma before oral propranolol therapy and laser therapy. (B) Involuted infantile hemangioma when the patient was admitted for acute bronchitis at the age of 15 months. (C) Infantile hemangioma showed a proliferation trend after 7 days of nebulized salbutamol treatment. (D) Infantile hemangioma worsened after receiving another 3 days of nebulized salbutamol therapy in the outpatient.*

Source: Chen Q, Zhang Y, Sun C, Liu L, Luo X, Wang H and Ni S (2022) Case report: Deterioration of infantile hemangioma related to oral or nebulized administration of β2-AR agonist: Three cases reports. Front. Oncol. 12:1000099. doi: 10.3389/fonc.2022.1000099.

7.1.1. Signs and Symptoms

It usually occurs in the first few weeks or months of life for infantile hemangiomas. They are more prevalent in Caucasians, females, premature infants weighing less than 3 pounds (1.4 kg), and twin pregnancies. Early lesions can have the appearance of a bruise, a white patch, or a red scratch or patch. Though they can happen practically anywhere, they usually happen on the head and neck. The IH's color and appearance are determined by its depth and location relative to the skin's surface.

Higher in the skin, superficial IHs are characterized by their bright red, erythematous to reddish-purple appearance. Flat and telangiectatic superficial lesions consist of a macule or patch of tiny, variably branching capillary blood vessels. Additionally, they have the ability to rise above the skin in the form of raised islands, papules, and confluent bright red plaques. Because raised superficial hemangiomas can resemble the side of a strawberry without seeds, infantile hemangiomas have historically been referred to as strawberry marks or strawberry hemangiomas. This term is still frequently used in lay language.

There is a chance that superficial IHs in specific areas, like the groin/perianal regions, neck folds, and posterior scalp, will become ulcerated. Painful erosions or ulcers, as well as black crusted papules or plaques, can be symptoms of ulcerated hemangiomas. Secondary bacterial infections, which can manifest as pain, drainage, odor, or yellow crusting, are common after ulcerations. Bleeding is another risk associated with ulcers, especially in deep or abrasive areas. Infants with more than five superficial hemangiomas may also have extracutaneous hemangiomas, the most common of which is a hepatic hemangioma of the liver, for which an ultrasound examination is necessary.

Deep infantile hemangiomas appear as poorly defined, bluish patches that can develop into bumps, lumps, or larger growths. These growing lesions are often compressible but firm to the touch. Some deep hemangiomas may show visible superficial capillaries around the main growth or nearby veins. Deep hemangiomas tend to appear later than superficial ones and may have longer and delayed growth phases. While they rarely open into sores, deep hemangiomas can cause issues depending on where they are located, how big they are, and how quickly they grow. Hemangiomas near delicate structures can press on surrounding tissues during the growth phase, such as the outer ear canal or eyelid. Mixed hemangiomas are simply a mix of superficial and deep types, which may not become noticeable until months later. Patients may have any combination of superficial, deep, or mixed infantile hemangiomas.

IHs are frequently categorized as segmental, indeterminate, or focal/localized. Focal IHs seem to be confined to a particular area and to originate from a single spot. Segmental hemangiomas are bigger and give the impression of encircling a specific body part. Larger or segmental hemangiomas that cover a significant area occasionally have underlying abnormalities that need to be looked into, particularly if they are on the face, sacrum, or pelvis.

An IH is usually painless and does not bleed unless ulceration occurs. If something is heavy and obstructs a vital orifice, discomfort could result.

7.1.1.1. Complications

Complications are almost never linked to IHs. Ulcerations, or their breakdown at the surface, can be uncomfortable and problematic. Deep ulcerations can cause severe discomfort, bleeding, and infection. Breathing may become difficult if a laryngeal hemangioma forms. A developing hemangioma close to the eye may obstruct or deviate the eye, which can result in amblyopia. Extremely big hemangiomas hardly ever result in high-output heart failure because of the volume of blood that has to be pumped to extra blood vessels. Bone erosion may result from lesions next to the bone.

Psychosocial complications are the reason for the majority of complaints regarding IHs. A person's appearance may be impacted by the condition, which may draw notice from others and elicit negative responses. If the lip or nose is affected, there are more issues because surgical correction of these deformities can be challenging. Psychological harm is a possibility as soon as a person reaches school age. In the event that sufficient spontaneous improvement has not happened, it is crucial to think about treatment before school starts. Because of the extreme stretching that causes alterations in surface texture, large IHs may leave visible skin changes.

PHACES syndrome is a condition that may be linked to large segmental hemangiomas of the head and neck. Large segmental hemangiomas covering the lumbar spine have been linked to LUMBAR syndrome, a disorder that is characterized by dysraphism, renal, and urogenital issues. Infants with multiple cutaneous hemangiomas may have liver hemangiomas. It is frequently advised to screen infants with five or more skin hemangiomas for liver involvement.

7.1.2. Causes

Although the exact cause of hemangiomas is still unknown, several studies have indicated that estrogen signaling plays a key role in proliferation. The stimulus could be a combination of increased circulating estrogen after birth and localized hypoxia of soft tissues. Additionally, researchers proposed the theory that hemangiomagenesis results from the maternal placenta embolizing to the fetal dermis during gestation. Nevertheless, this theory was refuted by a different team of researchers who performed genetic analyses of single-nucleotide polymorphism in hemangioma tissue in comparison to the mother's DNA. Additional research has demonstrated the part that elevated vasculogenesis and angiogenesis play in the development of hemangiomas.

7.1.3. Diagnosis

The majority of IHs are diagnosable through physical examination and history taking. Rarely, additional diagnostic tests such as cytology or histopathology, magnetic resonance imaging, or ultrasound with Doppler are required to confirm the diagnosis. IHs are typically absent at birth, though they can show up as a tiny patch of pallor, telangiectasias, or duskiness. Upon birth, a fully developed mass typically suggests an alternative diagnosis. Deep hemangiomas in the deep dermis and subcutis can appear blue and feel firm or rubbery to the touch. Superficial hemangiomas in the upper dermis are bright red in color. Both characteristics are possible in mixed hemangiomas. A rare kind of IH known as minimally proliferative IH is characterized by fine macular telangiectasias with sporadic bright-red, papular proliferative components. In the lower body, minimally proliferative IHs are more prevalent.

When diagnosing, a detailed history of the IH's growth characteristics can be highly beneficial. IHs grow quickly in the first 4 to 8 weeks of life, mostly through volumetric growth as opposed to radial growth. Usually, a slower growth phase lasting six to nine months ensues after this, with 80% of the growth finished in three months. Ultimately, IHs develop over many years. Large, deep IHs, whose discernible growth begins later and lasts longer, and minimally proliferative His, which do not significantly proliferate, are the exceptions to these growth characteristics. Imaging or histopathology can assist in confirming the diagnosis if the physical examination and growth history do not provide a clear diagnosis (which occurs frequently in deep hemangiomas with minimal cutaneous involvement). An IH in the proliferative phase typically lacks direct arteriovenous shunting and manifests on Doppler ultrasound as a high-flow, soft-tissue mass. IHs exhibit a well-circumscribed lesion on MRI with fast-flow vessels, an increase in signal intensity on T1- and T2-weighted sequences, and a strong enhancement following gadolinium injections. Excisional biopsy, skin biopsy, or fine-needle aspiration can all be used to obtain tissue for diagnosis. IHs are unencapsulated aggregates of densely packed, thin-walled capillaries that typically have an endothelium lining when viewed under a microscope. There is not much connective tissue separating blood-filled vessels. They could have an organized and thrombosed lumina. It is possible to see hemosiderin pigment deposition as a result of vessel rupture. When differentiating between IHs and other items on the differential diagnosis, like vascular malformations, the GLUT-1 histochemical marker can be useful (North et al, 2000).

7.1.3.1. Liver

Of all liver hemangiomas, 16% are infantile hemangiomas. Typically, its diameter is between one and two centimeters. Instead of the typical hemangioma's slow, centripetal, nodular filling of the lesions, it might exhibit a flash-filling phenomenon, in which the contrast material in the lesion is rapidly enhanced. It exhibits quick filling during the arterial phase on CT and MRI, with contrast retention during the venous and delayed phases.

7.1.4. Management of Infantile Hemangiomas

7.1.4.1. Treatment Indications

The type of hemangioma, stage of the lesion, location, and extent, number, and distribution of the lesion (segmental/non-segmental), associated systemic involvement, presence or absence of ulceration, and psychological distress of the child or parents are the factors that determine how IH is treated. Intervention is generally required for any IH that poses a threat to function (ocular, ear, nasal tip, lip, large disfiguring facial lesion, and genitalia involvement) or a threat to life (airway lesion), which accounts for 10–20% of cases. For the vast majority of cases that remain, active non-intervention is all that is required. This includes educating patients about treatment options, the natural course of the condition, and proactive guidance. Systemic steroids and propranolol are the two main drugs in the management of IH.

7.1.4.2. Pre-Treatment Evaluation

The majority of IH cases can be diagnosed clinically, but in questionable cases, imaging tests (MRI, Doppler ultrasound), or tissue biopsies, may be necessary. Depending on the site(s) and degree of involvement, more research might be needed.

Visceral hemangiomatosis may be linked to segmental hemangiomas, and the site of cutaneous involvement is frequently correlated with the location of visceral lesions. A comprehensive ophthalmological, cardiac, and neurological evaluation should be performed on infants with large segmental hemangiomas on the face as they are at risk for PHACES syndrome (Posterior fossa anomalies, Hemangiomas, Arterial anomalies, Coarctation of aorta and Cardiac defects, Eye abnormalities, Sternal clefting, and Supra-umbilical raphe). In these infants, magnetic resonance imaging (MRI) combined with head and neck angiography is typically recommended. Segmental hemangiomas in the perineal region are similar to PHACES syndrome in that they may be linked to anogenital or urogenital system malformations. These include PELVIS (perineal hemangioma, external genitalia malformations, lipomyelomeningocele, vesicorenal abnormalities, imperforate anus, and skin tag) syndrome and SACRAL (spinal dysraphism, anogenital, cutaneous, renal, and urologic anomalies, associated with an angioma of lumbosacral localization) and angioma of lumbosacral localization. Lumbosacral hemangiomas could be a sign of latent spinal dysraphism. As a screening test, a spinal MRI is recommended for all cases of lumbosacral hemangiomas.

If hemangiomas are found on the cervicofacial, mandibular, or "beard" distribution, laryngeal involvement may result. Infants affected by this should be referred for a laryngeal examination and monitored for indications of airway obstruction, such as stridor or hoarseness. Another group of infants at risk for visceral involvement is those with multiple cutaneous hemangiomas (diffuse neonatal hemangiomatosis), for which abdominal ultrasonography is usually advised to screen for hepatic involvement. Large proliferative hemangiomas have been shown to have elevated iodothyronine deiodinase levels, which may result in hypothyroidism. Although elevated iodothyronine deiodinase activity has also been found in certain large cutaneous lesions, the majority of hypothyroidism cases to date have been linked to hepatic hemangiomatosis. Therefore, it is advised that patients with large cutaneous hemangiomas or hepatic hemangiomatosis undergo serial thyroid function tests.

Following the decision to treat the hemangioma, pre-treatment studies ought to be customized for the selected therapeutic approach. The children should be evaluated for the following contraindications before starting propranolol therapy: bronchial asthma, heart failure, sinus bradycardia, hypoglycemia, hypotension, heart block, and known allergies to propranolol. A comprehensive cardiopulmonary assessment, including blood pressure, blood sugar, and pulse rate, should be part of the initial examination. Generally speaking, a baseline electrocardiogram (ECG) is advised. Echocardiography is not a routine test, but it might be necessary to rule out structural and functional heart conditions. Before beginning steroid therapy, a pre-treatment work-up is necessary to rule out active infection or primary immunodeficiency disease. This includes a baseline anthropometric examination (weight, height), blood pressure, serum biochemistry, chest X-ray, urine, and stool microscopy, and complete blood count with differential leucocyte count. These tests should be monitored on a serial basis.

7.1.4.3. Corticosteroids

Prednisolone, a type of systemic corticosteroid, has been the cornerstone of IH treatment for many years. Although the exact mechanism of action of steroids is unknown, it is believed that they inhibit the stem cells in hemangiomas from producing vascular endothelial growth factor A (VEGF-A). The early stages of the proliferative phase are when steroids work best. 2–4 mg/kg/day is the usual recommended dose, and it should be taken until the hemangioma stops growing or shrinking, at which point it should be gradually tapered. When oral steroids are taken at a dose of 2–3 mg/kg/day, 75% of patients respond, when the dose of >3 mg/kg/day 94% of patients respond but with more side effects, and when the dose of less than 2 mg/kg/day is taken, 70% of patients experience poor response and a rebound phenomenon. Bennett along with others. In their meta-analysis, 184 kids from a 10-case series were examined regarding the effectiveness of corticosteroids for IH. Prednisone was used for an average of 1.8 months (range: 0.5–5.4 months) at a mean dose of 2.9 mg/kg (1–4.5 mg/kg/day), according to statistical analysis, before the dose was tapered. The average rebound rate was 36% (range, 0–65%), and the overall response rate was 84% (range, 60–100%). In a recent study, oral prednisolone administered for a mean of 9.16 weeks (range, 3–15 weeks) at a mean dose of 3.1 mg/kg/day showed a response in the lesions in 20 children with IH. With the tapering dose applied, the mean total length of treatment was 29.9 weeks (range: 15–44 weeks). During the course of their six- to one-year follow-up, 90% of the cases demonstrated an improvement of more than 25% and no cases of rebound phenomenon.

High dose pulse corticosteroids, such as methyl prednisolone 30 mg/kg/day infused over an hour each day for three days, may be helpful in cases of IH that require an immediate therapeutic response, such as large airway hemangiomas causing respiratory difficulties or large peri-ocular IH with complete visual axis occlusion. Usually, a shorter oral steroid regimen is needed after three or more monthly doses. Pope and associates. They found that oral corticosteroids provide greater clinical and biological benefits than pulsed steroids in their randomized controlled trial comparing oral versus high-dose pulse steroids in 20 children with problematic IH. However, patients in the oral steroid group had a higher frequency of side effects such as hypertension (18% vs. 13%), abnormal cortisol levels (78% vs. 60%) and growth retardation (Table 7.1).

Numerous side effects are linked to long-term steroid use. Boon and associates found cushingoid facies in 44 out of 62 children who received systemic corticosteroid therapy for hemangiomas. The cushingoid facies started 1 to 2 months after the children started receiving a dose of 2–3 mg/kg/day. Throughout the last few months of reducing steroids, the cushingoid facies spontaneously resolved.

In the two weeks to 16 months (mean, seven months; median, four months) following treatment, 22 (35%) of the children fell off their weight growth curve. Of these, 91% of the children returned to their baseline. Additionally, they saw a brief decline in weight gain in 26 kids (42%).

Table 7.1. Papers concerning treatment of cutaneous infantile hemangioma (CIH)

Publication (authors and year)	Type of study	Study population and treatment outcomes
de Castro et al. (2017)	Retrospective cohort study	18 patients (9 female) with vascular lip anomalies underwent a single or double pentagonal-shaped wedgeresection of the involved upper or lower lip
Hutchins et al. (2017)	Case report	a 3-year-old girl presenting diffuse cutaneous, hepatic and pulmonary IHs with progressive pulmonary hypertension treated with oral sirolimus
Kim et al. (2017)	Clinical trial	34 patients (15 boys, 19 girls) randomized to receive either propranolol or steroid treatment (17 in each treatment group). The treatment response rate in the propranolol group was 95.65%, and that of the steroid group was 91.94%. Propranolol was considered noninferior. There was no difference between the groups in safety outcomes
Mashiah et al. (2017)	Retrospective cohort study	63 patients with a total of 75 IHs treated with topical propranolol 4%. Of the total number of IHs, 43 (57.3%) showed a good response to treatment, 19 (25.3%) a partial response, and 13 (17.33%) poor or no response
Yu et al. (2017)	Case report	A 1-month-old female infant with LUMBAR syndrome treated with oral propranolol (2 mg/day)
Wang et al. (2017)	Clinical trial	40 infants treated with 2% propranolol cream followed up for 12 months after 3-month treatment. Poor response was observed in 2 patients, moderate response in 15 patients, good response in 17 patients, and excellent response in 6 patients
Ying et al. (2017)	Clinical trial	21 patients with superficial IH. Each lesion was divided into two regions; one part was treated with 0.5% topical timolol cream four times daily, and the other part was treated monthly with PDL. Both treatments were continued for 2–6 months. Both treatments resulted in significant clinical improvements after 3.39 sessions in the 2-month follow up
Le Sage et al. (2018)	Case series	6 patients of which 1 with an infantile hemangioma on the right forehead without intracranial extension treated with topical sirolimus 0.1% without improvement
Xu et al. (2018)	Clinical trial	Thirty-five children achieved the treatment of Intralesional Compound Betamethasone, 134 children achieved the treatment of oral propranolol, and 16 children achieved the treatment of topical carteolol. In the follow-up, the treatment could be repeated or switched to oral propranolol if the tumor tended to grow again. At the end of follow- up, 89% of the patients' tumors shrinked or involuted completely, 5 patients switched to oral propranolol

Igarashi et al. (2018)	Case report	A case of an extremely low-birth-weight infant with massive cutaneous IH complicated with hypothyroidism, which had improvement of hypothyroidism and regression of cutaneous hemangioma after propranolol therapy
Xu et al. (2020)	Retrospective cohort study	Eighty-one lip infantile hemangiomas patients treated with systemic propranolol (2 mg/kg/die). Lesions showed the same outcomes and prognosis involving the upper lips as the lower lips. Lesions involving the vermillion border had longer treatment lengths, poorer outcomes, and prognosis than lesions confined to one side of the vermilion
Chen et al. (2019)	Research study	The inhibitory effects of itraconazole on IH and its underlying molecular mechanisms were explored usingthe endothelial cells of mouse hemangioendothelioma (EOMA) cell line and infantile primary hemangioma endothelialcell (HemEC)
Tani et al. (2020)	Case series	A3-month-old boy with cheek's hemangioma (mixed type), a 3-month-old boy with forehead and abdomen's hemangioma (mixed type), a 6-month-old girl with head's hemangioma (superficial type), a 4-month-old girl with buttock's hemangioma (superficial type), and a 4-month-old boy with forehead's hemangioma (deep type). All patients treated with oral propranolol (3 mg/kg/die)
Diociaiuti et al. (2020)	Retrospective cohort study	Seven patients with intracranial or intraspinal infantile hemangiomas were selected and treated with oral propranolol, without side-effects
Zeng et al. (2020)	Research study	PRH-CNPs were tested on abdominal skin from Sprague Dawley (SD) rats to evaluate skin permeation. PRH-CNPs cytotoxicity on endothelial cells of mouse hemangioendothelioma (EOMA) was also assessed
Cheng et al. (2020)	Clinical trial	Forty-two children received 12 months of 0.5% TTM solution (24 assigned to the TTM group and 17 to the no-TTM group) The TTM group had fewer complications than the no-TTM group (4.2% versus 29%). Mean IH volume percentage reduction was significantly more for the and no-TTM group at 3, 6 and 12 months

Source: Macca L, Altavilla D, Di Bartolomeo L, Irrera N, Borgia F, Li Pomi F, Vaccaro F, Squadrito V, Squadrito F and Vaccaro M (2022) Update on Treatment of Infantile Hemangiomas: What's New in the Last Five Years?. Front. Pharmacol. 13:879602. doi: 10.3389/fphar.2022.879602.

Among them, 23 kids (mean, 7.4 months; median, 6 months) got back to where they were before starting therapy. For a longer amount of time, three kids stayed in the lower percentile. It was discovered that children who received therapy during the first three months of life or for longer than six months were more likely to experience this brief halt in their growth in height. In 2 weeks of therapy, personality changes like irritability, depression, euphoria, insomnia, and restlessness were reported in 29% of their cases. These changes vanished the moment the medication was stopped. Other side effects included steroid myopathy (n = 1), oral, and/or perineal candidiasis

(6%, n = 4), and gastric irritation (n = 13). There was no increase in the overall risk of bacterial infection. No patient experienced severe side effects like cataracts, osteoporosis, or aseptic necrosis of the femur head. George along with others discovered that 16 (73%) of the 22 kids who received systemic steroid treatment were fussy, irritable, or had sleeplessness. 13 out of the 15 patients (87%) who underwent testing had abnormal morning cortisol levels, and 10 patients (45%) had hypertension. Furthermore, two out of the three infants tested had abnormal results from a low-dose corticotropin stimulation test. Only one case (6%) had adrenal insufficiency (on a corticotropin stimulation test) after therapy was completed, and that condition normalized three months later. This study involved 16 infants with hemangiomas who were treated with prednisolone at doses of 2–3 mg/kg/day for four weeks, followed by a tapering period (mean duration of steroid therapy: seven and a half months) (Lomenick et al., 2009).

7.1.4.4. Propranolol

Recently, propranolol, a non-selective -β adrenergic receptor blocker, has become a viable treatment option for IH. Leaute-Labreze and associates in 2008 revealed that a child receiving propranolol treatment for obstructive hypertrophic cardiomyopathy had a regression of a facial IH. Since then, many publications detailing its therapeutic effectiveness and adverse effects have been published. It is currently the most widely used therapeutic approach for IH, especially for complicated and ulcerated IH.

There are three distinct pharmacological effects of oral propranolol: immediate, intermediate, and long-term effects. Within one to three days of the start of therapy, the lesion begins to soften and exhibit a noticeable color change. This has to do with propranolol's β2 inhibitory action, which reduces the release of vasodilator transmitters like nitric oxide. The early alterations in hemangiomas are caused by the feeding capillaries' subsequent vasoconstriction. Propranolol is currently regarded as the most promising treatment for IH with ulceration or hemangiomas involving critical structures like the eyes, airways, genitalia, and so on because of its quick clinical effect.

Pro-angiogenic factors—specifically, vascular endothelial growth factor (VEGF) and basic fibroblast growth factor (bFGF)—are more expressed during the proliferative phase of IH. Propranolol's intermediate effects are caused by VEGF and bFGF downregulation, which inhibits the proangiogenic cascade and angiogenesis. Propranolol's long-term effects are caused by apoptosis, which causes hemangioma regression. Its application in the post-proliferative phase might be due to this.

Propranolol should ideally be started as soon as a decision is made. It is always preferable to begin propranolol therapy as soon as possible to prevent the tumor from growing rapidly, even though there is no proof in the literature that doing so causes less deforming residual skin changes. According to a recent meta-analysis, oral propranolol was started at a mean age of 6 months and varied from 3 days to 10 years, encompassing 1264 children across 41 studies. Propranolol was given to 174 children in a single-center prospective study at a mean age of 4.8 months (0.9–29 months). Propranolol was started in infancy at a mean age of 4.5 months (range, 27 days-12 months) in a recent review of 28 studies on IH. Propranolol was started after the age of 12 months in 11 cases.

A target dose of 1–3 mg/kg has been suggested in the consensus conference report on hemangiomas that was recently released. Numerous researchers, however, support a daily dosage of 2 mg/kg. Hermans along with others. In their large prospective study, patients with hemangiomas causing airway obstruction or associated with recurrent severe bleeding from ulcerations were given a higher dose of 3 mg/kg/day.

The length of therapy for hemangioma depends on the type of hemangioma, how extensive it is, and the reasons for treatment. Hogeling et al. suggest a treatment plan of at least 6 months, which can be adjusted based on the specific type of hemangioma. For example, deep, and mixed IH may continue to grow until the child is 1 year old, so treatment may need to be extended. The average duration of treatment typically ranges from 6 to 10 months. In a recent study on propranolol treatment for complicated IH, the mean duration of treatment was 10.7 months. For deep and mixed hemangiomas, treatment may continue until the child is 12–16 months old, for ulcerated lesions up to 9–12 months old, and for deep peri-orbital and airway lesions up to 15–18 months old. Marqueling et al. found in a meta-analysis that propranolol was typically given for an average of 6.4 months, but could range from 1 week to 15 months in different studies involving 1264 children.

Although propranolol administered orally is known to be beneficial during the rapid proliferative phase, several reports have demonstrated involution in which propranolol was started at the end of the growth phase or later. Hogeling and associates included a mix of growing, plateauing, and involuting lesions in their trial involving 40 children with IH.

The overall response rate, according to a meta-analysis, is 98% (82–100%). Comparable effectiveness has also been noted in a sizable prospective investigation. Most published studies base their assessment of the treatment response on visual changes in serial photograph color, volume, and quality. A small number of studies classified the response according to the reduction percentage. Price along with others determined a hemangioma clearance of 75% or higher by comparing the volume reduction percentage, a cosmetically acceptable outcome determined by the doctor and/or parent, and the absence of need for additional treatment. They report >75% clearance in 81% (48/59) of the cases over a mean duration of 7.9 months based on these criteria. Talaat along with others reported that of their 80 cases with IH in 5–8 months, 75% had clearance and 94% had clearance of >50% (mean 6.53 ± 0.75).

The therapeutic efficacy of propranolol therapy is evident right away. Sans et al. observed rapid color changes (within 24 hours) and softening in every case of 32 children with severe IH who received a daily dose of propranolol at a dose of 2–3 mg/kg. Within 48 hours, the symptoms of airway obstruction and hemodynamic compromise subsided, according to Hermans et al. additionally reported that respiratory symptoms in cases of airway hemangioma improved within hours of starting propranolol treatment. Another medication that appears to be promising for ulcerated hemangiomas is propranolol. It has been observed that painful hemangioma ulcerations heal fully in two months. Oral propranolol significantly reduced the duration of ulceration in a recent study involving 20 children with ulcerated IH when compared to the control group (8.7 vs. 22.4 per week, $P < 0.01$) (Figure 7.3).

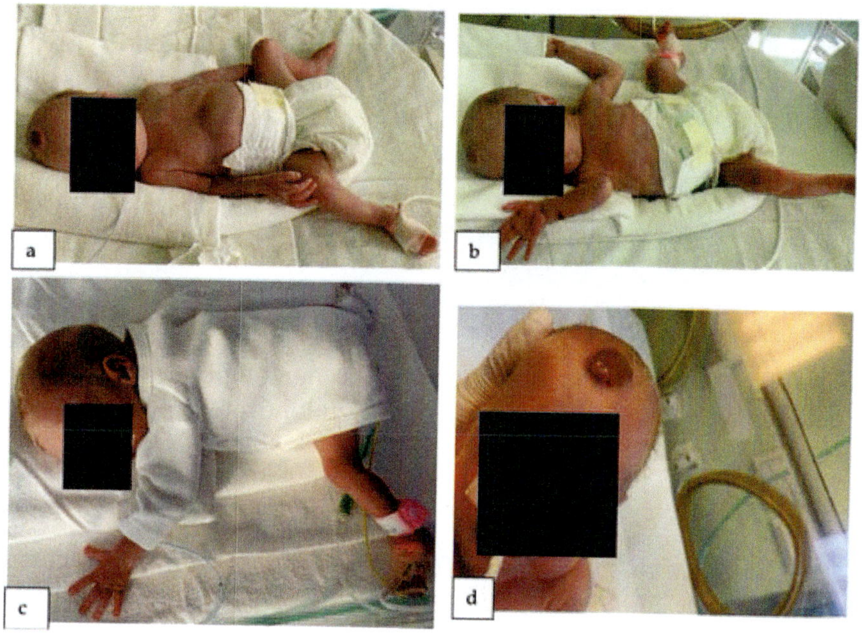

The infant in the intensive care unit. (**a**) The infant 30 days old. Notice the hemangioma on her forehead. The infant was being fed through gavage. (**b**) The infant is 40 days old. The hemangioma on the forehead increased its dimensions. Also notice the hemangioma on her right forearm. (**c**) the infant 45 days old. (**d**) the infant 50 days old. Close-up of the hemangioma on her forehead.

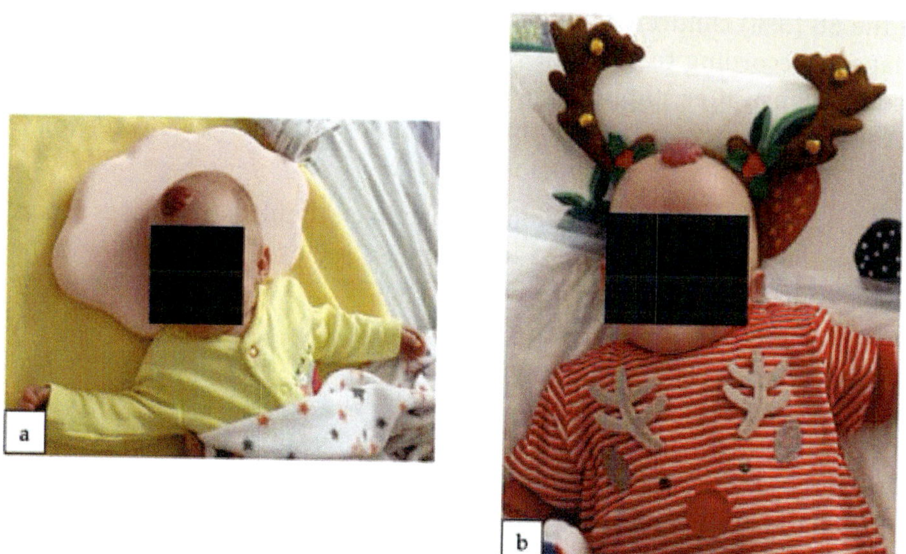

The infant at 2 months, 3 weeks (**a**), and 4 months (**b**). Notice the impressive forehead hemangioma.

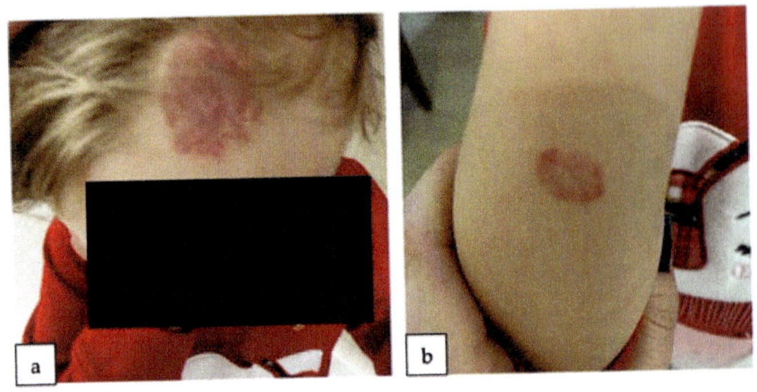

The patient, 2 years old. Notice the improvement of the hemangioma on her forehead (**a**) and forearm (**b**). The hemangiomas were treated with propranolol oral suspension for 10 months and afterwards with local ointment for 2 months.

Figure 7.3. *Case study*

Source: Sandru F, Petca A, Radu A-M, Preda AG, Turenschi A, Constantin AT, Miulescu R-G. Infantile Hemangioma: Risk Factors and Management in a Preterm Patient—A Case Report. Reports. 2024; 7(1):3. https://doi.org/10.3390/reports7010003.

Hemangioma regrowth, also known as rebound, can happen when treatment is stopped and the tumor grows larger, changes color, or does both. According to studies, there is a higher chance of rebound growth if propranolol is stopped before the age of one year. Because the proliferative phase of deeper hemangiomas may last longer, treating them early may increase the risk of rebound growth. Two of the 68 (3%) children who had propranolol started at 3 months and stopped at 10 months had relapsed, according to a recent retrospective analysis. In another study, 2 out of 32 cases experienced a relapse after stopping the medication before turning 1 year old. Menezes along with others. In their meta-analysis, they discovered that 14 out of 64 kids receiving treatment for an average of 51 months experienced a relapse.

Propranolol-resistant infantile hemangiomas have been identified as cases where there is no response to treatment with oral propranolol at a dosage of at least 2 mg/kg/day, either during the proliferative phase or in the post-proliferative phase, after a minimum of 4 weeks of treatment. This resistance has been reported to occur in approximately 0.9% of cases (10 out of 1130). The majority of these cases (8 out of 10) were found in France, with most of them located on the face. In five cases, children in the proliferative phase (under 4.2 months) showed continued growth despite treatment, while the remaining five cases (over 8 months) in the post-proliferative phase did not see any reduction in the size of the hemangioma. Further research on a larger scale is needed to better understand the factors that contribute to the success or failure of treatment in children with infantile hemangiomas.

As a beta blocker, propranolol adversely affects the cardiac inotropic and chronotropic functions. About two hours after the oral dose, the impact on the blood pressure and pulse rate becomes apparent. The most dangerous side effect is hypoglycemia, which is more common in babies under three months old who are not fed well. Pulmonary symptoms, sleep disturbances, somnolence, cold extremities, and gastrointestinal (GI) complaints are among the other potential side effects. These side effects are dose-dependent, reversible, and not very serious. 108 children (62.1%) out of 174 patients treated for IH at a single center experienced one or more adverse reactions. The two most prevalent issues were nocturnal restlessness (39, 22.5%) and cold extremities (63, 36.2%). During the day, 28 kids (16.1%) were less active. In six cases, there was a decrease in blood pressure (3.4%). Nine of the 16 patients (3.2%) who experienced pulmonary symptoms required medical attention. There were 12 children (6.9%) with documented GI complaints. 371 cases of 39 studies involving 1189 children experienced negative reactions in another meta-analysis. Sleep disturbances, including insomnia, nightmares, restlessness at night, exhaustion, and sleep disturbance in 136 cases, were the most frequent adverse events. In 61 cases, acrocyanosis occurred. 41 reports of gastrointestinal issues, such as reflux and diarrhea, were made. 35 patients experienced respiratory adverse events. There were 39 cases of bradycardia and 8 cases of hypotension, respectively. Only four cases of hypoglycemia were reported. Additional adverse effects documented in the literature include irritability, excessive perspiration, and transient hypotonia.

7.1.4.5. Steroids versus Propranolol

The effectiveness of these two medications has only been compared in a small number of retrospective and open RCT studies. 110 kids were examined in a recent multi-centric retrospective study comparing propranolol and corticosteroids for IH. For a mean duration of 7.9 months (range, 3.5–14 months), 68 children received a dose of propranolol (2 mg/kg/day), and 42 children received a dose of prednisolone (4 mg/kg/day) for a mean duration of 5.2 months (range, 2.5–8.0 months). Comparing the outcome parameters, only 12 of 42 (29%) patients in the steroid group achieved clearance of 75% or more, while 56 of 68 (82%) patients on propranolol achieved this ($P < 0.01$). Compared to every case in the steroid group, only 1 child in the propranolol group experienced side effects ($P < 0.01$). Additional outcome metrics, like the proportion of ulcerated cases [4 (6%) vs. 11(26%); $P < 0.01$] and the number of cases that needed to be referred for surgery [8 (12%) vs. Moreover, there was a significant decrease in the propranolol group compared to the steroid group (12 (29%); $P = 0.03$). A retrospective study was conducted wherein 12 infant pairs were chosen and compared. The steroid and propranolol groups had mean treatment durations of 12.7 months (range5–28 months) and 10.6 months (range7–13 months), respectively. After one, two, and six months of treatment, investigator ratings indicated that propranolol produced a much better response than steroids. After six months of treatment, the mean improvement using VAF was 44.8% and 78.7%, respectively ($P < 0.001$), for both groups.

The children were treated for a minimum period of 3 months. Group A received propranolol (2–3 mg/kg/day), group B received prednisolone (1–4 mg/kg/day) and group C was treated with both. Children in groups A and C had a significantly earlier response (mean initial response time in group A – 4.1 days; Group C – 4.7 days vs. Group B – 9.8 days; $P < 0.05$). Flattening of the hemangioma lesion was also sooner and more significant in groups A and C than in group B ($P < 0.05$). The mean reduction in the size was significant in groups A and C at 3, 6 and 12 months while in group B it was significant only at 6 months. Groups B and C had a higher number of complications. From these reports, oral propranolol appears to be a better drug than steroids. However, prospective blinded RCTs will provide a better understanding of its efficacy and safety.

7.1.4.6. Other Systemic Drugs

Treatment options such as vincristine, cyclophosphamide, and interferon α are reserved for life-threatening hemangiomas that do not respond to standard therapy.

7.2. Sturge–Weber Syndrome

Sturge-Weber syndrome, also known as encephalotrigeminal angiomatosis, is a rare congenital disorder affecting both the neurological system and the skin. It is classified as one of the phakomatoses, and is characterized by port-wine stains on the face, glaucoma, seizures, intellectual disability, and angiomas in the leptomeninges of the brain. There are three different types of Sturge-Weber syndrome: Type 1 involves facial and leptomeningeal angiomas, as well as potential glaucoma or choroidal lesions, mostly affecting one side of the brain. Type 2 includes a facial angioma with a risk of glaucoma, without brain involvement at first but symptoms may develop later on. Type 3 exclusively involves leptomeningeal angiomas, without facial angiomas or glaucoma typically present; this type is diagnosed solely through brain imaging. Further research is necessary to better understand this type of Sturge-Weber syndrome.

Sturge-Weber syndrome is a developmental anomaly that occurs due to errors in the development of mesodermal and ectodermal tissues. Unlike other neurocutaneous disorders, it is not hereditary and typically occurs sporadically. The syndrome is caused by a somatic activating mutation in the GNAQ gene, leading to various imaging findings such as tram track calcifications on CT scans, pial angiomatosis, and hemicerebral atrophy.

7.2.1. Signs and Symptoms

A port-wine stain on one side of the face, or the entire face, on the forehead and upper eyelid, is typically the first sign of Sturge-Weber syndrome. The birthmark is caused by an excess of capillaries surrounding the ophthalmic branch of the trigeminal nerve, which is located just beneath the surface of the face. It can range in color from light pink to deep purple. On the same side of the head as the birthmark, there is also blood vessel malformation in the pia mater that covers the brain. In the cerebral cortex, this leads to tissue calcification and nerve cell loss.

Seizures are one of the neurological symptoms, which start in infancy and can get worse with age. Convulsions can range in severity and typically occur on the side of the body across from the birthmark. Muscle weakness on the side of the body opposite the birthmark may also be present.

A small percentage of children will experience cognitive and developmental delays, and roughly 50% will develop glaucoma, which can develop later in life or be present from birth (optic neuropathy frequently linked to elevated intraocular pressure). Leukocoria, which is a manifestation of glaucoma, should prompt additional testing for retinoblastoma. The eyeball may grow and protrude out of its socket due to increased intraocular pressure (buphthalmos).

7.2.2. Cause

In the fetal stage, the blood vessel formations linked to SWS begin. A network of nerves begins to form around the region that will become a baby's head during the sixth week of development. This network typically disappears during the ninth week of development. This neural network remains in infants with SWS caused by GNAQ gene mutation. This lowers blood and oxygen flow to the brain, which may have an impact on the growth of brain tissue.

7.2.3. Diagnosis

The most common methods for detecting intracranial abnormalities are CT and MRI. To check for intracranial leptomeningeal angiomatosis, imaging should be done on a newborn with a facial cutaneous vascular malformation covering part of the upper or lower eyelids. Most often, the hemangioma on the surface of the brain occurs on the same side as the birthmark and causes atrophy in the affected area as well as calcification of the underlying brain over time.

7.2.4. History and Physical

The initial neurological symptom of Sturge-Weber syndrome is typically a seizure. 90% of the patients experience infantile spasms during the first year of life, which are followed by atonic, tonic, or myoclonic seizures. Seizures are frequently accompanied by increasing hemiparesis. Medication becomes increasingly ineffective in treating seizures. Another frequent finding is facial nevus, also known as port-wine stain nevus, which is usually observed along the ophthalmic or maxillary segment of the trigeminal nerve (forehead, cheeks). It is usually unilateral, present from birth, and remains constant as the patient ages. The infantile hemangioma, which is more common than a port-wine stain but absent at birth, is a stark contrast to this appearance. It expands gradually, and involution comes next. Brain involvement in a child with a facial port-wine stain ranges from 10% to 35%. The risk of glaucoma can rise by up to 50% when both the upper and lower eyelids are affected. Nearly invariably, glaucoma develops ipsilateral to the facial port-wine stain. Not every patient with port-wine stains has the syndrome of Sturge-Weber. Individuals with Sturge-Weber syndrome may exhibit cerebral symptoms in the absence of facial manifestations. Infancy-related ocular involvement can manifest as strabismus, increased tearing, eye enlargement, and increased conjunctival vascularity. Intellectual disability, early handedness, and gaze preferences are additional symptoms. About 20% of patients with Sturge-Weber syndrome have diffuse choroidal hemangioma, which is typically located on the same side as a facial port-wine stain. Slow-growing choroidal hemangiomas typically show no symptoms. The retina that covers the choroidal hemangioma may be normal, but it may also exhibit pathological changes like detachment, drusen formation, or epithelial atrophy/proliferation (Maraña Pérez et al., 2017).

7.2.5. Evaluation

Diagnosing Sturge-Weber syndrome involves identifying typical clinical symptoms, facial features, and brain MRI results. An eye exam is necessary to rule out glaucoma, while ocular ultrasound may reveal choroidal hemangioma. Skull radiographs can show gyriform calcifications known as the "tram-track sign." Although CT scans are useful for detecting calcifications, they involve radiation and are not recommended for routine use in children. Instead, brain MRI with contrast is the preferred imaging method, with commonly affected areas including the occipital and posterior parietal/temporal lobes. MRI findings vary depending on the disease stage, with early phases showing hyperperfusion, leptomeningeal enhancement, and restricted diffusion. Late stages display increased T2 signal in areas of gliosis, reduced pial enhancement, and cortical atrophy. The choroid plexus is enlarged and there are prominent deep medullary/subependymal veins instead of superficial cortical veins. Gyriform calcifications manifest as areas of signal loss along the gyri in a serpentine pattern and are best observed on T2* or SWI (susceptibility-weighted images). It is unlikely that patients with cutaneous and ocular symptoms who have a normal brain MRI at one year old will experience brain involvement later on. On MRI, choroidal angiomas appear as increased enhancement along the globe's posterior choroid layer. In patients with Sturge-Weber syndrome, fluorodeoxyglucose-positron emission tomography (FDG-PET) may be a helpful modality to study cerebral metabolism. Early on, the affected area is typically hypermetabolic, and later on, it is hypometabolic. When treating intractable seizures with cortical resection, PET may be helpful in surgical planning.

7.2.6. Treatment

Treatment for Sturge-Weber syndrome focuses on managing symptoms. Laser therapy can be used to reduce or remove birthmarks, while anticonvulsant medications may be prescribed to control seizures. Early monitoring for glaucoma is recommended, with surgery being an option for more severe cases. In situations where medication is ineffective and only one side of the brain is affected, neurosurgery such as hemispherectomy may be necessary. Physical therapy is beneficial for muscle weakness in infants and children, while educational therapy may help with intellectual disability and developmental delays. While there is no complete cure for delays, brain surgery to remove the affected area can greatly reduce seizure frequency and intensity. Surgeons may also consider disconnecting the affected side of the brain.

Patients with glaucoma associated with Sturge–Weber syndrome may experience a significant reduction in IOP (intraocular pressure) when using the prostaglandin latanoprost (Xalatan). In commercial formulations, latanoprost is prepared as an aqueous solution with a concentration of 0.005%, preserved with 0.02% benzalkonium chloride (BAC). One drop of latanoprost taken once a day in the evening is the recommended dosage, as it allows for better diurnal IOP control than does instillation in the morning. Its effects are age, gender, and ethnicity insensitive, and its side effects are minimal to nonexistent. A history of vitreous loss following cataract surgery, epiretinal membrane formation, branch retinal vein occlusion-related macular edema, anterior uveitis, diabetes mellitus, and cystic macular edema (CME) are among the contraindications. It's a good idea to inform patients that receiving treatment unilaterally may cause heterochromia or hypertrichosis, which could be unsightly from a cosmetic standpoint.

7.3. Pediatric Epidermolysis Bullosa

A rare group of hereditary disorders known as epidermolysis bullosa (EB) causes little to no apparent trauma to cause blistering or erosion of the skin and, in certain cases, the epithelial lining of other organs.

7.3.1. Signs and Symptoms

Conduct a thorough physical examination, paying particular attention to the areas of skin and mucosal surfaces. Determine the level at which the blister forms by assessing the blisters' size, location, and characteristics.

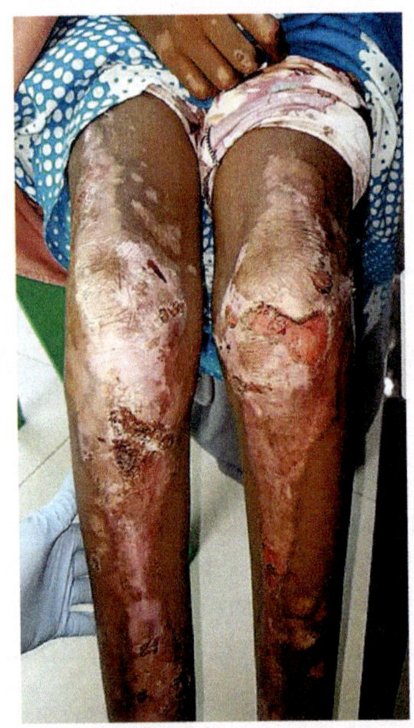

Figure 7.4. *Dystrophic epidermolysis bullosa (DEB) with multiple blisters and erosions.*

Examine the patient for involvement of the nails, hair, or teeth. Pressure, trauma, or overheating can cause blisters on the fingers, hands, elbows, feet, legs, and diaper area (in babies) (Figure 7.4) (Figure 7.5).

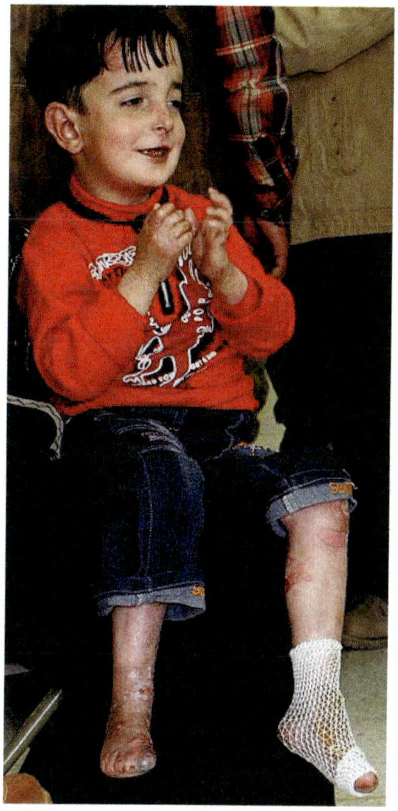

Figure 7.5. *Dystrophic epidermolysis bullosa (DEB) with generalized blistering and erosion.*

Source: By Master Sgt. Keith A. Milks – https://www.imef.marines.mil/News/News-Article-Display/Article/535004/marines-end-four-month-saga-that-brings-hope-to-iraqi-family/, Public Domain, https://commons.wikimedia.org/w/index.php?curid=6027506.

7.3.2. Diagnostics

7.3.2.1. Transmission Electron Microscopy

In addition to allowing for the visualization and semiquantitative evaluation of particular structures that are known to be altered in some epidermolysis bullosa subtypes, electron microscopy is used to assess the degree of skin cleavage in cases of epidermolysis bullosa (EB) (Figure 7.6).

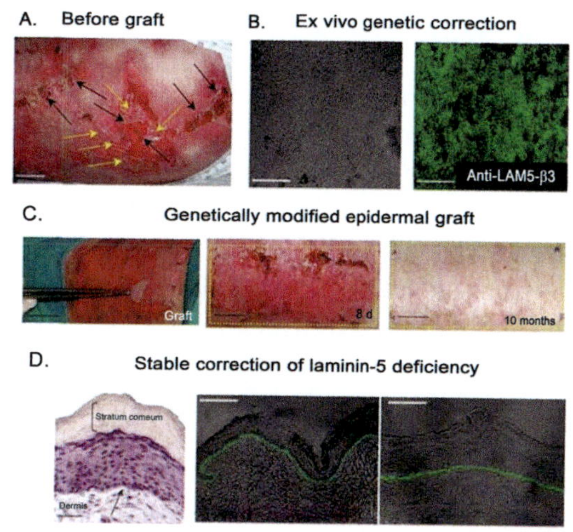

Figure 7.6. *Treatment of the epidermolysis bullosa.*

Source: By Gaelle, L. and Cédric, B., Medical applications of epidermal stem cells (November 15, 2008), StemBook, ed. The Stem Cell Research Community, StemBook, doi/10.3824/stembook.1.27.1, http://www.stembook.org. – [1] DirectStemBook Figure 3 Treatment of the epidermolysis bullosa by transplantation of laminin5 modified stem cells.Gaelle, L. and Cédric, B., Medical applications of epidermal stem cells (November 15, 2008), StemBook, ed. The Stem Cell Research Community, StemBook, doi/10.3824/stembook.1.27.1, http://www.stembook.org., CC BY 3.0, https://commons.wikimedia.org/w/index.php?curid=25463693.

Very few highly proficient electron microscopy laboratories are now available worldwide.

7.3.2.2. Immunofluorescence Mapping (IFM)

When it comes to diagnosing various types of epidermolysis bullosa, IFM is just as accurate as transmission electron microscopy. When combined with the use of particular monoclonal antibodies, IFM can shed light on the structural protein that is most likely mutated as well as the predominant type of epidermolysis bullosa.

7.3.2.3. Mutation Analysis

The most accurate method for identifying the type and exact location of molecular mutations, as well as the mode of inheritance, is mutation analysis. It is the method that is advised; preimplantation and fetal diagnosis can be carried out. It takes a lot of work and money to complete. Presently, this analysis can only be carried out in a small number of commercial or research laboratories.

7.3.3. Treatment

Studies have been focused on altering the production of keratins in the skin. There are a total of 54 known keratin genes, with 28 falling under type I intermediate filament genes and 26 under type II. These genes function as heterodimers and share similarities in structure and function, but are specific to certain cell types and conditions. By shifting the production balance from mutated, dysfunctional keratin genes to intact ones, symptoms could potentially be reduced. For instance, sulforaphane, a compound found in broccoli, was able to decrease blistering in a mouse model so significantly that affected pups could not be visually identified. This was achieved through injecting pregnant mice with 5 μmol/day (0.9 mg) and topically applying 1 μmol/day (0.2 mg in jojoba oil) to newborns.

A two-year-old child who is one of two brothers with EB is being treated by allogeneic bone marrow transplantation for RD and junctional EB as of 2008 as part of clinical research at the University of Minnesota. The child's elder brother has also undergone a second transplant. A five-year-old boy from Alabama and a boy from Missouri have both undergone the transplant procedure successfully. 12 transplants have been successful thus far. A baby from California is expected to receive another transplant. 30 subjects are intended for a clinical trial. On the other hand, there is a chance of severe infections, blisters on a large scale, and skin erosion due to the immunosuppressive nature of bone marrow transplantation. Indeed, out of the relatively small number of patients treated thus far, at least four have passed away during the planning or actualization of bone marrow transplantation for EB. The therapy's exact mechanism of action is unknown because it is believed that hematopoietic stem cells do not contribute to epithelial lineages. Rather, the observed clinical benefit may be attributed to cross-correction from immune cells derived from tissue-resident grafts.

According to a 2015 pilot study, patients with dystrophic EB may benefit from systemic granulocyte-colony stimulating factor (G-CSF) to facilitate faster wound healing. Research has shown that applying skin grown from genetically altered stem cells to the surfaces of wounds can improve outcomes in a single recipient.

In a 2017 clinical trial, type VII gene corrected keratinocytes (COL7A1 gene correction using retrovirus transduction) were successfully grafted onto male RDEB (recessive dystrophic EB) patients. The procedure was completed without any significant side effects. Significant amounts of Type VII collagen formation were seen at the dermis-epidermis junction.

A 2020 study showed that acellular dermal matrix/scaffolds could be safely allogenic grafted in EB patients without causing any infection or necrosis; instead, the patient's quality of life was improved overall, fewer dressing changes were needed, and wound healing was encouraged.

The European Union authorized the use of a pharmaceutical gel containing birch bark extract from *Betula pendula* and *Betula pubescens* in 2022 as a treatment for epidermolysis bullosa.

7.4. Ichthyosis in the Newborn

The ichthyoses are a broad category of cutaneous conditions that are connected by the discovery of aberrant epidermal differentiation. The term ichthyosis, which refers to the cutaneous scaling that is typical of these disorders and is said to resemble fish scales, is derived from the Greek word ichthys, which means fish. Scaling may be associated with a range of extracutaneous and/or systemic manifestations and can be localized or generalized. Even though these conditions are relatively uncommon, neonatologists, and perinatologists must have some understanding of them because the perinatal and early infancy periods are particularly crucial for patients with ichthyosis.

The skin's barrier function is weakened in ichthyosis patients, making it less able to fend off bacterial, chemical, and mechanical attacks as well as stop transepidermal water loss. The effects of this damaged barrier can be especially harmful, even fatal, to infants. They include heightened vulnerability to infection because of compromised skin integrity and markedly elevated metabolic demands because of increased epidermal turnover and evaporative heat and water loss.

7.4.1. Neonatal Presentations of Selected Ichthyoses

7.4.1.1. Collodion Baby

Collodion baby, also known as a "collodion fetus," is a common term for many congenital ichthyoses, the majority of which are inherited autosomally recessively. These include self-healing collodion baby, congenital ichthyosiform erythroderma (CIE), and lamellar ichthyosis (LI). When compared to harlequin ichthyosis, this phenotype is less severe, but it still has a high rate of associated morbidity and mortality. Collodion babies are frequently born before their due date and are covered in a shiny, taut membrane that resembles cellophane. Ectropion, or the turning out of the eyelids, and eclabium, or the eversion of the lips, are common conditions brought on by the taut skin around the mouth and eyes. Within the first few weeks of life, the membrane starts to dry out and crack after birth, which ultimately results in total shedding. At this point, the specific clinical symptoms of the underlying illness start to appear. Although they are much less common, trichothiodystrophy, neutral lipid storage disease, and Sjogren-Larsson syndrome are additional conditions that can manifest in collodion babies.

7.4.1.2. Harlequin Ichthyosis

Harlequin ichthyosis (HI), also known as "harlequin baby" or "harlequin fetus," is a very rare type of congenital ichthyosis with a distinctive appearance. It is caused by mutations in the ABCA12 gene and is inherited in an autosomal recessive manner. Babies born with HI have a thickened, hard outer layer of skin that cracks soon after birth, revealing deep red fissures and thick, yellow skin plates. They may also have features such as ectropion, eclabium, underdeveloped ears and nose, and swollen hands and feet. In the past, HI was often fatal, but with improved neonatal care and specialized skin treatment, many babies with HI now survive. Occasionally, HI may present with a milder phenotype resembling a collodion baby or with a less compact, vernix-like scale covering the body.

7.4.1.3. X-Linked Ichthyosis

As the name suggests, steroid sulfatase deficiency and recessive X-linked ichthyosis are other names for X-linked ichthyosis (XLI), which is inherited in an X-linked recessive manner. Steroid sulfatase is deficient in XLI due to either an inactivating mutation or a complete deletion of the STS gene, which occurs in most cases. A lack of steroid sulfatase in the placenta also causes low levels of estrogen secreted by the mother in her urine and in the amniotic fluid. This frequently results in inadequate cervical dilatation in females and a protracted or difficult labor that frequently requires medical assistance. At birth, the majority of affected male infants exhibit cutaneous manifestations, such as pink or red skin and large, translucent scales peeling off. With time, the scales darken and have a reduced propensity to desquamate. Males affected by this form of ichthyosis are more likely to develop cryptorchidism and ocular abnormalities, specifically corneal opacities, even though the skin findings at birth are relatively mild compared to other forms.

7.4.1.4. Epidermolytic Ichthyosis

Mutations in the genes KRT1 and KRT10, which encode keratin 1 and keratin 10, cause epidermolytic ichthyosis (EI), also known as bullous congenital ichthyosiform erythroderma or epidermolytic hyperkeratosis. This autosomal dominant disorder is brought on by these mutations. Blisters and skin thinning in certain places are how EI appears at birth. At first, this presentation might be mistaken for toxic epidermal necrolysis, staphylococcal scalded skin syndrome, or epidermolysis bullosa. Blisters tend to be smaller and form at trauma sites in infants with ichthyosis bullosa of Siemens, presenting similarly but mildly. With time, hyperkeratosis—characterized by thick, dark scales that frequently have a ridged or corrugated pattern—takes center stage in the cutaneous manifestation of EI, replacing the blistering and denudation that initially appeared.

7.4.1.5. Netherton Syndrome

Mutations in the SPINK5 gene6 cause the autosomal recessive disorder Netherton syndrome. Those that are affected exhibit generalized redness, or erythroderma, and peeling either from birth or soon after. Additional defining characteristics include elevated IgE levels and abnormalities of the hair shaft, most commonly trichorrhexis invaginata, also known as "bamboo" hair. When separating Netherton syndrome from other conditions that share similar clinical presentations, like congenital ichthyosiform erythroderma, abnormalities of the hair shaft can be especially useful.

7.4.2. Complications

Infants with harlequin ichthyosis, collodion babies, epidermolytic ichthyosis, and Netherton syndrome are among the neonates with congenital ichthyosis who are most at risk for complications in the postnatal period. Aside from prematurity-related issues, the main cause of morbidity and mortality during this period is compromised barrier function. Hypernatremic dehydration, other electrolyte imbalances, impaired thermoregulation, and malnutrition from excess transepidermal water and heat loss are caused by this. Microorganisms may enter through fissuring and denudation, which can result in sepsis and skin infections. Immobilization can lead to pneumonia, hypoxia, and impaired ventilation in neonates with collodion membrane or harlequin ichthyosis. It can also cause difficulties sucking or feeding. Furthermore, skin bands that contract can occasionally impair perfusion, resulting in peripheral edema and ischemia. Finally, exposure keratitis is a risk factor for infants with ectropion.

7.4.3. Management

A multidisciplinary approach is required for the management of neonates with ichthyosis, involving active participation from family members, nursing staff, neonatologists, dermatologists, and, in certain cases, other specialists. When an ichthyosis diagnosis is made during pregnancy, it is imperative to educate the staff and family as much as possible. Education is, after all, the cornerstone of good management. While infants with milder forms, like XLI, are unlikely to require intensive care and may not even need to stay longer in the hospital, those with collodion membrane, HI, erythroderma, or widespread blisters will require admission to the neonatal intensive care unit. Since prematurity is often the primary cause of risks or complications for infants with ichthyosis rather than skin conditions, many of the medical issues are similar to those that neonatologists regularly handle. Beyond the problems associated with preterm, as was previously mentioned, infants also face difficulties because of compromised barrier function. In this sense, management can be primary or secondary, meaning that efforts can be focused on enhancing barrier function while also attending to potential side effects like infection, malnourishment, or dehydration that may occur from it being compromised.

Most treatments targeted at enhancing barrier function are quite basic and easy to use. The cornerstones of management include bathing every day in lukewarm water or with a mild cleanser, applying copious amounts of bland emollients like petrolatum-based products, and providing a humidified, temperature-controlled environment through the use of an isolette. The following is a list of management techniques for several common complications (Table 7.2).

Table 7.2. *Clinical Classification of Ichthyoses*

Vulgar ichthyosis, isolated
Ichthyosis vulgaris
X-linked recessive ichthyosis
Vulgar ichthyosis, syndromic
Refsum syndrome
Multiple sulfatase deficiency
Congenital ichthyosis, isolated
Keratinopathic ichthyosis
Autosomal recessive congenital ichthyosis (ARCI)
Harlequin ichthyosis (subtype of ARCI)
Autosomal dominant lamellar ichthyosis
Congenital reticular ichthyosiform erythroderma (CRIE, Confetti ichthyosis)
Ichthyosis hystrix type Curth-Macklin
Peeling skin disease
Erythrokeratodermia
and others
Congenital ichthyosis, syndromic
HID/KID syndrome
Netherton syndrome
CHILD syndrome
SAM syndrome
Conradi-Hünermann-Happle syndrome
Sjögren-Larsson syndrome
Chanarin-Dorfmann syndrome
Trichothiodystrophy
IFAP syndrome
and others

Source: Metze D, Traupe H, Süßmuth K. Ichthyoses—A Clinical and Pathological Spectrum from Heterogeneous Cornification Disorders to Inflammation. Dermatopathology. 2021; 8(2):107-123. https://doi.org/10.3390/dermatopathology8020017.

7.4.3.1. Dehydration, Electrolyte Imbalances, and Increased Metabolic Demands

It is recommended to keep infants suffering from ichthyosis in a humidified incubator. Weight, electrolyte replacement, and urine output should all be closely monitored and treated as needed with intravenous hydration or electrolyte replacement. Determining calorie requirements may be aided by a nutrition consultation. Many advise putting an umbilical line when significantly thicker skin makes it difficult to obtain transcutaneous monitoring or peripheral intravenous access.

7.4.3.2. Infection

It is imperative to closely monitor for infection. When there is temperature instability, hemodynamic instability, lethargy, irritability, or inadequate feeding, blood cultures should be taken. Superficial wound cultures ought to be saved for situations where there is noticeable purulent discharge or significant erosions. All infections need to be treated vigorously as soon as they are suspected or confirmed. The application of preventive antibiotics in infants suffering from ichthyosis is still debatable because there are no published controlled trials supporting this treatment. Prophylactic antibiotics appear to favor *Pseudomonas aeruginosa* growth in burn patients, a population with a similarly compromised barrier. Some data suggest a beneficial effect, but others indicate no benefit or even a detrimental effect. Therefore, prophylactic antibiotics ought to be saved for situations involving extensive fissuring or denudation, and they ought to be given only after carefully weighing the advantages and disadvantages. Topical antibiotics like mupirocin can be applied to more isolated cutaneous fissures and erosions.

7.4.3.3. Skin Fragility, Risk of Systemic Absorption of Topical Medications, and Pain Control

Neonatals with ichthyosis frequently have delicate skin that makes them more prone to harm from even small trauma. It is advised to handle conventional adhesives carefully and to steer clear of them to reduce this risk. Whenever feasible, self-adherent wraps (like Coban™) or gauze should be used to secure lines and tubing rather than tape, especially for newborns with blisters or skin devoid of pigment. These infants are also at a higher risk of transcutaneous absorption, especially if they have Netherton syndrome or EI, which both have extensive skin denudation. Some topical medications carry a significant risk. These include topical calcineurin inhibitors, such as tacrolimus ointment and pimecrolimus cream, which can reach detectable serum levels and cause toxicity, and silver sulfadiazine cream, which has been connected to agranulocytosis. Furthermore, topical salicylic acid has been connected to salicylate intoxication and topical lactic acid preparations to lactic acidosis. Chlorhexidine and other antibacterial soaps and washes have the potential to be toxic. For this reason, babies should only be bathed in water or with very mild soaps or cleansers like Dove® or Cetaphil®, and only bland emollients like white petrolatum, Vaseline®, or Aquaphor® ointment should be used. Lastly, pain, and discomfort can also be felt through the skin, especially in cases of severe fissuring or denudation. As a result, it's best to give acetaminophen, non-steroidal anti-inflammatory drugs, or narcotics for adequate pain management.

7.4.3.4. Flexibility

Babies with hypohidrosis (HI) and occasionally collodion babies are susceptible to issues arising from reduced suppleness, especially during the initial stages of infancy when the dense covering has not yet started to crack. These side effects could include contractures, trouble eating or sucking, restricted lung movement and the ensuing risk of pneumonia, and, in certain HI cases, compartment syndrome. Emollients should be liberally applied to promote pliability; however, for infants with HI and for some who present as collodion babies, nasogastric feeding and ventilatory support will be necessary at first. A consultation with an orthopedist, plastic surgeon, or dermatologist may be required to help monitor for compartment syndrome. If perfusion is being compromised, it may be necessary to release contractures or constricting bands of skin, such as those commonly observed on the fingers and toes of infants with HI. Finally, topical or systemic retinoids (such as acitretin or tazarotene, respectively) may be taken into consideration for infants with HI or, less frequently, collodion babies. Retinoids have the potential to hasten the shedding of thick scale, which makes them useful. However, due to the possibility of systemic side effects, they should only be used cautiously and under the guidance of a dermatologist with experience.

7.4.3.5. Ocular Complications

It is important to assess infants for the possibility of ectropion, which is frequently observed in collodion baby or HI cases. It is advised to consult an ophthalmologist if present. Because ectropion puts infants at risk for exposure keratitis, it's critical to keep the eyes well lubricated. Artificial tears or ocular lubricant can help achieve this. Treatment for corneal abscess or conjunctivitis may involve topical antibiotics.

Certain situations, such as XLI cases, which can result in low unconjugated estriol levels that are measured during maternal serum screening in the second trimester, may indicate a diagnosis of ichthyosis prior to delivery. Based on the results of ultrasonography, HI may be found. Preimplantation testing, fetal skin biopsies, and chorionic villus sampling are additional techniques for diagnosing ichthyosis in utero (Fassihi et al., 2006).

Clinical criteria alone can frequently be used to determine a likely diagnosis in the neonatal period. Notably, though, treatment is usually not based on the specific type of ichthyosis that is present, so a definitive diagnosis is not required at this time. When a patient exhibits the characteristic cutaneous phenotype, as in EI or lamellar ichthyosis, or develops associated findings, such as neurologic findings in the setting of Sjögren-Larsson syndrome, many cases that were unclear at birth become more clinically recognizable within the first year of life.

At times, relatively straightforward diagnostic tests can confirm the diagnosis during the neonatal period. Although the results of a skin biopsy are frequently nonspecific and therefore only helpful in a small percentage of cases, the procedure is minimally invasive and occasionally yields useful information; e.g., EI frequently exhibits characteristic histologic findings. A hair mount can be done to check for abnormalities in cases of suspected Netherton syndrome. These abnormalities include trichorrhexis nodosa (nodes along the hair shaft), pili torti (twisted hair), and trichorrhexis invaginata (bamboo hair, most common). However, these abnormalities are not always present in infants. The presence of lipid-containing vacuoles in white blood cells in circulation is indicative of neutral lipid storage disease, a condition linked to cataracts, myopathy, and sensorineural deafness. Under the supervision of a dermatologist or geneticist, genetic testing can be carried out in situations where a diagnosis is unclear or to confirm a suspected diagnosis.

Most commercial genetic testing laboratories offer testing for mutations known to cause ichthyosis. When it comes to future family planning, genetic diagnosis becomes especially helpful. As pathogenesis-based therapies are developed and the genetics of these disorders become better understood, we believe that genetic diagnosis will become more prevalent and significant in the years to come.

7.5. Irritant Diaper Dermatitis

Diaper or nappy rash, also known as irritant diaper dermatitis (IDD), is a general term for skin rashes around the diaper area that are brought on by a variety of skin conditions and/ or irritants. The hallmarks of generic irritant diaper dermatitis are convex surfaces with united areas of erythema and scaling; the skin folds are largely unaffected. When secondary bacteria or fungi are involved, diaper dermatitis typically spreads to concave surfaces (i.e., skin folds), convex surfaces, and frequently shows a red, beefy erythema in the center surrounded by satellite pustules.

Typically, it is regarded as a type of irritant contact dermatitis. The reason the word diaper appears in the name isn't because the diaper itself causes the rash; rather, it's because using a diaper is linked to the rash, which is brought on by the materials the diaper traps (typically feces). There isn't much proof to support the theory that allergic contact dermatitis is the cause. The rash in adults with fecal, urinary, or both types of incontinence is sometimes referred to as incontinence-associated dermatitis (IAD).

When a fungal origin is found, the condition is referred to as diaper candidiasis. Because the treatment is different (antifungals), the distinction is significant (Figure 7.7).

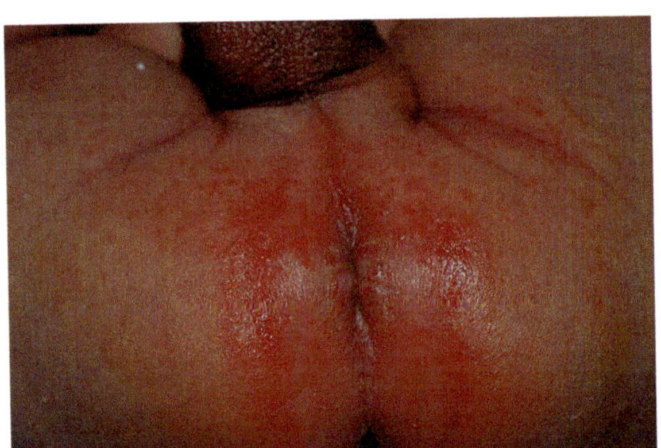

Figure 7.7. *A boy with diaper rash.*

Source: By Dailyboth - Own work, CC0, https://commons.wikimedia.org/w/index.php?curid=25252319.

7.5.1. Causes

When the skin is exposed to prolonged wetness, elevated skin pH brought on by the combination and subsequent reactions of urine and feces, and the subsequent breakdown of the stratum corneum, or outermost layer of the skin, irritant diaper dermatitis develops. This could be the result of allergic reactions, diarrhea, frequent stools, tight diapers, or excessive ammonia exposure. Adult stratum corneum consists of 25–30 layers of dead keratinocytes that have been flattened; these layers are constantly being shed and replaced from below. Lipids secreted by the stratum granulosum just beneath these dead cells act as an impermeable barrier, contributing to the skin's barrier function. Reducing water loss, repelling water, shielding the deeper skin layers from damage, and preventing microbial invasion of the skin are the functions of the stratum corneum. This layer of skin is much thinner and more easily disrupted in infants (Chiou et al., 2004).

7.5.1.1. Urine

Urine affects skin pH, which has an additional effect on skin integrity even though wetness alone has the effect of macerating the skin, softening the stratum corneum, and greatly increasing susceptibility to friction injury. Even though research indicates that ammonia by itself only slightly irritates the skin, the breakdown of urea in the presence of fecal urease raises pH because ammonia is released, which in turn stimulates the activity of fecal enzymes like lipase and protease. These fecal enzymes act as skin irritants by increasing the skin's permeability to bile salts and its level of hydration.

When using reusable cloth diapers as opposed to conventional disposable diapers, there is no discernible difference in the incidence of diaper rash. When compared to their cloth diaper counterparts, babies who use superabsorbent disposable diapers with a central gelling material experience fewer episodes of diaper dermatitis. However, be aware that dyes found in superabsorbent diapers have been linked to allergic contact dermatitis (ACD). Even if they don't feel wet, babies should have regular diaper changes to avoid diaper rash, whether they are in cloth or disposable diapers. Disposable diapers are designed with synthetic, non-biodegradable gel to draw moisture away from the baby's skin, lowering the risk of diaper rash. Currently, available superabsorbent microfiber cloth that is placed in a pocket with a layer of light-permeable material that comes into contact with the skin can be used with cloth diapers. This pattern draws moisture into the microfiber cloth from the skin. Nowadays, many commercial pocket cloth diaper brands in developed markets use this technology.

7.5.1.2. Diet

Since the diet also affects fecal enzymes, the relationship between fecal enzyme activity and IDD explains the observation that diaper rash and infant diet are related. For example, breastfed infants experience fewer cases of diaper rash; this may be due to the higher pH and lower enzymatic activity of their stools. Additionally, infants 8 to 12 months old are the most likely to be diagnosed with diaper rash; this could be due to an increase in the consumption of solid foods and dietary modifications that alter the makeup of their feces at that age. Diaper rash seems to be more common when an infant's diet drastically changes (such as switching from breast milk to formula or from milk to solids).

The observation that infants are more prone to diaper rash following antibiotic treatment, which alters the intestinal microflora, further supports the link between feces and IDD. Additionally, diaper rash is more common in babies who have had diarrhea within the last 48 hours. This could be due to the fact that fecal enzymes like lipase and protease are more active in feces that have moved quickly through the digestive system.

7.5.1.3. Secondary Infections

There is ongoing debate regarding the importance of secondary infection in IDD. Microbiological counts and the existence or absence of IDD do not appear to be related. The severity of the diaper rash observed seems to positively correlate with the likelihood of secondary involvement, even though seemingly healthy infants can occasionally culture positive for Candida and other organisms without displaying any symptoms. There have been reports of many different infections, such as *Pseudomonas aeruginosa*, *Proteus mirabilis*, *Streptococcus pyogenes*, *Staphylococcus aureus*, and enterococci, but it seems that Candida is the most frequent opportunistic invader in diaper areas.

7.5.2. Diagnosis

Clinical observation of the erythematous eruption's restriction to the convex surfaces of the buttocks and genital region allows for the diagnosis of IDD. Diaper candidiasis can be identified by looking for the beefy red, sharply marginated patches that indicate a Candida albicans colonization if the dermatitis lasts longer than three days.

7.5.2.1. Differential Diagnosis

Additional rashes that can appear in the diaper area are atopic dermatitis and seborrheic dermatitis. Atopic dermatitis and seborrheic dermatitis both need customized care; they are not the topic of this article. Though it can also occur in the inguinal folds, greasy, thick yellowish scales are the hallmark of seborrheic dermatitis, which is most frequently observed on the scalp (cradle cap).

Eczema, also known as atopic dermatitis, is linked to allergic reactions, which are frequently inherited. This group of rashes is characterized by extreme itching and can occur anywhere on the body.

7.5.3. Treatments

Reducing the use of diapers as well as applying barrier creams, low-dose topical cortisones, and antifungal medications are all potential treatments. The diaper area can experience a range of additional inflammatory and infectious processes. It is helpful to recognize these secondary types of diaper dermatitis so that patients can be accurately diagnosed and treated.

Overall, there is not enough high-quality evidence to be certain about the various treatments' efficacy. Skin cleansers and washcloths with hydrating, cleansing, and protective qualities might be superior to soap and water, but there is very little proof to support the claims made for other treatments.

7.5.3.1. Diaper Changing

Giving up diapers and letting the affected skin air out is the most effective treatment, albeit not the most practical one. Just changing diapers more frequently is an additional option. It is a good idea to completely dry the skin before changing diapers because excess moisture from sweating or urine and feces creates the ideal environment for diaper rash to develop.

7.5.3.2. Diaper Type

According to some reports, using cloth diapers increases the risk of diaper rash. Some argue that the diaper's material matters because it can wick moisture away from the baby's skin and stop a secondary Candida infection. Nevertheless, there might not be enough information from high-caliber randomized controlled trials at this time to confirm or deny the use of disposable diapers. Public policy should also be concerned about the impact of non-biodegradable diapers on the environment.

7.5.3.3. Creams, Ointments

An alternative method involves preventing moisture from penetrating the skin. Commonly suggested treatments utilizing this method include barrier creams or oil-based protectants, petroleum jelly, dimethicone, and other oils, as well as different over-the-counter diaper creams. When the skin is not completely dry, these sealants can have the opposite effect and help to keep moisture inside the skin instead of outside.

Because they have a drying and astringent effect on the skin and are mildly antiseptic without causing irritation, zinc oxide-based ointments like zinc and castor oil cream, Sudocrem, or Pinxav can be effective treatments, especially in prevention. A 2005 meta-analysis found no evidence to support the use of topical vitamin A to treat the condition.

7.5.3.4. Dangers of Using Powders

While some moisture-absorbing powders, like talcum or starch, absorb moisture, they can also cause other issues. Any type of powder that is released into the air can irritate lung tissue. The American Academy of Dermatology does not advise using powders derived from starchy plants like corn or arrowroot because they serve as a food source for fungi.

7.5.3.5. Antifungals

Antifungal creams are frequently required for rashes that are particularly severe or persistent. When the rash is more irritating than inflammatory, a topical corticosteroid preparation such as hydrocortisone cream is used. Since it can be challenging to distinguish between a fungal infection and a simple skin irritant, many doctors prefer combination creams that contain corticosteroids and antifungals, like hydrocortisone/miconazole.

A Closer Look

A Closer Look at Oral Propranolol as First-Line Treatment in Infantile Hemangioma

Due to the tendency of infantile hemangiomas to spontaneously regress, the majority of cases do not require therapy; however, oral propranolol has emerged as the preferred treatment for the few infants with complicated cases.

Led by Christine Léauté-Labrèze, M.D., of Pellegrin Children's Hospital in Bordeaux, France, researchers reviewed studies published between 2008 and 2015 finding that 2–3 mg/kg of propranolol daily for six months, resulted in a response rate of 96–98% of 1264 cases. 60% of cases experienced a complete or nearly complete regression.

It has been demonstrated that propranolol works well for both ulcerated infantile hemangioma and obstructive, potentially fatal airway infantile hemangioma. Although propranolol's precise modes of action are still unclear, it may control the proliferation of hemangioma cells by acting through the VEGF pathway or catecholamines.

In the past 10 years, research on infantile hemangiomas has made "tremendous progress.." Propranolol has been thoroughly examined in the scientific literature, risk factors have been identified, more is understood about its pathophysiology, and more clinical presentations have been reported.

It has been demonstrated that propranolol works well in the most severe situations. The primary indications for treatment include ulceration; severe anatomic distortion, particularly on the face; and life-threatening infantile hemangiomas that result in heart failure or respiratory distress. Tumors posing functional risks include visual obstruction, amblyopia, or feeding difficulties.

Propranolol, a beta-blocker, should be started as soon as possible to prevent potential complications, according to the literature search results.

The most frequent side effects of treatment, including somnolence, irritability, and sleep disturbances, affect 20–25% of patients. Thankfully, side effects are mostly harmless and reversible. Asymptomatic hypotension and bronchospasm or bronchiolitis are less frequent side effects (>1%). More uncommon are the potentially fatal consequences of undiagnosed atrioventricular blocks, hypoglycemia, and more severe bradycardia side effects. Most side effects can be effectively resolved by stopping the treatment; however, recurrence after stopping the treatment happens in 10–15% of cases, mainly in segmental and deep infantile hemangiomas. In cases of diarrhea, obstructive bronchitis, and poor oral feeding, temporary cessation is advised.

The blood-brain barrier can be crossed by propranolol, which makes it a highly lipophilic β blocker. This means that propranolol may have effects on cognition or neurodevelopment that are relevant.

Referring Patients

Given that 80% of all hemangiomas reach their final size by three months of age, and that infantile hemangiomas are the most common soft-tissue tumors of infancy, with a prevalence of 4% to 5% in the overall infantile population, the article recommends close follow-up in the first weeks of life to identify at-risk hemangiomas.

Hypoxia is the most likely initiating factor that causes the HIF-1 alpha pathway to become activated. Precursor lesions manifest as a telangiectatic red macule or as a pale area of vasoconstriction during the early neonatal period. They can also be present at birth.

The best course of action for a patient with an infantile hemangioma who is at risk of complications is to send them to a multidisciplinary team for assessment and targeted diagnostic procedures. MRIs and tests for coagulation problems or hypothyroidism are some of these interventions.

The Hemangioma Dynamic Complication Scale and the Hemangioma Severity Scale are two additional scores that can be used to access severity.

It has also been demonstrated that other beta-blockers, such as acebutolol, atenolol, and nadolol, are beneficial in the treatment of infantile hemangioma. Additionally, because these beta-blockers are hydrophilic and do not cross the blood-brain barrier like propranolol does, there may be a decreased chance of side effects related to the central nervous system (CNS), including bronchospasm, hypoglycemia, and disturbed sleep.

Summary

- Childhood dermatological problems contribute about one-third of all consultations in the setting of both pediatrics and dermatology outpatient services.
- An infantile hemangioma (IH), sometimes called a strawberry mark due to appearance, is a type of benign vascular tumor or anomaly that affects babies.
- Infantile hemangiomas typically develop in the first few weeks or months of life. They are more common in Caucasians, in premature children whose birth weight is less than 3 pounds (1.4 kg), in females, and in twin births.
- Sturge–Weber syndrome, sometimes referred to as encephalotrigeminal angiomatosis, is a rare congenital neurological and skin disorder. It is one of the phakomatoses and is often associated with port-wine stains of the face, glaucoma, seizures, intellectual disability, and ipsilateral leptomeningeal angioma (cerebral malformations and tumors).
- Epidermolysis bullosa (EB) is a rare group of inherited disorders that manifests as blistering or erosion of the skin and, in some cases, the epithelial lining of other organs, in response to little or no apparent trauma.
- The ichthyoses represent a large group of cutaneous disorders linked by the common finding of abnormal epidermal differentiation.
- Collodion baby, sometimes referred to as "collodion fetus," is a common presentation of several congenital ichthyoses, most of which are inherited in an autosomal recessive manner, including lamellar ichthyosis (LI), congenital ichthyosiform erythroderma (CIE) and self-healing collodion baby.
- Irritant diaper dermatitis (IDD, also called a diaper or nappy rash) is a generic term applied to skin rash in the diaper (in British and Australian English "nappy") area that are caused by various skin disorders and/or irritants.

References

1. Akiyama, M., Sugiyama-Nakagiri, Y., Sakai, K., et al. (2005). Mutations in lipid transporter ABCA12 in harlequin ichthyosis and functional recovery by corrective gene transfer. *Journal of Clinical Investigation, 115*, 1777–1784.
2. Bonifas, J. M., Morley, B. J., Oakey, R. E., Kan, Y. W., & Epstein, E. H. Jr. (1987). Cloning of a cDNA for steroid sulfatase: Frequent occurrence of gene deletions in patients with recessive X chromosome-linked ichthyosis. *Proceedings of the National Academy of Sciences, 84*, 9248–9251.
3. Chang, L. C., Haggstrom, A. N., Drolet, B. A., Baselga, E., Chamlin, S. L., Garzon, M. C., et al. (2008). Hemangioma Investigator Group. Growth characteristics of infantile hemangiomas: Implications for management. *Pediatrics, 122*, 360–367.
4. Chen, Q., Zhang, Y., Sun, C., Liu, L., Luo, X., Wang, H., & Ni, S. (2022). Case report: Deterioration of infantile hemangioma related to oral or nebulized administration of β2-AR agonist: Three cases reports. *Frontiers in Oncology, 12*, 1000099. https://doi.org/10.3389/fonc.2022.1000099.
5. Chiou, Y. B., & Blume-Peytavi, U. (2004). Stratum corneum maturation: A review of neonatal skin function. *Skin Pharmacology and Physiology, 17*(2), 57–66.
6. Darrow, D. H., Greene, A. K., Mancini, A. J., & Nopper, A. J. (2015). Diagnosis and management

of infantile hemangioma. *Pediatrics, 136*(4), e1060–e104. https://doi.org/10.1542/peds.2015-2485.

7. Drolet, B. A., Dohil, M., Golomb, M. R., Wells, R., Murowski, L., Tamburro, J., et al. (2006). Early stroke and cerebral vasculopathy in children with facial hemangiomas and PHACE association. *Pediatrics, 117*, 959–964.

8. Fassihi, H., Eady, R. A., Mellerio, J. E., et al. (2006). Prenatal diagnosis for severe inherited skin disorders: 25 years' experience. *British Journal of Dermatology, 154*, 106–113.

9. Haggstrom, A. N., Drolet, B. A., Baselga, E., Chamlin, S. L., Garzon, M. C., Horii, K. A., et al. (2006). Prospective study of infantile hemangiomas: Clinical characteristics predicting complications and treatment. *Pediatrics, 118*, 882–887.

10. Kelsell, D. P., Norgett, E. E., Unsworth, H., et al. (2005). Mutations in ABCA12 underlie the severe congenital skin disease harlequin ichthyosis. *American Journal of Human Genetics, 76*, 794–803.

11. Kilcline, C., & Frieden, I. J. (2008). Infantile hemangiomas: How common are they? A systematic review of the medical literature. *Pediatric Dermatology, 25*, 168–173.

12. Li, J., Chen, X., Zhao, S., Hu, X., Chen, C., Ouyang, F., et al. (2011). Demographic and clinical characteristics and risk factors for infantile hemangioma: A Chinese case-control study. *Archives of Dermatology, 147*, 1049–1056.

13. Lomenick, J. P., Reifschneider, K. L., Lucky, A. W., Adams, D., Azizkhan, R. G., Woo, J. G., et al. (2009). Prevalence of adrenal insufficiency following systemic glucocorticoid therapy in infants with hemangiomas. *Archives of Dermatology, 145*, 262–266.

14. Maraña Pérez, A. I., Ruiz-Falcó Rojas, M. L., Puertas Martín, V., Domínguez Carral, J., Carreras Sáez, I., Duat Rodríguez, A., & Sánchez González, V. (2017). Analysis of Sturge-Weber syndrome: A retrospective study of multiple associated variables. *Neurología, 32*(6), 363–370.

15. Metry, D. W., Hawrot, A., Altman, C., & Frieden, I. J. (2004). Association of solitary, segmental hemangiomas of the skin with visceral hemangiomatosis. *Archives of Dermatology, 140*, 591–596.

16. North, P. E., Waner, M., Mizeracki, A., & Mihm, M. C. Jr. (2000). GLUT1: A newly discovered immunohistochemical marker for juvenile hemangiomas. *Human Pathology, 31*(1), 11–22. https://doi.org/10.1016/S0046-8177(00)80192 6.

17. Thomas, A. C., Cullup, T., Norgett, E. E., et al. (2006). ABCA12 is the major harlequin ichthyosis gene. *Journal of Investigative Dermatology, 126*, 2408–2413.

18. de Castro, D. K., Ng, Z. Y., Holzer, P. W., Waner, M., Cetrulo, C. L., and Fay, A. (2017). One-Stage Supramaximal Full-Thickness Wedge Resection of Vascular Lip Anomalies. *J. Oral Maxillofac. Surg.* 75, 2449–2455. doi:10.1016/j.joms.2017.03.020

19. Hutchins, K. K., Ross, R. D., Kobayashi, D., Martin, A., and Rajpurkar, M. (2017). Treatment of Refractory Infantile Hemangiomas and Pulmonary Hypertension with Sirolimus in a Pediatric Patient. *J. Pediatr. Hematol. Oncol.* 39, e391. doi:10.1097/MPH.0000000000000961

20. Kim, K. H., Choi, T. H., Choi, Y., Park, Y. W., Hong, K. Y., Kim, D. Y., et al. (2017). Comparison of Efficacy and Safety between Propranolol and Steroid for Infantile Hemangioma: A Randomized Clinical Trial. *JAMA Dermatol.* 153, 529–536. doi:10.1001/jamadermatol.2017.0250

21. Mashiah, J., Kutz, A., Rabia, S. H., Ilan, E. B., Goldberg, I., Sprecher, E., et al. (2017). Assessment of

the Effectiveness of Topical Propranolol 4% Gel for Infantile Hemangiomas. *Int. J. Dermatol.* 56, 148–153. doi:10.1111/ijd.13517

22. Yu, X., Zhang, J., Wu, Z., Liu, M., Chen, R., Gu, Y., et al. (2017). LUMBAR Syndrome: A Case Manifesting as Cutaneous Infantile Hemangiomas of the Lower Extremity, Perineum and Gluteal Region, and a Review of Published Work. *J. Dermatol.* 44, 808–812. doi:10.1111/1346-8138.13763

23. Wang, Y., Zhang, X., Yang, Y., Zhang, J., Yang, Y., and Lu, Y. (2017). Efficacy and Safety of 2% Topical Propranolol Cream for the Treatment of Proliferating Infantile Strawberry Hemangiomas. *Indian J. Pediatr.* 84, 425–429. doi:10.1007/s12098-017-2303-7

24. Ying, H., Zou, Y., Yu, W., Qiu, Y., Ma, G., Chang, L., et al. (2017). Prospective, Open-Label, Rater-Blinded and Self-Controlled Pilot Study of the Treatment of Proliferating Superficial Infantile Hemangiomas with 0.5% Topical Timolol Cream versus 595-nm Pulsed Dye Laser. *J. Dermatol.* 44, 660–665. doi:10.1111/1346-8138.13747

25. le Sage, S., David, M., Dubois, J., Powell, J., McCuaig, C. C., Théorêt, Y., et al. (2018). Efficacy and Absorption of Topical Sirolimus for the Treatment of Vascular Anomalies in Children: A Case Series. *Pediatr. Dermatol.* 35, 472–477. doi:10.1111/pde.13547

26. Xu, M. N., Zhang, M., Xu, Y., Wang, M., and Yuan, S. M. (2018). Individualized Treatment for Infantile Hemangioma. *J. Craniofac. Surg.* 29, 1876–1879. doi:10.1097/SCS.0000000000004745

27. Igarashi, A., Hata, I., Yuasa, M., Okuno, T., and Ohshima, Y. (2018). A Case of an Infant with Extremely Low Birth Weight and Hypothyroidism Associated with Massive Cutaneous Infantile Hemangioma. *J. Pediatr. Endocrinol. Metab.* 31, 1377–1380. doi:10.1515/jpem-2018-0369

28. Xu, P., Yu, Q., Huang, H., Zhang, W., and Li, W. (2020). Lip Infantile Hemangiomas Involving the Vermillion Border Have Worse Outcomes and Prognosis to Oral Propranolol Than Lesions Confined to One Side of the Vermillion. *J. Oral Maxillofac. Surg.* 78, 446–454. doi:10.1016/j.joms.2019.09.010

29. Chen, S., Zhuang, K., Sun, K., Yang, Q., Ran, X., Xu, X., et al. (2019). Itraconazole Induces Regression of Infantile Hemangioma via Downregulation of the Platelet-Derived Growth Factor-D/PI3K/Akt/mTOR Pathway. *J. Invest. Dermatol.* 139, 1574–1582. doi:10.1016/j.jid.2018.12.028

30. Tani, S., Kunimoto, K., Inaba, Y., Mikita, N., Kaminaka, C., Kanazawa, N., et al. (2020). Change of Serum Cytokine Profiles by Propranolol Treatment in Patients with Infantile Hemangioma. *Drug Discov. Ther.* 14, 89–92. doi:10.5582/ddt.2020.03014

31. Diociaiuti, A., Carnevale, C., Torres, E. B., Léauté-Labrèze, C., Neri, I., Rotunno, R., et al. (2020). Cutaneous Infantile Haemangiomas with Intracranial and Intraspinal Involvement: A European Multicentre Experience and Review. *Acta Derm. Venereol.* 100, adv00255. doi:10.2340/00015555-3608

32. Zeng, L., Tao, C., Liu, Z., Zhang, J., Zhang, M., Zhang, J., et al. (2020). Preparation and Evaluation of Cubic Nanoparticles for Improved Transdermal Delivery of Propranolol Hydrochloride. *AAPS PharmSciTech* 21, 266. doi:10.1208/s12249-020-01809-7

33. Cheng, J. W. C. H., Lam, Y. Y., Fung, G. P. G., Sin, C., Luk, D. C. K., Chan, B. H. B., et al. (2020). Randomised Controlled Trial: Can Topical Timolol Maleate Prevent Complications for Small Superficial Infantile Haemangiomata in High-Risk Areas? *Pediatr. Res.* 88, 756–760. doi:10.1038/s41390-020-0917-3

Chapter

PLASMA DERMATOLOGY: SKIN THERAPY USING COLD ATMOSPHERIC PLASMA

8

Contents

Introduction

The range of specializations in cold atmospheric plasma-based plasma medicine has been increasing. As a burgeoning field, plasma dermatology capitalizes on the advantageous complexity of plasma constituents (such as UV photons, electromagnetic radiation, reactive oxygen and nitrogen species), technical adaptability (such as indirect aqueous treatment and direct irradiation), and practical viability (such as a compact, hand-held device and clinician-friendly operation). This chapter's goal is to provide an overview of the most recent developments in CAP-dominated skin therapy by focusing on three main areas. Starting with plasma optimization of intact skin, we go into detail about how CAP affects blood flow, cells, lipids, and histology in the skin. The treatment of various skin diseases with CAP is then thoroughly dissected and clinically oriented, with special attention to wound healing, inflammatory disorders, infectious conditions, parasitic infestations, cutaneous malignancies, and alopecia. We wrap up with a quick review of the safety aspects of CAP treatment and a suggestion for reducing any possible risks.

Orientation and Directional Terms

Term	Definition	Illustration
Onychomycosis	Onychomycosis, also known as tinea unguium, is a fungal infection of the nail. Symptoms may include white or yellow nail discoloration, thickening of the nail, and separation of the nail from the nail bed.	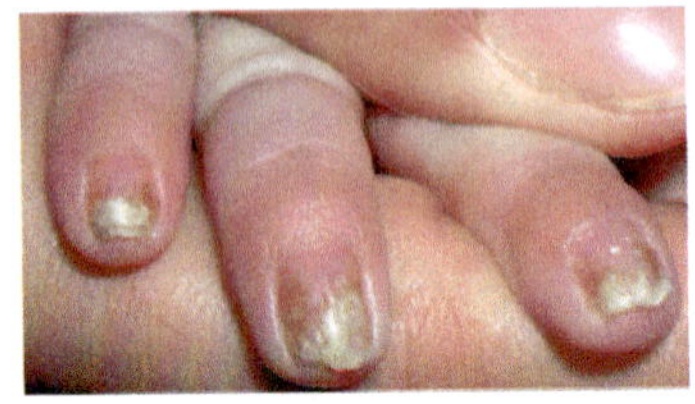
Dermatophytosis	Dermatophytosis is an infection of the hair, skin, or nails caused by a dermatophyte, which is most commonly of the Trichophyton genus and less commonly of the Microsporum or Epidermophyton genera.	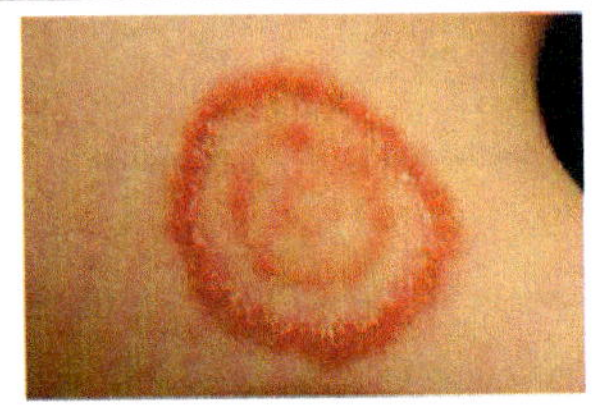
Demodicosis	The term demodicosis refers to a group of disorders caused by Demodex folliculorum and characterized by variable degree of spinulosis, erythema, and papules of the face, generally accompanied by a burning or pruritic sensation.	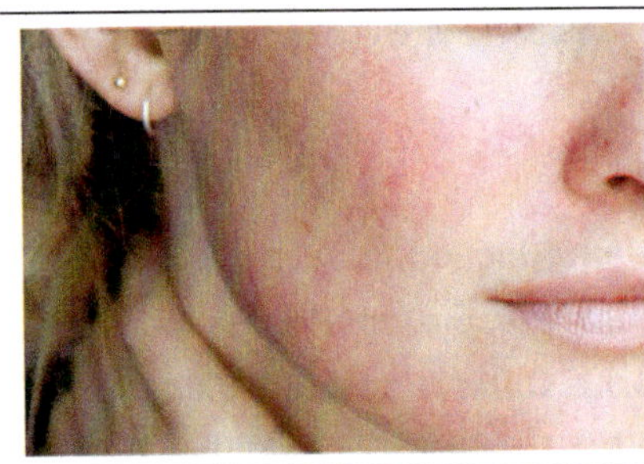
Mitogen-activated protein (MAP) kinases	Mitogen-activated protein (MAP) kinases are a group of protein kinases that regulate cellular responses to stimuli like mitogens, heat shock, and osmotic stress.	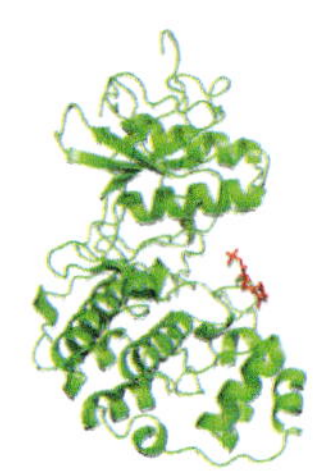
Epidermal growth factor (EGF)	Epidermal growth factor (EGF) is a protein that stimulates cell growth and differentiation by binding to its receptor, EGFR. Human EGF is 6-kDa and has 53 amino acid residues and three intramolecular disulfide bonds.	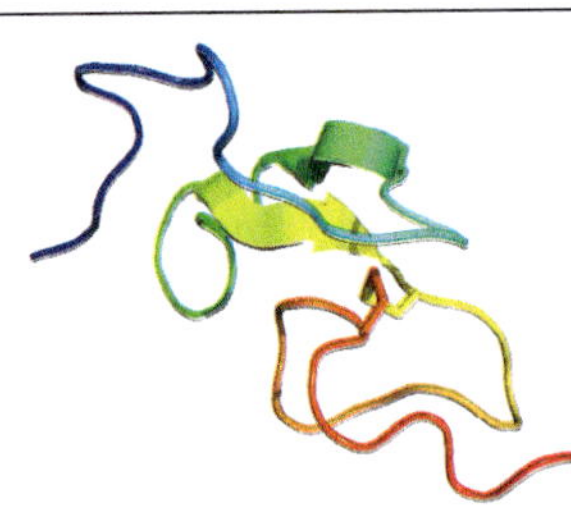

8.1. Plasma and Plasma Medicine

8.1.1. Cold Atmospheric Plasma

Plasma is sometimes referred to as the fourth state of matter (physical plasma) or the majority of human blood (physiological plasma), depending on the context. Electrons, ions, photons, metastables, and electromagnetic fields are the constituents of plasma as defined by physics. In the past, high pressure and temperatures were used to create plasma. These days, room temperature and atmospheric pressure can be used to create cold atmospheric plasma (CAP).

Piezoelectric direct discharge (PDD) and pulsed atmospheric arc (PAA) technologies are two examples of the technologies that have been used to create atmospheric plasma. For instance, a PDD CAP generator is a singular device that combines plasma generation and voltage transformation into one small, incredibly effective unit. Numerous benefits are offered by its piezoelectric radiofrequency (RF) plasma generator, including a high ionization speed, multi-gas ignition, low power consumption, and an efficient rate of reactive oxygen and nitrogen species (RONS) generation (Figure 8.1).

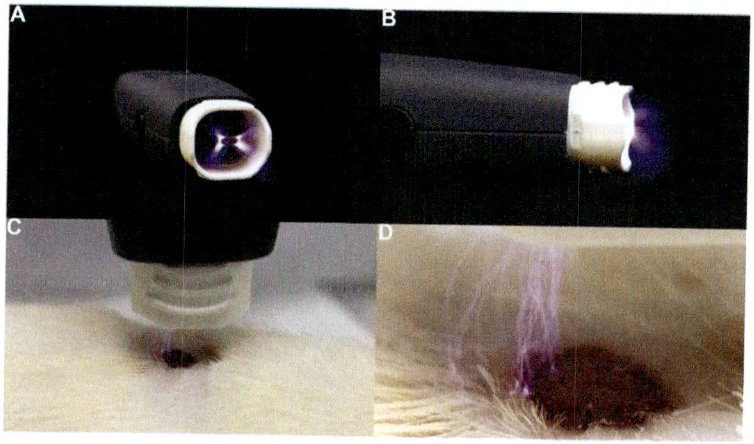

Figure 8.1. *Demonstration of a hand-held CAP generator and its direct application on the skin. The PDD (piezoelectric direct discharge) technology-based plasma instrument, PZ3, was used to generate plasma on the cutaneous wound of a Sprague-Dawley rat's dorsum. (A) axial view of the PZ3 outlet. (B) sagittal view of the PZ3 body. (C) Skin therapy using PZ3. (D) Close-up of PZ3 in operating mode.*

Source: Tan F, Wang Y, Zhang S, Shui R and Chen J (2022) Plasma Dermatology: Skin Therapy Using Cold Atmospheric Plasma. Front. Oncol. 12:918484. doi: 10.3389/fonc.2022.918484.

8.1.2. Plasma Medicine

The utilization of RONS in the medical field has been made easier by the fact that they are essential to numerous biological and cellular processes as a result of CAP's hierarchical reaction with surrounding air. Furthermore, the transient electric fields and UV light may be significant for biomedical applications. The term "plasma medicine," which was recently created, refers to an interdisciplinary field that combines chemistry, biology, medicine, and physics. There are two main categories of applications for plasma medicine: direct applications and indirect applications. While the latter suggests delivering the reactive species of the CAP to a living recipient via an intermediary carrier, the former refers to subjecting a living recipient to a gaseous plasma plume.

Numerous medical specialties have seen the direct medical applications of CAP. These cover a wide range of fields, such as dentistry (such as root canal disinfection and tooth bleaching), neurology (such as promoting neural cell differentiation into neurons *in vitro* and *in vivo*), oncology (such as causing immunogenic cancer cell death and collaborating with other anti-neoplastic agents), infection control (such as managing microbial biofilm), and so on. Conversely, the indirect uses of CAP are accomplished by means of a mixture (such as a stem cell niche), a liquid object (such as plasma-activated medium), or a solid object (such as a surgical implant). The biological impact of CAP permeates through cellular, protein, and even DNA/mRNA levels, regardless of the operating mode.(Isbary et al., 2012).

8.1.3. Plasma Dermatology

A growing field of plasma medicine is plasma dermatology, partly due to the fact that skin is the largest and most superficial organ in the human body, making plasma treatment comparatively simple. Chronic wounds were the main focus of the initial round of clinical randomized controlled trials (RCTs) utilizing CAP in dermatology. Their achievement was complex.

First of all, chronic wounds are a common skin condition, particularly in patients with impaired immune systems and the elderly population. Second, there are still very few available treatment options for this illness. Finally, CAP's antimicrobial and anti-inflammatory properties make it a perfect tool for a wound that is persistently colonized.Several reviews have been published on the topic, each with its own strengths and weaknesses. Some have oversimplified the disease spectrum, while others have not effectively balanced clinical findings with scientific interpretation (Tan et al., 2022).

8.2. Optimizing Intact Skin Using Cap

8.2.1. Clinical Anatomy of Human Skin

The human skin has a surface area of 2 m^2, making up to 20% of the body weight. It is a unique structure. The skin serves as a barrier of defense, a sensory organ, a means of transferring nutrients and metabolites, a means of controlling body temperature, and a site of immunological activity. The epidermis, dermis, and hypodermis are the three layers of skin that make up the skin's depths, arranged superficially (Figure 8.2).

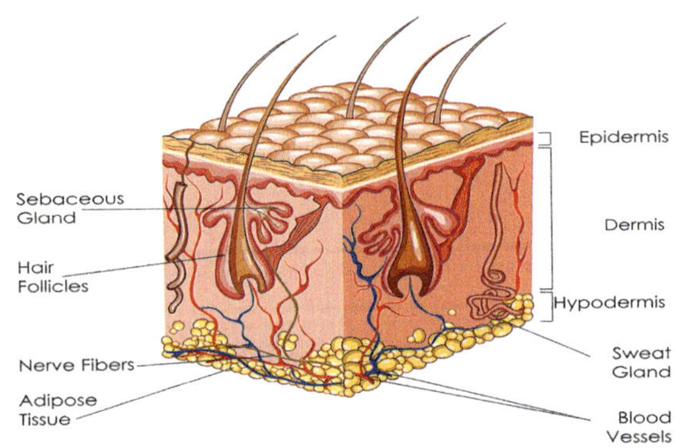

Figure 8.2. *Schematic diagram of the skin: its three layers and accessory structures.*

Source: Tan F, Wang Y, Zhang S, Shui R and Chen J (2022) Plasma Dermatology: Skin Therapy Using Cold Atmospheric Plasma. Front. Oncol. 12:918484. doi: 10.3389/fonc.2022.918484.

The stratum corneum, stratum lucidum, stratum granulosum, stratum spinosum, and stratum basale are the five sublayers that make up the epidermis. Melanocytes, Langerhans cells, and keratinocytes are the three main cell types that make up the epidermis. Originating from the ectoderm, keratinocytes are specialized cells that produce keratin. The neural crest gives rise to melanocytes, which produce melanin. Dendritic cells called Langerhans cells have the ability to identify, interpret, and present antigens to lymphocytes during an allergic reaction.

The basement membrane zone connects the dermis to the epidermis. The reticular region (deep area) and the papillary region (superficial area) make up the two regions of the dermis. Adnexal structures like sweat glands, hair follicles, sebaceous glands, and nails are found within it. Collagen, especially type I collagen, which is the main substance in the skin that is resistant to stress, makes up the majority of the dermis.

The skin is attached to the underlying muscles and bones by the hypodermis, or subcutaneous tissue, which is made up of adipose tissue and loose connective tissue. The three primary cell types present here are lipocytes, macrophages, and fibroblasts. The larger blood vessels and nerves that supply the skin are also found in the hypodermis.

8.2.2. The Effect of CAP on Skin Cells

In vitro research on the impact of CAP solely on healthy skin cells has been the subject of numerous studies in the past few years. HaCaT human immortalized keratinocytes were primarily used as the cellular model in these studies. It was discovered that, despite some variances in the cellular changes induced by plasma, the corresponding changes at the cellular level were also mirrored at the protein and gene levels (Table 8.1).

Arndt et al. conducted a relatively early study. applied the MicroPlaSter β plasma torch system to primary keratinocytes from human skin. Their primary novel discovery was the upregulation of β-defensin family antimicrobial peptides following CAP treatment. Defensins are cationic proteins with a high cysteine content that exhibit antibacterial, antifungal, and antiviral properties. They may be present in atopic dermatitis and other inflammatory skin disorders. Important regulators of inflammation and wound healing, including transforming growth factor beta (TGF-β) and interleukin 8 (IL-8), were also made to express their genes in response to CAP. CAP did not, however, affect keratinocyte migration, proliferation, or apoptosis. Using CAP treatment, it was possible to alter cell proliferation, motility, and apoptosis, leading to different outcomes in subsequent HaCaT cell studies.(Schmidt et al., 2017).

Choi and associates used a dielectric barrier discharge (DBD)-based low-frequency argon plasma device. At the cellular level, CAP accelerated the G1 cell cycle phase and sped up the S and G2 phases, which in turn promoted keratinocyte proliferation. At the protein level, CAP moved β-catenin from the cytosol to the nucleus and distributed E-cadherin-mediated cell-to-cell interactions. CAP treatment boosted c-MYC and cyclin D1 transcription and expression at the gene level. Thus, these findings of increased epidermal cell proliferation suggested that CAP could be applied as a novel skin-regenerating device.

Conversely, a number of research projects carried out by Schmidt et al. The atmospheric argon plasma jet using kINPen 09 produced suppressive results instead. First, following direct CAP exposure, human keratinocytes showed decreased cell proliferation, a brief increase in cell migration, and the secretion of immunomodulatory signal proteins.

Table 8.1. *The Effect of CAP on Skin Cells*

Novelty	Cell type	Cellular level	Molecular level	Gene level
Skin renewal activity ***via*** activation of β-catenin	HaCaT keratinocytes	Increases cell proliferation *via* cell cycle change	Translocation of β-catenin to nucleus	Enhances gene expression of c-MYC & cyclin D1
CAP modulates p53 & activates MAPK signaling	HaCaT keratinocytes	Reduction in cell proliferation, transient increase in cell migration	Induces accumulation & nuclear translocation of p53	Upstream ATM & ATR, downstream MAP, Hsp27, IL-6 & IL-8
Transcriptomic microarray, periodic long-term Tx with PAM	HaCaT keratinocytes	Reduces cell motility & induces morphological changes	Selective protein validation	260 genes in inflammation & redox homeostasis
Role of ambient gas composition on CAP-elicited cell signaling	HaCaT keratinocytes	O_2 shielding provides stronger apoptotic effects than N_2, & induces cell response more efficiently	Modulates cell-signaling molecules, alters ROS & RNS compositions in liquids	Pathway-specific microarray, IL-6, HMOX1, VEGFA, HBEGF, CSF2, & MAPK
CAP promotes cell growth ***via*** NF-κB signaling pathway	L929 fibroblasts	Increases cell proliferation *via* cell cycle change	Secretion of EGF & TGF-β1, upregulates P-p65 & cyclin D1, but downregulates IkB	N/A
Activation of antimicrobial peptides of β-defensin family	Primary skin keratinocytes	Does not modulate cellular proliferation, migration & apoptosis	Induces IL-8, activates TGF-β, promotes β-defensins	Induces key regulators

Source: Tan F, Wang Y, Zhang S, Shui R and Chen J (2022) Plasma Dermatology: Skin Therapy Using Cold Atmospheric Plasma. Front. Oncol. 12:918484. doi: 10.3389/fonc.2022.918484.

The aforementioned alterations were focused on the p53 regulatory axis, whereby ATM and ATR were phosphorylated upstream and checkpoint kinases Chk and mitogen-activated protein (MAP) kinases were activated downstream. Consequently, it was established that plasma had proapoptotic, proinflammatory, and pro-survival effects. Second, keratinocyte motility was suppressed and cell size was increased by intermittent, continuous, indirect therapy with plasma-activated medium (PAM). Using transcriptome microarray technology, the researchers found differential expression of 260 genes related to redox homeostasis and inflammation. These dysregulated genes produce a variety of cytokines, growth factors, antioxidant enzymes, and targets for apoptotic signaling as protein products. Finally, the same research team modulated the ambient gas composition from pure nitrogen to pure oxygen, changing the generation of reactive species in the plasma effluent. Compared to its nitrogen counterpart, the oxygen-shielding plasma induced keratinocyte response more effectively and had a stronger apoptotic effect. The study of gene expression demonstrated the upregulation of various antioxidative molecules and signaling and communication proteins, including immunomodulatory interleukin 6 (IL-6).

In summary, the inconsistency in plasma-induced cellular change in healthy skin cells, such as cell proliferation, cell migration, and cell apoptosis are multifactorial. CAP-generating technology (e.g., DBD or others), treatment modality (e.g., direct jet or indirect PAM), plasma parameters (e.g., duration, and gas composition), and target skin cell type (e.g., keratinocytes vs. fibroblasts, human vs. murine) all could be contributing factors. More dedicated studies are required to expand our understanding on the effect of CAP on healthy skin cells.

8.2.3. The Effect of CAP on Skin Histology

The cellular effects of CAP have been investigated further at the histological level. Using different histological staining techniques, such as Masson's trichrome staining, immunohistochemical (IHC) analysis, and hematoxylin and eosin (HandE) staining, more architectural information was discovered. The two studies that Choi et al. demonstrated that giving HRM2 mice a brief CAP treatment led to a significant increase in dermal collagen density and epidermal thickness. Activating β-catenin in the epidermal cells, repeated CAP treatment not only caused epidermal expansion but also accelerated dermal remodelling. Conversely, the skin tissue expression of several growth factors, including TGF, VEGF, GM-CSF, and epidermal growth factor (EGF), was elevated by plasma. It's interesting that. Remarkably, Hasse et al. added greater clinical value because they treated patients with plasma using human skin biopsies from nine different patients. The pro-proliferative effect of CAP in the current work occurred as deep as the stratum basale, while the epidermal integrity and keratin expression remained unchanged. This is in contrast to what was previously demonstrated, where plasma-generated species only penetrated the first few layers of the epidermis. All of these *in vivo* research point to CAP as a novel tool with potential for skin anti-aging.

8.2.4. The Effect of CAP on Cutaneous Blood Vessels

For intact skin, CAP generally improves cutaneous microcirculation. 2016 saw Kisch et al. conducted a controlled, prospective cohort study utilizing the radial forearm skin of 20 healthy patients. Their DBD CAP device was effective for at least eight minutes and raised the cutaneous tissue oxygen saturation by 24%. Furthermore, there was a 73% increase in cutaneous capillary blood flow, which persisted for 11 minutes at a fast rate. Additionally, patients with lower body mass index (BMI) showed an even more pronounced elevation of these parameters.

By contrast, Borchardt, and colleagues carried out a similar study with fewer patients, but for a longer monitoring period, assessed a greater number of circulation parameters. First, there was a plasma duration-dependent improvement in tissue oxygen saturation and blood flow. Second, skin temperature and moisture did not change following CAP treatment; instead, skin pH dropped by 0.3. Most notably, it was discovered that the improvement in skin microcirculation associated with CAP was unique to the plasma treatment and was not brought on by the mechanical pressure that was applied.

Arndt et al. conducted experiments both *in vitro* and *in vivo* using the MicroPlaSter β plasma torch system to investigate how CAP influences vascularization-involved molecules in skin-related cells. The results showed that CAP significantly increased the expression of various molecules such as artemin, EGF, EG-VEGF, endothelin-1, bFGF, IL-8 in human epidermal keratinocytes, and angiogenin, endostatin, MCP-1, MMP-9, TIMP-1, and VEGF in human dermal fibroblasts. In addition, CAP also enhanced the expression of Ang-2, angiostatin, amphiregulin, endostatin, bFGF, and angiogenic receptors in HUVECs. These findings suggest that CAP plays a role in modulating angiogenesis-related factors through autocrine and paracrine mechanisms.

8.2.5. The Effect of CAP on Skin Chemical Components

One of the most crucial elements of the skin barrier is the stratum corneum's lipids. Marschewski's team was among the first to analyze CAP-induced alterations in the physiological skin lipid composition using X-ray photoelectron spectroscopy (XPS). The authors found that using human forearms with their skin lipids removed, the total carbon amount decreased from 84.4% to 76.7%, the oxygen amount increased from 10.8% to 16.5%, and the nitrogen amount slightly increased from 4.8% to 6.8%. Reduced C-C bonds and increased C-O, C=O, C-N, and N-C-O bonds were the cause of these chemical alterations. Striesow's *in vitro* experiment, which used an argon plasma jet to treat collected human forehead lipids, solidified this proof-of-principle study. Minimal CAP-driven oxidation of triacyclglycerols, ceramides, and cholesteryl esters was detected by the liquid chromatography-tandem mass spectroscopy (RP-LC/MS2) and direct-infusion high-resolution tandem mass spectroscopy (DI-MS2). Functionally speaking, the epidermal lipid overlay might be adequately shielded, and mild CAP treatment would have little detrimental effects on the dermal tissue. Moreover, Schmidt, and colleagues performed an *in vivo* investigation on mouse skin and used reversed-phase liquid chromatography/mass spectroscopy to find oxidative modification in the relative abundance of lipid classes. In conclusion, Kartaschew et al. employed Raman vibrational microspectroscopy and infrared spectroscopy to analyze chemically the changes in skin components caused by plasma, including keratin and lanolin, which are similar to human sebum. The authors proposed that an antibacterial and regenerative milieu in the stratum corneum where plasma interacted may have originated from the resulting acidic and NO-containing functional groups.

Even though the investigational hardware mentioned, including different forms of mass spectroscopy, has made studying the effect of CAP on skin chemistry much easier, there are limitations in the analytical software's capacity to detect unexpected oxidized lipids. This could result in an underestimation of CAP's influence on skin lipids, highlighting the necessity for software improvements (Tan et al., 2022).

8.3. Treatment of Skin Disease Using CAP

The target skin diseases that can be treated with CAP in dermatology include alopecia, wound healing, inflammatory, and infectious skin disorders, parasite infestation, skin cancer, and genetic and skin disorders. Preclinical animal research, human clinical trials, and laboratory cellular experiments make up the studies that are summarized here (Table 8.2).

Table 8.2. *Skin Disease-Specific Application of CAP*

Category	Subgroup	Disease	Test Model	Synopsis
Wound healing	Cutaneous wound	Acute wound	Keratinocytes, fibroblasts, mice	Accelerates full-thickness re-epithelialization & gap closure
			Mice	Combined Tx of Ar & He plasma needle
			Mice	Dual effects, low dose boosts but high dose suppresses
			Mice	Differential galectin expression in CAP & electrocoagulation
			Mice	Enhances burn wound neovascularisation *via* eNOS signaling
			Mice	Nrf2 signaling & inflammation are key events
			Mice	Enhances ECM formation in skin graft recipient site
			Bacteria, mice	PAW inactivates bacteria, promotes healing & suppresses inflammation
			Rats	Multimodal Tx with CAP & aFGF for multi-tissue regeneration
			Human	RCT on skin graft donor sites
		Chronic wound	MRSA, P. aeruginosa	Multi-device inactivation of multi-microbe
			Fibroblasts, mice	Activates genes for key cytokines & growth factors
			Rats	Higher mechanical strength of CAP-repaired wound in pressure ulcer
			Human	Comparable immediate antimicrobial effect to OCT, but limited coverage

			Human	Promotes various types of superficial skin erosion wounds healing
			Human	RCT, 2-min Tx of 2 CAP devices reduce bacterial load
			Human	RCT, higher antibacterial effect, ulcer reduction & applicability, lower pt pain
		Diabetic wound	Rats	PAW treats STZ-induced diabetic wound
			Keratinocytes, mice	Reduces inflammation & oxidative stress, without systemic toxic effects
			glycated GPx, mice	Increases enzyme & antioxidant activity, and reduces inflammation
			Human, foot ulcer	RCT, accelerates healing by decreasing bacterial load & inflammatory phase
			Human, foot ulcer	RCT, beneficial in wound surface reduction & time to wound closure
	Neural wound		Astrocytes	PAM, CNS injury
Inflammatory disorder	Dermatitis	Allergic contact dermatitis	Mice	Humidified argon plasma
		Atopic dermatitis	Mast cells, mice	PAM inhibits mast cell activation, ameliorates HDM-induced AD
		Diaper dermatitis	Human	case report
	Psoriasis		Keratinocytes	Induces cellular apoptosis & reduces IL-12
			Keratinocytes, mice	Inhibits pro-inflammatory molecules and increases PD-L1 expression
			Keratinocytes, mice	Exerts antiproliferative & proapoptotic effects
		Palmo-plantar psoriasis	Human	PCC instrument, case report

		Inverse psoriasis	Human	Case reports
	Lichen planus		Human, mucosal tissue	Decreased T-cell infiltrate & inflammatory markers
Infectious disease	Fungal infection	Dermatophytosis	Fungal isolates	Lower sensitivity to bacteria and yeast
			Fungal isolates	He/O_2 suppresses ergosterol biosynthesis, increases keratinase activity
			Guinea pigs	Course of infection was a week shorter and milder
			Fungal isolates, guinea pigs	Combined Tx of Ag NPs and CAP, comparable with fluconazole
		Onychomycosis	Human, nail plate model	Cadaver nails and agarose media
			Human, toenail	Good clinical cure rate and high patient satisfaction
			Human	Synergistic effect of CAP and NPAR
		Alternariosis	dogs	Immunocompromised
	Viral infection	HPV	Human	Adult case reports
			Human	Pediatric case series
		HSV-1	Vero cells, neuroblastoma cells	Low but measurable antiviral effect
Infestation	Parasitic bites	Pediculosis	Human	Comb-like plasma device
		Demodicosis	Human, mite isolates	Potential in papulopustular rosacea
Skin malignancy	Melanoma		Melanoma cells	SMD plasma induces senescence
			Melanoma cells, mice	Flexible capillary CAP slows progression of cancer
			Melanoma cells, mice	Comparison of direct & indirect CAP treatment
			Melanoma cells	Comparison of target genes by ROS & non-ROS

			Melanoma cells	EM emission from CAP kills *via* transbarrier contactless method
			Melanoma cells	PpIX-loaded polymersome-mediated PDT with CAP posttreatment
			Mice	CAP alone & combined with ECT
			Melanoma cells, mice xenograft	CAP & SN synergistically inhibits *via* HGF/c-MET pathway
	SCC		HNSCC cells	CAP selectively impairs cancer cells
			HNSCC cells	Reduces cell viability & induces apoptosis
			Oral SCC cells	Selective killing effect with NO-induced dysfunction of EGFR
			Oral SCC cells	N_2 CAP inhibits cell migration & invasion most potently *via* decreased FAK & MMP
			Oral SCC cells	Synergistic effect of cisplatin & CAP
			Cutaneous SCC cells	PAM induces apoptosis & decreases proliferation
			Cutaneous SCC cells, mice	CAP limits cancer development
	BCC		BCC cells	PAM induces apoptosis *via* MAPK pathway
	Premalignant lesions	Actinic keratosis	Human	Case series
			Human	Seven patients
			Human	Various plasma devices
			Human	Clinical & ultrasound evaluation
Genetic disorder	Keratinization issue	Hailey disease	Human	Case report

Alopecia			Human dermal hair follicle papilla cells	PAM regulates cell cycle and proliferation
			Human	Long-term, PAM
			Wistar rats	N_2 plasma increases hair follicle diameter
Symptom of skin disease	Pruritus		Human	Various etiologies, VAS similar to Ar

Source: Tan F, Wang Y, Zhang S, Shui R and Chen J (2022) Plasma Dermatology: Skin Therapy Using Cold Atmospheric Plasma. Front. Oncol. 12:918484. doi: 10.3389/fonc.2022.918484.

8.3.1. Wound Healing

8.3.1.1. Cutaneous Wound

Through a number of mechanisms, such as its pro-angiogenic and antiseptic properties, stimulation of cell migration and proliferation, and modulation of topical inflammation, CAP can accelerate the healing of skin wounds. CAP treatment can help promote the healing of wounds of different kinds, including diabetic, chronic, and acute wounds.

1. **Acute Wound:** Several studies have provided additional mechanistic information regarding the treatment of acute skin wounds with CAP, based on the aforementioned known phenomena. By downregulating connexin 43, E-cadherin, and multiple integrins that are involved in adherence junctions and cytoskeletal dynamics, CAP may hasten the closure of wound gaps. Through the modulation of VEGF signaling and endothelial nitric oxide synthase (eNOS), CAP may improve wound neovascularization. Additionally, by controlling the nuclear E2-related factor (Nrf2) pathway and redox-sensitive p53 signaling, CAP may be able to balance the inflammatory and antioxidant responses. However, not many other studies provided useful cues. Since argon and helium plasma were found to be more effective for coagulation and healing, respectively, CAP treatment could be tailored to the various stages of wound healing. Galectins could be used as a marker to track the impact of CAP in contrast to electrocoagulation since they were increased in the latter treatment modality and inhibited in the former. However, the length of CAP must be carefully regulated while treating wounds because an excessive amount of plasma may inhibit wound healing by causing excessive necrosis or apoptosis. In the work above, full-thickness surgical incisions and third-degree burns are the two most frequently used models of acute wounds. In a novel procedure known as skin grafting, healthy skin from one part of the body is taken out and transplanted to a damaged area. At the site of donation, Heinlin et al. carried out a randomized placebo-controlled trial and found that following CAP treatment, there were fewer fibrin layers and blood crusts, as well as better wound re-epithelialisation. At the location of the recipient, Frescaline, and co. discovered that by triggering the canonical SMAD-dependent TGF-β1 pathway, CAP could improve the formation of extracellular matrix (ECM).(Frescaline et al., 2020) Lastly, the multimodality of CAP treatment for acute skin wounds has been shown to be flexible. CAP could be

employed indirectly in a PAM form in addition to directly in a plasma jet. Xu and others. found that PAM had the same ability to suppress inflammation, inactivate bacteria, and accelerate wound healing. Most recently, Tan, and co. observed that during wound healing and other tissue regenerative processes, CAP could cooperate with acidic FGF.

2. **Chronic Wounds:** Even though a chronic wound begins as an acute wound, it takes longer to heal because it does not go through the stages of wound healing as expected. The three main categories of chronic wounds that will be covered in separate sections are diabetic, pressure, and vascular ulcers. Some characteristics are similar among them, including an exaggerated phase of inflammation, an ongoing infection, and the development of drug-resistant biofilm. The most desired aspect of CAP's chronic wound care is its antimicrobial effect. First, the Mohd Nasir group. discovered that two common bacteria found in clinically recalcitrant chronic wounds, *Pseudomonas aeruginosa* and methicillin-resistant *Staphylococcus aureus* (MRSA), can both be inactivated by CAP generated using the capillary guided corona discharge (CGCD) and parallel plate dielectric barrier discharge (DBD) technologies. Although for different strains of the aforementioned bacteria, these two plasma designs' antibacterial efficacy varied. Furthermore, Ulrich et al. found that CAP had an instantaneous antimicrobial effect similar to that of octenidine, a contemporary antiseptic used for cutaneous and mucous wounds. Long-term efficacy of octenidine over CAP was observed, despite the fact that patients with chronic leg ulcers tolerated both treatments well. Finally, during the course of treating chronic wounds with CAP, two randomized controlled trials (RCTs) demonstrated a strong antimicrobial effect. Isbary and associates proved that, regardless of the type of bacteria, a two-minute argon plasma treatment was adequate to dramatically lower the bacterial load. In contrast, Brehmer et al. showed that plasma treatment resulted in a subjective increase in patient and physician satisfaction in addition to an objective reduction in the bacterial load and ulcer size in chronic venous leg ulcers. Apart from the vascular ulcer model utilized in the previous experiments, Chatraie's recent work also employed a pressure ulcer model. This intriguing study concentrated on how CAP closes wounds that are chronic. The outcomes demonstrated that the repaired wound's mechanical strength in the group receiving plasma treatment was noticeably greater than that of the control. This suggested that during the chronic wound healing process, CAP could provide enhanced tissue strength and maturity.

3. **Diabetic Wound:** Diabetic wounds are more common than vascular and pressure chronic ulcers, and they have unique pathologies like neuropathy, microangiopathy, and hyperglycemia. A small number of animal studies consistently reported benefits from CAP for diabetic wound healing, including decreased oxidative stress and inflammation, enhanced angiogenesis, and improved wound closure. Additionally, each of these studies offered more details. Antioxidants like glutathione peroxidase (GPx) were

found in wound tissue at higher levels following indirect plasma treatment (PAM), but the antioxidant activity of glycated GPx induced by diabetes was significantly increased following direct plasma treatment. Most importantly, biochemical results from routine blood tests indicated that CAP treatment did not result in systemic toxic effects.

8.3.1.2. Neural Wound

The focus of recent CAP-facilitated wound healing research has shifted from cutaneous to other tissues, including neural tissue. In Sardella et al.'s pilot study. PAM was discovered to have the ability to control astrocyte migration and growth in response to RONS. In particular, PAM that was enriched with $H_2O_2^-$ and nitrite had a negative and neutral effect on cell growth, respectively, whereas PAM that was balanced could promote the growth of astrocytes and improve the healing of neural wounds. This may expand the application of CAP-assisted wound healing to injuries to the central nervous system (CNS), including Parkinson's disease (PD) and Alzheimer's disease (AD).

8.3.2. Inflammatory Skin Disorder

8.3.2.1. Dermatitis

Skin inflammation is what dermatitis is. In the early stages of dermatitis, symptoms like itching, redness, and rash may be present; in the more advanced stages, edema, and blisters may occur. Pathophysiologically speaking, dermatitis is distinguished by spongiosis, which permits the accumulation of inflammatory cells and mediators. Atopic, seborrheic, and allergic dermatitis are common forms of dermatitis.

Firstly, using a mouse model of allergic contact dermatitis (ACD), Xiong et al. found that humidified CAP is better than oxygen or nitrogen plasma when treating mild and severe ACD. This was mainly because active species delivered by water-containing argon plasma became adhesive to the dry skin of ACD leading to good penetration of ROS. Secondly, Lee et al. discovered that PAM could inhibit mast cell activation by inhibiting the expression of IL-6, tumor necrosis factor (TNF)-α, and nuclear factor kappa B (NF-κB). In addition, direct CAP treatment could ameliorate house dust mite (HDM)-induced atopic dermatitis in mice by suppressing the recruitment of mast cells and eosinophils as well as differentiation of Th2 cells. Finally, in a case report on a 14-month-old girl with diaper dermatitis with urinary and faecal bacterial infection, who failed topical and oral medical treatment, Zhang et al. presented satisfactory therapeutic effect of CAP. After six sessions of treatment, patient's pain and genital ulcer completely resolved without any adverse reactions or disease recurrence.

8.3.2.2. Psoriasis

Psoriasis is a multisystem autoimmune syndrome characterized by well-defined, pink, scaly, itchy patches, mostly on the body's extensor surfaces, like the scalp, knees, and elbows. Psoriasis is primarily caused by two pathogenic processes: secondary epidermal proliferation and immune suppression combined with dermal inflammation.

Zhong et al. used a cellular model of psoriasis. discovered that CAP could lower the expression of IL-12 and cause lysosomal leakage, apoptosis, and mitochondrial dysfunction in human keratinocytes. Overall, by inhibiting keratinocyte hyperproliferation and focusing on T-cell activation, these effects have implications for managing the exacerbation of skin inflammation.

Gan et al. used a mouse model of imiquimod-induced psoriasis and demonstrated that repeated CAP administration could lessen epidermal proliferation and improve the appearance of psoriasis. Conversely, Lee, and colleagues observed that plasma treatment could increase the expression of programmed cell death ligand 1 (PD-L1) and suppress the expression of pro-inflammatory molecules.

According to case reports of psoriasis patients, Gareri et al. as well as Zheng and others demonstrated that CAP had a good preventing or even curing effect on palmo-plantar psoriasis and inverse psoriasis, respectively. These subtypes of psoriasis are typically resistant to conventional therapies.

8.3.2.3. Lichen Planus

The primary tissues affected by lichen planus (LP), a chronic inflammatory and immune-mediated disorder, are the skin and oral mucosa. A purple papule or plaque that is pruritic and polygonal in shape, with white striae covering it, is indicative of cutaneous lipomatosis. The pathophysiology of LP may involve basal cell damage and liquefaction caused by an inflammatory infiltrate mediated by T cells.

Seebauer and associates used mucosal tissue samples from oral LP patients in an *ex vivo* experiment and CAP treatment. The oral LP tissue exhibited elevated levels of GM-CSF, IL-1β, IL-6, and IL-8, as well as an increased infiltrate of $CD8^+$ and $CD45\text{-}R0^+$ T cells. When CAP was applied to this diseased mucosal tissue, it dramatically lowered the T-cell infiltrate as well as the production of inflammatory cytokines and chemokines (Tan et al., 2022).

8.3.3. Infectious Skin Disease

Gram-positive bacteria like streptococci and staphylococci are responsible for the majority of bacterial skin infections. Treatment of bacterial skin disease will not be elaborated here, as the antibacterial effect of CAP has already been discussed in "Cutaneous wound healing" and other reviews. CAP therapy is receiving more attention for viral and fungal skin diseases.

8.3.3.1. Fungal Infection

A fungal infection of the skin called dermatophytosis is brought on by dermatophytes, which take up nutrients from keratin in the stratum corneum. Usually, it appears as a circular, red, scaly, itchy rash. Numerous *in vitro* and *in vivo* investigations have examined the antifungal potential of CAP recently. Scholtz and others tested CAP on four human pathogenic dermatophytes: geophilic *Microsporum gypseum*, zoophilic *Arthroderma benhamiae*, and anthropophilic *Trichoderma rubrum* and *Trichoderma interdigitale*. A 25-minute CAP exposure could result in total fungal spore inactivation and consequent decontamination, although the susceptibility of dermatophytes to CAP treatment appeared to be genus-specific and lower than that of bacteria and yeast. Moreover, Shapourzadeh, and colleagues. applied a 98% oxygen/2% helium CAP to *Trichopteron rubrum*. In a plasma dose-dependent manner, CAP treatment markedly inhibited fungal growth by up to 91%, decreased ergosterol biosynthesis by up to 54%, and increased keratinase activity by up to 21%. Once more, Scholtz et al. tested the CAP on guinea pigs infected with the dermatophyte *Trichophyton mentagrophytes* SK 3286. Their specialized plasma device not only reduced the number of fungal colony-forming units (CFU), but it also shortened and mildened the infection's week-long duration. Lastly, Ouf, and associates applied a combination of CAP therapy and silver nanoparticles (AgNPs) to an animal model of dermatophytosis. In terms of antifungal efficacy, combinatorial therapy was found to be superior to standalone treatment and on par with fluconazole.

Onychomycosis is a fungal infection of the nail plate and the nail bed, and is more commonly found in toenails than in fingernails. Its symptoms include discolored and thickened nail plate, subungual debris, and onycholysis. In an *in vitro* study using a novel toenail-plate model using cadaver nails and fungi-inoculated agarose mold, Bulson et al. found that direct CAP exposure resulted in the complete killing of *Candida albicans* and *Trichophyton mentagrophytes* at a low dose, and CAP treatment through the nail plate reduced viability of *C. albicans* at a higher dose. In 2017, Lipner et al. recruited 19 patients with toenail onychomycosis. The overall clinical cure and mycological cure were 53.8% and 15.4%, respectively, after CAP treatment. In 2020, Lux et al. significantly improved the above indices to 70% and 85.7% using the synergistic combination of CAP and nail plate abrasion and refreshment (NPAR).

8.3.3.2. Viral Infection

Only two years have passed since the antiviral potential of CAP has been studied, and there are very few studies that are pertinent to this topic. Herpes simplex virus (HSV) is a common and contagious virus that spreads through direct skin or mucosal contact, where it causes watery blisters. HSV-1 can cause encephalitis and conjunctivitis in addition to producing the majority of herpes labialis. Bunz and associates used Vero cells, a common HSV research cell line, and SH-SY5Y cell line from neuroblastoma as models for neuronal infection to infect them with HSV-1. They showed that CAP had a negligible but discernible antiviral effect on HSV-1.

Warts on the skin or mucous membrane are caused by the human papilloma virus (HPV), and they are believed to be caused by the proliferating basal keratinocytes that are infected. Two adult patients and five pediatric patients were included in the two small case series that Friedman's group recently published. Both patient groups reported remarkable resolutions of verruca vulgaris, periungual warts, and palmoplantar warts.

8.3.4. Parasitic Infestation

Demodex folliculorum mites are the usual cause of demodecosis in humans, and they may also contribute to or exacerbate papulopustular rosacea. Rosacea is a deformity that usually affects the skin in the midface and is a chronic condition. Daeschlein and others effectively rendered a patient's isolated *Demodex folliculorum* inactive using CAP *in vitro*, a non-antimicrobial treatment. The antiparasitic effectiveness of CAP may indicate a treatment option for Rosacea (Arndt et al., 2013).

There are three types of lice infestations known as pediculosis: pediculosis capitis (infestation of the head louse), pediculosis corporis (infestation of the body louse), and pediculosis pubis (infestation of the pubic louse). 10 Bosch along with others created a comb-like CAP device intended to treat pediculosis capitis physically. Their findings demonstrated that high rates of *Pediculus humanus* and parasitic egg mortality were caused by a single plasma stroke over a hair strand. Three other areas, such as ozone concentration, UV emission, and patient leakage current, were satisfactorily verified as safe for this innovative pesticide-free option.

8.3.5. Skin Malignancy

The three primary forms of skin cancer are melanoma, squamous cell carcinoma (SCC), and basal cell carcinoma (BCC), which are ranked in decreasing order of aggressiveness and increasing order of prevalence, respectively. The capacity of CAP to kill cancer cells while sparing nearby healthy cells is a key component of plasma oncology. Recent research that is pertinent is mostly animal and cellular in nature.

8.3.5.1. Melanoma

Melanoma, the most deadly kind of skin cancer, arises from melanocytes. Both horizontal and vertical spread, such as into the epidermis or hypodermis, contribute to its local invasiveness.

Malignant melanoma warning signs include irregular borders, variegated color, asymmetry, diameter greater than 6 mm, and evolving.

The effectiveness of standalone CAP treatment in inhibiting melanoma cells has been proven. Arndt et al. discovered that different levels of CAP dosages using a novel CAP device based on surface micro discharge (SMD) technology resulted in differential induction of apoptosis or senescence of melanoma cells. Binenbaum et al. adapted the conventional plasma jet system to create a hand-held elongated flexible capillary for precise delivery of CAP to target tumors. The treatment significantly reduced the tumor volume of cutaneous melanoma in a dose-dependent manner. In Saadati's research, the antineoplastic effects of direct and indirect CAP treatments for melanoma were compared in both *in vitro* and *in vivo* studies. While direct plasma treatment was more effective than the indirect method, combining PAM with a chemotherapeutic drug proved to be the most potent approach.

As a result, an increasing number of studies are focusing on combining cold atmospheric plasma (CAP) with other treatment methods such as electrochemotherapy (ECT), photodynamic therapy (PDT), and nanomedicine. In a study using a melanoma mouse model, Daeschlein et al. demonstrated that CAP combined with ECT effectively suppressed tumor growth and improved mouse survival rates. Wang et al. successfully used polymersomes loaded with protoporphyrin IX to kill 50% of melanoma cells through PDT and found that adding CAP posttreatment further reduced melanoma cell viability. Additionally, Adhikari et al. discovered that a combination of CAP and silymarin nanoemulsion could synergistically inhibit melanoma tumorigenesis by targeting the HGF/c-Met pathway in human melanoma cells and mice xenografts. Some researchers have recently looked again at CAP's antitumor potential from a different angle—that is, from the non-RONS component of CAP. Yan and others showed that melanoma cells could be killed by the electromagnetic (EM) radiation from CAP using a transbarrier contactless technique. Because of a different mode of cell death, EM had a greater inhibitory effect than RONS on the reactive species-resistant melanoma cell line B16F10. Conversely, Ji, and colleagues compared the target genes of the ROS and non-ROS components of CAP across the entire genome in cancer cells, including melanoma cells (Tan et al., 2022).

8.3.5.2. Squamous Cell Carcinoma

The malignant keratinocyte tumor known as cutaneous SCC typically manifests as a firm, hard nodule or a red, crusted, and scaling patch after infiltrating the dermis. Under the microscope, the tissue is frequently invaded, there is focal and aberrant keratinization, and there is cellular and nuclear heterogeneity.

Numerous studies have confirmed that CAP is more selective for SCC cells than healthy cells, each with unique additional findings. Guerrero-Preston et al. discovered that helium CAP specifically targeted head and neck SCC cells through a non-apoptotic mechanism. Welz et al. showed that SMD CAP could produce anticancer effects similar to those seen in studies utilizing DBD-based plasma. Lee et al. delved deeper into CAP's selectivity by revealing that only EGFR-overexpressing SCC cells showed degradation and dysfunction of epidermal growth factor receptors after CAP treatment, while normal human fibroblasts did not. Furthermore, pre-treatment with a nitric oxide scavenger prevented these EGFR abnormalities, suggesting that CAP could potentially be a valuable treatment for SCC by inducing EGFR dysfunction through NO radicals. Meanwhile,

Pasqual-Melo et al. confirmed CAP's selectivity *in vivo*, demonstrating that CAP hindered the progression of SCC without harming non-SCC skin tissue, with Nrf2 expression decreased in the lesion but increased in non-lesion tissue.

In addition to its effectiveness in treating SCC, CAP has shown its technical flexibility. PAM, a form of indirect CAP management, has proven to have a strong anti-cancer impact on cutaneous SCC cells. Research by Lee et al. demonstrated a synergistic relationship between CAP and cisplatin chemotherapy in fighting SCC cells. Kang et al. found that nitrogen CAP, when optimized, was the most effective in inhibiting SCC cell migration and invasion by reducing the expression of focal adhesion kinase (FAK) and MMP.

8.3.5.3. Basal Cell Carcinoma

BCC is a basaloid cell skin cancer that is locally invasive but rarely spreads. A pearly, translucent appearance, telangiectasia, and occasionally central ulceration are characteristics of a typical nodular BCC. Yang and associates showed that PAM, such as CAP-activated phosphate-buffered saline (PBS) and Dulbecco's modified Eagle's Medium (DMEM), could cause BCC cells to undergo apoptosis *in vitro* and impair their ability to survive. The authors demonstrated increased MAPK, TNF, and IL-17 signaling pathways using next-generation RNA sequencing, which may be closely linked to PAM-induced apoptosis.

8.3.5.4. Premalignant Lesions

The most prevalent precancerous condition in skin damaged by prolonged sun or UV exposure is actinic keratosis (AK). It usually manifests as thick, crusty, scaly plaques that are more tactile than visual. When AK is examined histopathologically, abnormal keratinocytic proliferation that begins in the basal layer and is limited to the epidermis is typically seen.

Two separate research groups have recently published case series that demonstrate the successful use of CAP in the treatment of AK. Later on, Friedman, and colleagues outlined the key distinctions between the two studies, taking into account the number of lesions treated, the plasma treatment regimen, and the treatment measurement grading system. The authors suggested that rather than focusing solely on reducing clinical thickness, treatment efficacy should be assessed based on the complete elimination of AK. Arisi and associates carried out a more extensive investigation utilizing CAP to treat AK and skin field cancerization last year. The number of AKs, the actinic keratosis area and severity index (AKASI) score, and the cumulative AK area were all found to be decreased by plasma irradiation. Furthermore, CAP treatment improved features of chronic photodamage of the skin surrounding and beneath the AK spots, according to high-frequency ultrasound (Tan et al., 2022).

8.3.6. Hair Loss

Lee et al. conducted an *in vitro* cellular study. Dermal papilla cells (DPCs) from human hair follicles were subjected to controlled cell cycle progression using CAP-activated medium. Mesenchymal cells isolated from the hair papilla of healthy scalp hair follicles are known as human DPCs. The hair papilla in adult hair follicles is essential for regulating hair growth and production. DPCs' cell cycle and proliferation were found to be stopped by PAM treatment at the right concentration and length, after which they were able to gradually recover (Gay-Mimbrera et al., 2016).

In a study conducted on Wistar rats *in vivo*, Babossalam et al. used a novel pulsed nitrogen plasma touch to achieve skin rejuvenation. Skin collagenesis, fibroblast proliferation, and epidermal thickness were found to be significantly increased. Most notably, in the skin that was treated, CAP also caused an increase in the diameter of the primary and secondary hair follicles.

In a study conducted by Khan et al., 14 patients with androgenic alopecia were given long-term CAP treatment using PAM. The study was based on CAP's potential to stimulate stem cell differentiation in different cell types and its inconsistent penetration depth, particularly in thick human scalp skin. Patients underwent PAM washing every six months, which was well received with most reporting subjective improvements in hair quality, as observed by both patients and clinicians.

8.4. Improving Drug Absorbance Into Skin Using CAP

Transdermal drug delivery (TDD) is a technique for administering topical drugs for both local and systemic therapeutic purposes by passing through the stratum corneum and into the deeper skin and blood circulation. To overcome the obstacle of drug penetration, several techniques have been developed, including iontophoresis, electroporation, and microneedles. The drawbacks of the aforementioned approaches might be addressed by CAP, which could act as an effective and non-invasive pretreatment to enhance TDD. The precise process involves multiple factors. First off, CAP may improve the transdermal penetration of medications like cyclosporine and galantamine hydrochloride. Second, CAP may change the makeup of lipids in the skin and other places. Since the stratum corneum is made up of keratinocytes and intercellular lipid matrix, CAP may alter how the skin barrier functions. Thirdly, E-cadherin expression may be downregulated by CAP, which would temporarily hinder the tight junction's ability to open up intercellular pores. Current developments on CAP-facilitated TDD have concentrated on two areas: testing novel medications as a downstream strategy and adjusting plasma parameters as an upstream strategy.

In two research projects that Gelker et al. the electrical properties of plasma could be engineered to induce differentiable permeabilization of human skin that has been removed in its entirety. DBD plasma with both μs and ns pulses has the potential to greatly lower the transepithelial electrical resistance (TEER). Furthermore, in comparison to the ns-pulsed DBD, the μs-pulsed CAP caused more noticeable pore formation in the stratum corneum and skin permeabilization of a test drug. The results were more noticeable when the plasma power was increased, but this could also raise the possibility of skin side effects. This emphasizes the significance of safety and risk assessment prior to the clinical application of CAP-aided TDD.

In a series of consecutive studies conducted by Xin et al., it was found that pre-treatment with capsaicin (CAP) enhanced the transdermal delivery of lidocaine, a local anesthetic drug. Using a mouse model, the researchers observed that the flux of lidocaine through the skin was nearly doubled, allowing the drug to penetrate deeper layers. The study also showed that transepidermal water loss (TEWL) significantly increased immediately after CAP treatment but returned to normal levels within 3 hours, indicating a temporary and reversible alteration in skin barrier function. In a randomized split-face study involving 20 patients, the authors demonstrated that topical lidocaine had a more effective analgesic effect after CAP pre-treatment. The visual analog scale (VAS) scores for pain were significantly lower in the CAP group compared to the control group. Importantly, there were no serious adverse events reported, with only minor disruptions in skin sensation noted (Tan et al., 2022).

8.5. Safety and Risk Assessment in Plasma Dermatology

While it is true that CAP has shown potential as a treatment option for clinical dermatology, it is vital to thoroughly assess its safety before using it. The various elements present in CAP, including electrons, ions, RONS, electromagnetic emission, and UV radiation, make it likely that overtreating with plasma could lead to negative side effects like sensory disturbances, physical harm, and thermal injuries.

The impact of plasma factors was the main focus of the short-term safety analysis. To begin with, Daeschlein et al. examined the dangers associated with three distinct plasma sources: DBD plasma, non-pulsed plasma jet, and pulsed plasma jet. Every plasma treatment was well received and did not result in skin dryness or damage to the skin barrier. Furthermore, Wiegand et al. used a 3D skin model to find the time- and dose-dependent cellular effects of CAP. Negative effects resulted from increasing plasma input power or treatment intervals, and nitrogen was not as damaging as air as a working gas. Lastly, additional dissections of skin damage related to plasma overtreatment were performed by Kos and colleagues. As treatment times and gas flow rates increased, the direct skin damage caused by released heat and reactive oxygen species (RONS) worsened and mostly took the form of skin burns. Conversely, the localized edema that was indicative of indirect skin damage did not become apparent until after two days of plasma overtreatment, regardless of plasma parameters.

The long-term safety analysis of the CAP treatment produced positive findings. Schmidt and associates. examined in a rodent model with a full-thickness skin wound the long-term side effects of repeated argon plasma treatment over a period of 14 days. Blood tests, quantitative PCR, and IHC analysis did not identify any systemic or local side effects, such as tumor formation or chronic inflammation, after a year. Moreover, Rutkowski, and colleagues finished a 5-year clinical follow-up with five patients who had initially taken part in a study on CAP treatment-assisted wound healing. There were no indications of a malignant tumor, an inflammatory response, or a pathological alteration in the plasma-treated regions, according to a comprehensive imaging diagnostic evaluation.

Overall, CAP treatment is considered safe for both normal and diseased skin as long as excessive plasma exposure is prevented. The specific threshold for plasma dosage that distinguishes between safety and potential risks is still unknown due to the diversity of plasma devices and their settings. Additional clinical research is needed to establish dosage recommendations tailored to specific conditions (Tan et al., 2022).

A Closer Look

Platelet Rich Plasma Therapy

Recently, Platelet Rich Plasma (PRP) therapy, also known as the "vampire facial," has garnered significant attention from the media. During this treatment, approximately 30–60mL of the client's blood is extracted, processed, and then the platelet-rich plasma is reinjected into the skin, typically the face. PRP therapy offers a less invasive alternative to procedures such as surgery and may also be referred to as plasma facial, plasma needling, PRP lift, or collagen induction therapy.

PRP as a Beauty Therapy

PRP therapy has grown in popularity as an anti-aging treatment for damaged, sagging, or wrinkled skin because it reduces fine lines and increases collagen production. The jaw, neck, hands, décolletage, and face, especially the area around the eyes, are the body parts where this kind of therapy is usually advised. Customers are informed that although the treatment enhances the skin's tone and texture, the results take time to manifest. Beauty therapists usually advise monthly treatments spread out over three to four months to achieve long-lasting results.

Description of PRP Therapy

The procedure begins with the client having blood drawn from their arm, which is then centrifuged to separate the platelets and plasma from other blood components. The platelet-rich plasma is then reintroduced to the client's skin through either microneedling or injection using a syringe. Microneedling is considered a dual therapy, as the needling helps the skin resurface while the PRP introduces collagen and elastin to promote cell growth.

Potential Side Effects

It is possible to experience some or all of the following skin-related side effects up to a week after the therapy:

- bruising.
- burning.
- intense itching.
- swelling.
- dryness.
- puffiness.
- redness.

There may also be side effects like slight nausea, fainting, and dizziness. Infection, nerve injuries, pain, and tissue damage are possible injection side effects.

Summary

- As an emerging branch, plasma dermatology takes advantage of the beneficial complexity of plasma constituents (e.g., reactive oxygen and nitrogen species, UV photons, and electromagnetic emission), technical versatility (e.g., direct irradiation and indirect aqueous treatment), and practical feasibility (e.g., hand-held compact device and clinician-friendly operation).
- Plasma dermatology has emerged as an attractive specialty of plasma medicine, partially because the skin is the largest and most superficial organ in the human body, which makes plasma treatment relatively easy.
- The lipids of the stratum corneum are one of the most important components of the skin barrier.
- The dermatological applications of CAP can be categorized according to the types of target skin disease, including wound healing, inflammatory skin disorder, infectious skin disease, parasite infestation, skin malignancy, genetic skin disorder, and alopecia.
- From a pathophysiological viewpoint, dermatitis is characterized by spongiosis which allows inflammatory cells and mediators to accumulate. Common types of dermatitis include allergic, atopic, and seborrheic dermatitis.
- Psoriasis is a multisystem autoimmune syndrome that presents with well-defined, pink, itchy scaly patches predominantly on the extensor surface of the body, such as elbows and knees, back, and scalp.
- Dermatophytosis is a fungal infection of the skin caused by dermatophytes which absorb nutrients from keratin in the stratum corneum.
- Demodicosis in humans is usually caused by *Demodex folliculorum* mites, which may be a cause or exacerbating factor in papulopustular rosacea.
- Actinic keratosis (AK) is the most common precancerous condition found in skin that's damaged by chronic solar or ultraviolet exposure. It tends to appear as thick, scaly, or crusty plaques that are better felt than seen.
- Transdermal drug delivery (TDD) is a method to deliver topical medications through the stratum corneum into the deeper skin and blood circulation for local and systemic therapeutic purposes.

References

1. Akimoto, Y., Ikehara, S., Yamaguchi, T., Kim, J., Kawakami, H., Shimizu, N., et al. (2016). Galectin expression in healing wounded skin treated with low-temperature plasma: Comparison with treatment by electronical coagulation. *Archives of Biochemistry and Biophysics, 605*, 86–94. https://doi.org/10.1016/j.abb.2016.01.012.
2. Amini, M. R., Sheikh Hosseini, M., Fatollah, S., Mirpour, S., Ghoranneviss, M., Larijani, B., et al. (2020). Beneficial effects of cold atmospheric plasma on inflammatory phase of diabetic foot ulcers; a randomized clinical trial. *Journal of Diabetes and Metabolic Disorders, 19*, 895–905. https://doi.org/10.1007/s40200-020-00577-2.

3. Arisi, M., Soglia, S., Guasco Pisani, E., Venturuzzo, A., Gelmetti, A., Tomasi, C., et al. (2021). Cold atmospheric plasma (CAP) for the treatment of actinic keratosis and skin field cancerization: Clinical and high-frequency ultrasound evaluation. *Dermatology Therapy (Heidelberg), 11*(4), 855–866. https://doi.org/10.1007/s13555-021-00514-y.

4. Arndt, S., Unger, P., Berneburg, M., Bosserhoff, A. K., & Karrer, S. (2018). Cold atmospheric plasma (CAP) activates angiogenesis-related molecules in skin keratinocytes, fibroblasts, and endothelial cells and improves wound angiogenesis in an autocrine and paracrine mode. *Journal of Dermatological Science, 89*, 181–190. https://doi.org/10.1016/j.jdermsci.2017.11.008.

5. Arndt, S., Wacker, E., Li, Y. F., Shimizu, T., Thomas, H. M., Morfill, G. E., et al. (2013). Cold atmospheric plasma, a new strategy to induce senescence in melanoma cells. *Experimental Dermatology, 22*, 284–289. https://doi.org/10.1111/exd.12127.

6. Babossalam, S., Abdollahimajd, F., Aghighi, M., Mahdikia, H., Dilmaghanian, A., Toossi, P., et al. (2020). The effect of nitrogen plasma on the skin and hair follicles: A possible promising future for the treatment of alopecia. *Archives of Dermatological Research, 312*(4), 361–371. https://doi.org/10.1007/s00403-019-02020-w.

7. Brehmer, F., Haenssle, H. A., Daeschlein, G., Ahmed, R., Pfeiffer, S., Gorlitz, A., et al. (2015). Alleviation of chronic venous leg ulcers with a hand-held dielectric barrier discharge plasma generator (PlasmaDerm((R)) VU-2010): Results of a monocentric, two-armed, open, prospective, randomized and controlled trial (NCT01415622). *Journal of the European Academy of Dermatology and Venereology, 29*, 148–155. https://doi.org/10.1111/jdv.12490.

8. Bulson, J. M., Liveris, D., Derkatch, I., Friedman, G., Geliebter, J., Park, S., et al. (2020). Non-thermal atmospheric plasma treatment of onychomycosis in an *in vitro* human nail model. *Mycoses, 63*, 225–232. https://doi.org/10.1111/myc.13030.

9. Bunz, O., Mese, K., Funk, C., Wulf, M., Bailer, S. M., Piwowarczyk, A., et al. (2020). Cold atmospheric plasma as antiviral therapy: Effect on human herpes simplex virus type 1. *Journal of General Virology, 101*, 208–215. https://doi.org/10.1099/jgv.0.001382.

10. Busco, G., Robert, E., Chettouh-Hammas, N., Pouvesle, J. M., & Grillon, C. (2020). The emerging potential of cold atmospheric plasma in skin biology. *Free Radical Biology and Medicine, 161*, 290–304. https://doi.org/10.1016/j.freeradbiomed.2020.10.004.

11. Chatraie, M., Torkaman, G., Khani, M., Salehi, H., & Shokri, B. (2018). *In vivo* study of non-invasive effects of non-thermal plasma in pressure ulcer treatment. *Scientific Reports, 8*, 5621. https://doi.org/10.1038/s41598-018-24049-z.

12. Choi, B. B. R., Choi, J. H., Ji, J., Song, K. W., Lee, H. J., & Kim, G. C. (2018). Increment of growth factors in mouse skin treated with non-thermal plasma. *International Journal of Medical Sciences, 15*, 1203–1209. https://doi.org/10.7150/ijms.26342.

13. Choi, J. H., Nam, S. H., Song, Y. S., Lee, H. W., Lee, H. J., Song, K., Hong, J. W., et al. (2014). Treatment with low-temperature atmospheric pressure plasma enhances cutaneous delivery of epidermal growth factor by regulating E-cadherin-mediated cell junctions. *Archives of Dermatological Research, 306*(6), 635–643. https://doi.org/10.1007/s00403-014-1463-9.

14. Classen, J., Dengler, B., Klinger, C. J., Bettenay, S. V., Rickerts, V., & Mueller, R. S. (2017). Cutaneous alternariosis in an immunocompromised dog successfully treated with cold plasma

and cessation of immunosuppressive medication. *Tierärztliche Praxis Ausgabe K, Kleintiere/ Heimtier, 45*, 337–343. https://doi.org/10.15654/TPK-160851.

15. Daeschlein, G., Scholz, S., Ahmed, R., Majumdar, A., von Woedtke, T., Haase, H., et al. (2012). Cold plasma is well-tolerated and does not disturb skin barrier or reduce skin moisture. *Journal of the German Society of Dermatology, 10*(7), 509–515. https://doi.org/10.1111/j.1610-0387.2012.07857.x.
16. Daeschlein, G., Scholz, S., Arnold, A., von Woedtke, T., Kindel, E., Niggemeier, M., et al. (2010). *In vitro* activity of atmospheric pressure plasma jet (APPJ) plasma against clinical isolates of *Demodex folliculorum. IEEE Transactions on Plasma Science, 38*, 2969–2973. https://doi.org/10.1109/TPS.2010.2061870.
17. Daeschlein, G., Scholz, S., Lutze, S., Arnold, A., von Podewils, S., Kiefer, T., et al. (2013). Comparison between cold plasma, electrochemotherapy, and combined therapy in a melanoma mouse model. *Experimental Dermatology, 22*, 582–586. https://doi.org/10.1111/exd.12201.
18. Dai, X., Bazaka, K., Richard, D. J., Thompson, E. R. W., & Ostrikov, K. K. (2018). The emerging role of gas plasma in oncotherapy. *Trends in Biotechnology, 36*, 1183–1198. https://doi.org/10.1016/j.tibtech.2018.06.010.
19. Demidova-Rice, T. N., Hamblin, M. R., & Herman, I. M. (2012). Acute and impaired wound healing: Pathophysiology and current methods for drug delivery, part 1: Normal and chronic wounds: Biology, causes, and approaches to care. *Advances in Skin & Wound Care, 25*(6), 304–314. https://doi.org/10.1097/01.ASW.0000416006.55218.d0.
20. Duchesne, C., Banzet, S., Lataillade, J. J., Rousseau, A., & Frescaline, N. (2019). Cold atmospheric plasma modulates endothelial nitric oxide synthase signalling and enhances burn wound neovascularisation. *The Journal of Pathology, 249*, 368–380. https://doi.org/10.1002/path.5323.
21. Frescaline, N., Duchesne, C., Favier, M., Onifarasoaniaina, R., Guilbert, T., Uzan, G., et al. (2020). Physical plasma therapy accelerates wound re-epithelialisation and enhances extracellular matrix formation in cutaneous skin grafts. *The Journal of Pathology, 252*, 451–464. https://doi.org/10.1002/path.5546.
22. Friedman, P. C. (2020). Cold atmospheric pressure (physical) plasma in dermatology: Where are we today? *International Journal of Dermatology, 59*, 1171–1184. https://doi.org/10.1111/ijd.15110.
23. Friedman, P. C., Fridman, G., & Fridman, A. (2020). Using cold plasma to treat warts in children: A case series. *Pediatric Dermatology, 37*, 706–709. https://doi.org/10.1111/pde.14180.
24. Friedman, P. C., Miller, V., Fridman, G., & Fridman, A. (2019). Use of cold atmospheric pressure plasma to treat warts: A potential therapeutic option. *Clinical and Experimental Dermatology, 44*, 459–461. https://doi.org/10.1111/ced.13790.
25. Friedman, P. C., Miller, V., Fridman, G., Lin, A., & Fridman, A. (2017). Successful treatment of actinic keratoses using nonthermal atmospheric pressure plasma: A case series. *Journal of the American Academy of Dermatology, 76*(2), 349–350. https://doi.org/10.1016/j.jaad.2016.09.004.
26. Gan, L., Jiang, J., Duan, J. W., Wu, X. J. Z., Zhang, S., Duan, X. R., et al. (2019). Cold atmospheric plasma ameliorates imiquimod-induced psoriasiform dermatitis in mice by mediating

antiproliferative effects. *Free Radical Research, 53*, 269–280. https://doi.org/10.1080/10715762.2018.1564920.

27. Gan, L., Zhang, S., Poorun, D., Liu, D., Lu, X., He, M., et al. (2018). Medical applications of nonthermal atmospheric pressure plasma in dermatology. *Journal der Deutschen Dermatologischen Gesellschaft, 16*, 7–13. https://doi.org/10.1111/ddg.13373.

28. Gao, J., Wang, L., Xia, C., Yang, X., Cao, Z., Zheng, L., et al. (2019). Cold atmospheric plasma promotes different types of superficial skin erosion wounds healing. *International Wound Journal, 16*, 1103–1111. https://doi.org/10.1111/iwj.13161.

29. Garcia-Alcantara, E., Lopez-Callejas, R., Morales-Ramirez, P. R., Pena-Eguiluz, R., Fajardo-Munoz, R., Mercado-Cabrera, A., et al. (2013). Accelerated mice skin acute wound healing *in vivo* by combined treatment of argon and helium plasma needle. *Archives of Medical Research, 44*, 169–177. https://doi.org/10.1016/j.arcmed.2013.02.001.

30. Gay-Mimbrera, J., Garcia, M. C., Isla-Tejera, B., Rodero-Serrano, A., Garcia-Nieto, A. V., & Ruano, J. (2016). Clinical and biological principles of cold atmospheric plasma application in skin cancer. *Advances in Therapy, 33*(5), 894–909. https://doi.org/10.1007/s12325-016-0338-1.

31. Gelker, M., Mrotzek, J., Ichter, A., Muller-Goymann, C. C., & Viol, W. (2019). Influence of pulse characteristics and power density on stratum corneum permeabilization by dielectric barrier discharge. *Biochimica et Biophysica Acta–General Subjects, 1863*(7), 1513–1523. https://doi.org/10.1016/j.bbagen.2019.05.014.

32. Gelker, M., Muller-Goymann, C. C., & Viol, W. (2020). Plasma permeabilization of human excised full-thickness skin by micros- and ns-pulsed DBD. *Skin Pharmacology and Physiology, 33*(2), 69–76. https://doi.org/10.1159/000505195.

33. Gherardi, M., Tonini, R., & Colombo, V. (2018). Plasma in dentistry: Brief history and current status. *Trends in Biotechnology, 36*, 583–585. https://doi.org/10.1016/j.tibtech.2017.06.009.

34. Gilmore, B. F., Flynn, P. B., O'Brien, S., Hickok, N., Freeman, T., & Bourke, P. (2018). Cold plasmas for biofilm control: Opportunities and challenges. *Trends in Biotechnology, 36*, 627–638. https://doi.org/10.1016/j.tibtech.2018.03.007.

35. Guerrero-Preston, R., Ogawa, T., Uemura, M., Shumulinsky, G., Valle, B. L., Pirini, F., et al. (2014). Cold atmospheric plasma treatment selectively targets head and neck squamous cell carcinoma cells. *International Journal of Molecular Medicine, 34*, 941–946. https://doi.org/10.3892/ijmm.2014.1849.

36. Haertel, B., von Woedtke, T., Weltmann, K. D., & Lindequist, U. (2014). Non-thermal atmospheric-pressure plasma possible application in wound healing. *Biomolecules & Therapeutics (Seoul), 22*(6), 477–490. https://doi.org/10.4062/biomolther.2014.105.

37. Hasse, S., Duong Tran, T., Hahn, O., Kindler, S., Metelmann, H. R., von Woedtke, T., et al. (2016). Induction of proliferation of basal epidermal keratinocytes by cold atmospheric-pressure plasma. *Clinical and Experimental Dermatology, 41*, 202–209. https://doi.org/10.1111/ced.12735.

38. He, R., Li, Q., Shen, W., Wang, T., Lu, H., Lu, J., et al. (2020). The efficacy and safety of cold atmospheric plasma as a novel therapy for diabetic wound *in vitro* and *in vivo*. *International Wound Journal, 17*, 851–863. https://doi.org/10.1111/iwj.13341.

39. Heinlin, J., Isbary, G., Stolz, W., Zeman, F., Landthaler, M., Morfill, G., et al. (2013). A randomized

two-sided placebo-controlled study on the efficacy and safety of atmospheric non-thermal argon plasma for pruritus. *Journal of the European Academy of Dermatology and Venereology, 27*(3), 324–331. https://doi.org/10.1111/j.1468-3083.2011.04395.x.

40. Heinlin, J., Morfill, G., Landthaler, M., Stolz, W., Isbary, G., Zimmermann, J. L., et al. (2010). Plasma medicine: Possible applications in dermatology. *Journal der Deutschen Dermatologischen Gesellschaft, 8*, 968–976. https://doi.org/10.1111/j.1610-0387.2010.07495.x.

41. Heinlin, J., Zimmermann, J. L., Zeman, F., Bunk, W., Isbary, G., Landthaler, M., et al. (2013). Randomized placebo-controlled human pilot study of cold atmospheric argon plasma on skin graft donor sites. *Wound Repair and Regeneration, 21*, 800–807. https://doi.org/10.1111/wrr.12078.

42. Hubner, N. O., Siebert, J., & Kramer, A. (2010). Octenidine dihydrochloride, a modern antiseptic for skin, mucous membranes and wounds. *Skin Pharmacology and Physiology, 23*(5), 244–258. https://doi.org/10.1159/000314699.

43. Isbary, G., Heinlin, J., Shimizu, T., Zimmermann, J. L., Morfill, G., Schmidt, H. U., et al. (2012). Successful and safe use of 2 min cold atmospheric argon plasma in chronic wounds: Results of a randomized controlled trial. *British Journal of Dermatology, 167*, 404–410. https://doi.org/10.1111/j.1365-2133.2012.10923.x.

44. Isbary, G., Morfill, G., Schmidt, H. U., Georgi, M., Ramrath, K., Heinlin, J., et al. (2010). A first prospective randomized controlled trial to decrease bacterial load using cold atmospheric argon plasma on chronic wounds in patients. *British Journal of Dermatology, 163*, 78–82. https://doi.org/10.1111/j.1365-2133.2010.09744.x.

45. Isbary, G., Morfill, G., Zimmermann, J., Shimizu, T., & Stolz, W. (2011). Cold atmospheric plasma: A successful treatment of lesions in Hailey-Hailey disease. *Archives of Dermatology, 147*(3), 388–390. https://doi.org/10.1001/archdermatol.2011.57.

46. Isbary, G., Zimmermann, J. L., Shimizu, T., Li, Y. F., Morfill, G. E., Thomas, H. M., et al. (2013). Non-thermal plasma—More than five years of clinical experience. *Clinical Plasma Medicine, 1*, 19–23. https://doi.org/10.1016/j.cpme.2012.11.001.

47. Kang, S. U., Seo, S. J., Kim, Y. S., Shin, Y. S., Koh, Y. W., Lee, C. M., et al. (2017). Comparative effects of non-thermal atmospheric pressure plasma on migration and invasion in oral squamous cell cancer, by gas type. *Yonsei Medical Journal, 58*(2), 272–281. https://doi.org/10.3349/ymj.2017.58.2.272.

48. Keidar, M., Yan, D., Beilis, I. I., Trink, B., & Sherman, J. H. (2018). Plasmas for treating cancer: Opportunities for adaptive and self-adaptive approaches. *Trends in Biotechnology, 36*, 586–593. https://doi.org/10.1016/j.tibtech.2017.06.013.

49. Khan, A., Malik, S., Walia, J., Fridman, G., Fridman, A., Friedman, P. C., et al. (2020). Tolerability of six months indirect cold (physical) plasma treatment of the scalp for hair loss. *Journal of Drugs in Dermatology, 19*(11), 1177–1180. https://doi.org/10.36849/JDD.2020.5186.

50. Kisch, T., Helmke, A., Schleusser, S., Song, J., Liodaki, E., Stang, F. H., et al. (2016). Improvement of cutaneous microcirculation by cold atmospheric plasma (CAP): Results of a controlled, prospective cohort study. *Microvascular Research, 104*, 55–62. https://doi.org/10.1016/j.mvr.2015.12.002.

51. Lee, M. H., Lee, Y. S., Kim, H. J., Han, C. H., Kang, S. U., Kim, C. H., et al. (2019). Non-thermal plasma inhibits mast cell activation and ameliorates allergic skin inflammatory diseases in NC/Nga mice. *Scientific Reports, 9*, 13510. https://doi.org/10.1038/s41598-019-49938-9.

52. Lipner, S. R., Friedman, G., & Scher, R. K. (2017). Pilot study to evaluate a plasma device for the treatment of onychomycosis. *Clinical and Experimental Dermatology, 42*, 295–298. https://doi.org/10.1111/ced.12973.

53. Marschewski, M., Hirschberg, J., Omairi, T., Hofft, O., Viol, W., Emmert, S., et al. (2012). Electron spectroscopic analysis of the human lipid skin barrier: Cold atmospheric plasma-induced changes in lipid composition. *Experimental Dermatology, 21*, 921–925. https://doi.org/10.1111/exd.12043.

54. Mohd Nasir, N., Lee, B. K., Yap, S. S., Thong, K. L., & Yap, S. L. (2016). Cold plasma inactivation of chronic wound bacteria. *Archives of Biochemistry and Biophysics, 605*, 76–85. https://doi.org/10.1016/j.abb.2016.03.033.

55. Ouf, S. A., El-Adly, A. A., & Mohamed, A. H. (2015). Inhibitory effect of silver nanoparticles mediated by atmospheric pressure air cold plasma jet against dermatophyte fungi. *Journal of Medical Microbiology, 64*, 1151–1161. https://doi.org/10.1099/jmm.0.000133.

56. Schmidt, A., Bekeschus, S., Jablonowski, H., Barton, A., Weltmann, K. D., & Wende, K. (2017). Role of ambient gas composition on cold physical plasma-elicited cell signaling in keratinocytes. *Biophysical Journal, 112*, 2397–2407. https://doi.org/10.1016/j.bpj.2017.04.030.

57. Schmidt, A., Bekeschus, S., Wende, K., Vollmar, B., & von Woedtke, T. (2017). A cold plasma jet accelerates wound healing in a murine model of full-thickness skin wounds. *Experimental Dermatology, 26*, 156–162. https://doi.org/10.1111/exd.13156.

58. Schmidt, A., Liebelt, G., Striesow, J., Freund, E., von Woedtke, T., Wende, K., et al. (2020). The molecular and physiological consequences of cold plasma treatment in murine skin and its barrier function. *Free Radical Biology and Medicine, 161*, 32–49. https://doi.org/10.1016/j.freeradbiomed.2020.09.026.

59. Schmidt, A., von Woedtke, T., Vollmar, B., Hasse, S., & Bekeschus, S. (2019). Nrf2 signaling and inflammation are key events in physical plasma-spurred wound healing. *Theranostics, 9*, 1066–1084. https://doi.org/10.7150/thno.29754.

60. Scholtz, V., Souskova, H., Hubka, V., Svarcova, M., & Julak, J. (2015). Inactivation of human pathogenic dermatophytes by non-thermal plasma. *Journal of Microbiological Methods, 119*, 53–58. https://doi.org/10.1016/j.mimet.2015.09.017.

61. Scholtz, V., Souskova, H., Hubka, V., Svarcova, M., & Julak, J. (2017). Inactivation of dermatophyte infection by nonthermal plasma on an animal model. *Medical Mycology, 55*, 422–428. https://doi.org/10.1093/mmy/myw094.

62. Seebauer, C., Freund, E., Hasse, S., Miller, V., Segebarth, M., Lucas, C., et al. (2020). Effects of cold physical plasma on oral lichen planus: An *in vitro* study. *Oral Diseases, 27*, 1728–1737. https://doi.org/10.1111/odi.13697.

63. Shapourzadeh, A., Rahimi-Verki, N., Atyabi, S. M., Shams-Ghahfarokhi, M., Jahanshiri, Z., Irani, S., et al. (2016). Inhibitory effects of cold atmospheric plasma on the growth, ergosterol biosynthesis, and keratinase activity in *Trichophyton rubrum*. *Archives of Biochemistry and Biophysics, 608*, 27–33. https://doi.org/10.1016/j.abb.2016.07.012.

64. Shi, X. M., Xu, G. M., Zhang, G. J., Liu, J. R., Wu, Y. M., Gao, L. G., et al. (2018). Low-temperature plasma promotes fibroblast proliferation in wound healing by ROS-activated NF-kappaB signaling pathway. *Current Medical Science, 38*, 107–114. https://doi.org/10.1007/s11596-018-1853-x.

65. Shimizu, K. (2015). Biological effects and enhancement of percutaneous absorption on skin by atmospheric microplasma irradiation. *Plasma Medicine, 5*(4), 205–221. https://doi.org/10.1615/PlasmaMed.2016015688.

66. Taghiabadi, E., Nilforoushzadeh, M. A., & Aghdami, N. (2020). Maintaining hair inductivity in human dermal papilla cells: A review of effective methods. *Skin Pharmacology and Physiology, 33*(5), 280–292. https://doi.org/10.1159/000510152.

67. Tan, F., & Al-Rubeai, M. (2021). A multifunctional dexamethasone-delivery implant fabricated using atmospheric plasma and its effects on apoptosis, osteogenesis, and inflammation. *Drug Delivery and Translational Research, 11*, 86–102. https://doi.org/10.1007/s13346-019-00700-8.

68. Tan, F., Fang, Y., Zhu, L., & Al-Rubeai, M. (2021). Cold atmospheric plasma as an interface biotechnology for enhancing surgical implants. *Critical Reviews in Biotechnology, 41*, 425–440. https://doi.org/10.1080/07388551.2020.1853671.

69. Tan, F., Wang, Y., Zhang, S., Shui, R., & Chen, J. (2022). Plasma dermatology: Skin therapy using cold atmospheric plasma. *Frontiers in Oncology, 12*, 918484. https://doi.org/10.3389/fonc.2022.918484.

70. Ulrich, C., Kluschke, F., Patzelt, A., Vandersee, S., Czaika, V. A., Richter, H., et al. (2015). Clinical use of cold atmospheric pressure argon plasma in chronic leg ulcers: A pilot study. *Journal of Wound Care, 24*, 198–200, 202–193. https://doi.org/10.12968/jowc.2015.24.5.196.

71. Wang, L., Yang, X., Yang, C., Gao, J., Zhao, Y., Cheng, C., et al. (2019). The inhibition effect of cold atmospheric plasma-activated media in cutaneous squamous carcinoma cells. *Future Oncology, 15*(5), 495–505. https://doi.org/10.2217/fon-2018-0419.

72. Wang, M., Geilich, B. M., Keidar, M., & Webster, T. J. (2017). Killing malignant melanoma cells with protoporphyrin IX-loaded polymersome-mediated photodynamic therapy and cold atmospheric plasma. *International Journal of Nanomedicine, 12*, 4117–4127. https://doi.org/10.2147/IJN.S129266.

73. Wen, X., Xin, Y., Hamblin, M. R., & Jiang, X. (2020). Applications of cold atmospheric plasma for transdermal drug delivery: A review. *Drug Delivery and Translational Research, 11*(3), 741–747. https://doi.org/10.1007/s13346-020-00808-2.

74. Wiegand, C., Fink, S., Beier, O., Horn, K., Pfuch, A., Schimanski, A., et al. (2016). Dose- and time-dependent cellular effects of cold atmospheric pressure plasma evaluated in 3D skin models. *Skin Pharmacology and Physiology, 29*(5), 257–265. https://doi.org/10.1159/000450889.

75. Xin, Y., Wen, X., & Jiang, X. (2021). Analgesic effect of topical lidocaine is enhanced by cold atmospheric plasma pretreatment in facial CO2 laser treatments. *Journal of Cosmetic Dermatology, 20*(11), 2794–2799. https://doi.org/10.1111/jocd.13983.

76. Xin, Y., Wen, X., Hamblin, M. R., & Jiang, X. (2021). Transdermal delivery of topical lidocaine in a mouse model is enhanced by treatment with cold atmospheric plasma. *Journal of Cosmetic Dermatology, 20*(2), 626–635. https://doi.org/10.1111/jocd.13581.

77. Xiong, Q., Wang, X., Yin, R., Xiong, L., Chen, Q., Zheng, M. X., et al. (2018). Surface treatment with non-thermal humid argon plasma as a treatment for allergic contact dermatitis in a mouse model. *Clinical Plasma Medicine, 12*, 10–16. https://doi.org/10.1016/j.cpme.2018.09.002.

78. Xiong, Z. (2018). Cold atmospheric plasmas: A novel and promising way to treat neurological diseases. *Trends in Biotechnology, 36*, 582–583. https://doi.org/10.1016/j.tibtech.2018.04.003.

79. Xu, G. M., Shi, X. M., Cai, J. F., Chen, S. L., Li, P., Yao, C. W., et al. (2015). Dual effects of atmospheric pressure plasma jet on skin wound healing of mice. *Wound Repair and Regeneration, 23*, 878–884. https://doi.org/10.1111/wrr.12364.

80. Yan, D., Sherman, J. H., & Keidar, M. (2017). Cold atmospheric plasma, a novel promising anti-cancer treatment modality. *Oncotarget, 8*, 15977–15995. https://doi.org/10.18632/oncotarget.13304.

81. Yan, D., Wang, Q., Adhikari, M., Malyavko, A., Lin, L., Zolotukhin, D. B., et al. (2020). A physically triggered cell death via transbarrier cold atmospheric plasma cancer treatment. *ACS Applied Materials & Interfaces, 12*, 34548–34563. https://doi.org/10.1021/acsami.0c06500.

82. Yang, X., Yang, C., Wang, L., Cao, Z., Wang, Y., Cheng, C., et al. (2020). Inhibition of basal cell carcinoma cells by cold atmospheric plasma-activated solution and differential gene expression analysis. *International Journal of Oncology, 56*(5), 1262–1273. https://doi.org/10.3892/ijo.2020.5009.

83. Zhong, S. Y., Dong, Y. Y., Liu, D. X., Xu, D. H., Xiao, S. X., Chen, H. L., et al. (2016). Surface air plasma-induced cell death and cytokine release of human keratinocytes in the context of psoriasis. *British Journal of Dermatology, 174*, 542–552. https://doi.org/10.1111/bjd.14236.

Chapter 9

LOW-LEVEL LASER (LIGHT) THERAPY (LLLT) IN SKIN: STIMULATING, HEALING, AND RESTORING

Contents

Introduction

A rapidly developing technology, low-level laser (light) therapy (LLLT) is used to treat a wide range of conditions that call for inflammation and pain relief, function restoration, and stimulation of healing. The skin reacts well to red and near-infrared wavelengths, despite being the organ that is naturally exposed to light the most. Skin cells' mitochondrial chromophores absorb the photons. As a result, several signaling pathways are activated, blood flow, nitric oxide release, electron transport, adenosine triphosphate (ATP), and reactive oxygen species are increased. Activating stem cells can promote tissue healing and repair. In the field of dermatology, LLLT is beneficial for wrinkles, hypertrophic scars, acne scars, and burn healing. As a preventative measure as well as a treatment, LLLT can lessen UV damage. By promoting melanocyte proliferation and suppressing autoimmunity, LLLT can improve pigmentation in pigmentary disorders like vitiligo and decrease depigmentation. Acne and other inflammatory conditions like psoriasis can also be helped. Further research in dermatology is encouraged by the nearly total lack of side effects and non-invasive nature of the procedure.

Non-invasive treatments for skin disorders and skin rejuvenation are becoming more and more popular, particularly in Western nations where social pressures to have an ideal appearance combine with comparatively high disposable incomes. The skin responds well to red and near-infrared wavelengths when they are applied therapeutically within the appropriate parameters, despite being the organ that is naturally exposed to the greatest amount of light. Although low-level laser therapy (LLLT) was developed in the late 1960s, dermatologists have only recently begun to use it extensively. Since the advent of light-emitting diode (LED) devices, many of the issues surrounding lasers have been resolved, including cost, safety, and the requirement for skilled personnel to operate them. In actuality, a large number of LED products are offered for sale online and are intended for domestic use.

Orientation and Directional Terms

Term	Definition	Illustration
Photorejuvenation	Photorejuvenation is a skin treatment that uses lasers, intense pulsed light, or photodynamic therapy to treat skin conditions and remove effects of photoaging such as wrinkles, spots, and textures. The process induces controlled wounds to the skin. This prompts the skin to heal itself, by creating new cells.	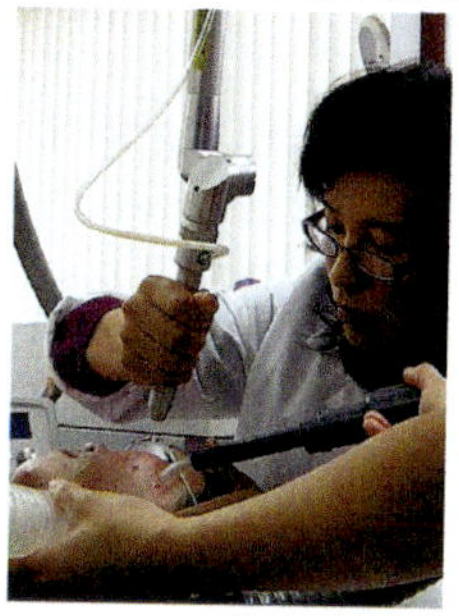
Adenosine triphosphate (ATP)	Adenosine triphosphate (ATP) is a molecule that stores and transfers energy in cells, making it possible for organisms to live. It's often called the cell's "energy currency" because it provides energy that can be easily released.	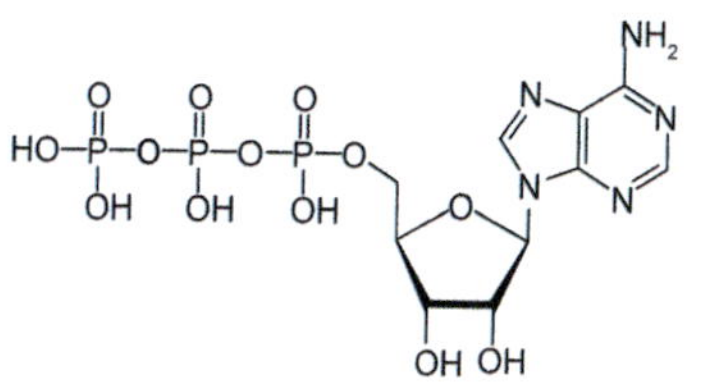
Photobiomodulation (PBM)	Photobiomodulation (PBM) is a non-invasive medical treatment that uses red or near-infrared (NIR) light to stimulate cells and tissues. It's also known as low-level laser therapy, cold laser therapy, or red-light therapy.	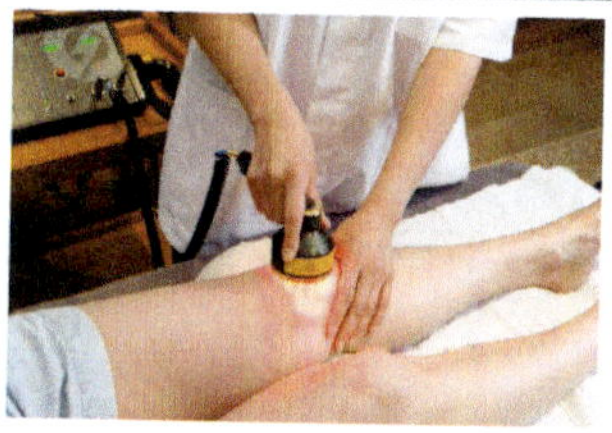
Tissue regeneration	Tissue regeneration is the process by which organisms repair or replace damaged or lost tissue. It's a complex process that involves the synergistic effects of inflammatory cells, signaling molecules, and secreted cytokines.	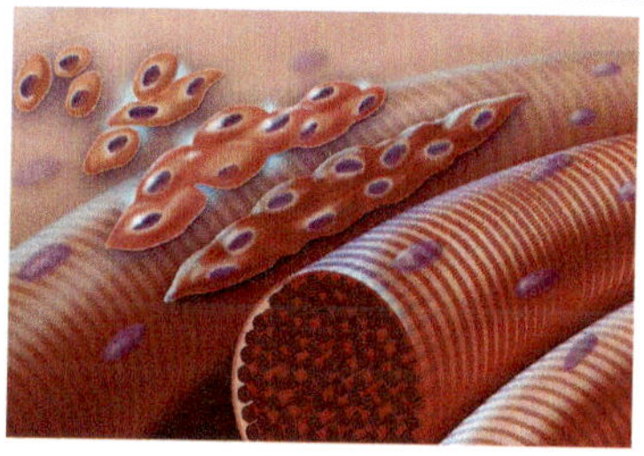
Acne	Acne is a common skin condition that happens when hair follicles under the skin become clogged. Sebum—oil that helps keep skin from drying out—and dead skin cells plug the pores, which leads to outbreaks of lesions, commonly called pimples or zits.	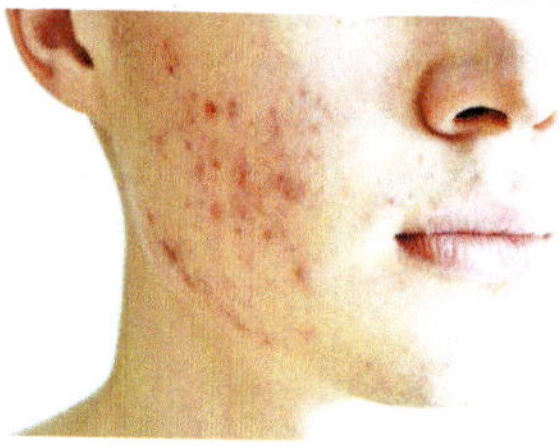

9.1. Low-Level Laser (Light) Therapy and its Mechanism of Action

The term "photobiomodulation" "phototherapy" or "LLLT" describes the application of photons at a non-thermal irradiance to modify biological activity. Depending on the situation, LLLT may employ non-coherent light sources like light-emitting diodes (LEDs) or filtered lamps in addition to coherent light sources like lasers. The primary uses of LLLT in medicine include lowering pain and inflammation, enhancing tissue repair, encouraging the regeneration of various tissues and nerves, and averting tissue damage in circumstances where it is likely to happen. Photorejuvenation, the aesthetic treatment of fine wrinkles, photoaged skin, and scars, has been made more popular in recent decades by non-ablative laser therapies. This method has also been applied more recently to treat inflammatory acne. Red and near-infrared (NIR) light at low levels are applied to cells or tissue during LLLT. Because the energy or power densities used in this procedure are lower than in other types of laser therapy, such as ablation, cutting, and thermally coagulating tissue, it is known as "low-level." It has recently been discovered that LLLT therapy, at different intensities, can either stimulate or inhibit a variety of cellular functions (Table 9.1).

Table 9.1. *Examples of LLLT Devices for Dermatological Applications*

Supplier	Product name	Wavelength (nm)	Power Density (mW/cm^2)	Standard Dose(J/cm^2)	Application
PhotoMedex (Manchester, UK)	Omnilux	415 (±5)	40	48	Acne, photodamage, non-melanoma skin cancers, skin rejuvenation, vitiligo, and wound healing post elective surgery
		633 (±6)	105	126	
		830 (±5)	55	66	
Edge Systems (Signal Hill, CA)	Delphia del Sol	420		7.4 J per treatment area	Acne, improving skin texture, firmness, and resilience, increasing lymphatic system activity, fine lines, wrinkles, and superficial hyperpigmentation
		600–700			
		700–1000			
Flip 4 (Sainte-Julie, Quebec, Canada)	Max7	420–700	≤4		Acne, rejuvenation, injured skin healing including the shortening of the post skin resurfacing erythema duration
Light BioSciences (Virginia Beach, VA)	Gentlewaves	588 (±10)	Variable		Anti-aging

OPUSMED (Montreal, Canada)	LumiPhase-R	660	150		Skin firmness, rhytid depth, wrinkles
Revitalight (Chicago, IL)	Revitalight 747	420	80	7.2 J per 90 sec. per treatment area	Fine lines, wrinkles, and age spots on the face, neck, and hands
	Hand Spa	590	80		
	Food Spa	625	80		
	Evolution	940	80		
Soli-Tone (Woburn, MA)	LumiFacial	470	84		Acne, anti-aging, hyperpigmentation, rosacea
	Lumilift	525	27		
		590	10		
		640	89		
DUSA (Wilmington, MA)	BLU-U	417	10		Acne
Curelight (Rehovot, Israel)	iClearXL	405–420		60	Acne, anti-aging, skin rejuvenation, acceleration of healing of post peel and post surgical suture sites
	Clear100XL	890–900			
Lumenis (Santa Clara, CA)	ClearLight	405–420	200	60	Acne
	Clear100				
LIGHTWAVE Technologies (Phoneix, AZ)	LIGHTWAVE Professional Deluxe LED System	417			Anti-aging, skin rejuvenation
		630			
		880			
Dynatronics (Salt Lake City, UT)	Synergie LT2	660	500 mW (total power)	6 J per treatment area	Anti-aging, skin firmness, wrinkles, skin tone and texture for face and neck
		880			

Source: https://www.ncbi.nlm.nih.gov/pmc/articles/PMC4126803/table/T1/?report=objectonly.

The exact mechanism by which LLLT induces cellular photobiostimulation remains unclear. Based on observations, it seems that LLLT affects molecules, cells, and tissues in a variety of ways. Red and NIR light absorption by mitochondrial chromophores, specifically cytochrome c oxidase (CCO), which is found in the respiratory chain inside the mitochondria, and possibly by photoacceptors in the cell plasma membrane, is considered to be the fundamental biological mechanism underlying the effects of LLLT. As a result, a series of events take place in the mitochondria that cause different processes to be biostimulated. It was discovered that the absorption spectra for CCO in various oxidation states, which were measured, closely matched the action spectra for biological reactions to the light. Theoretically, this light energy absorption could lead to the photodissociation of inhibitory nitric oxide from CCO, which would increase the activity of enzymes, electron transport, mitochondrial respiration, and the synthesis of adenosine triphosphate (ATP). As a result, LLLT modifies the cellular redox state, which triggers the activation of multiple intracellular signaling pathways and modifies the affinity of transcription factors involved in tissue regeneration, cell proliferation, and survival (Figure 9.1).

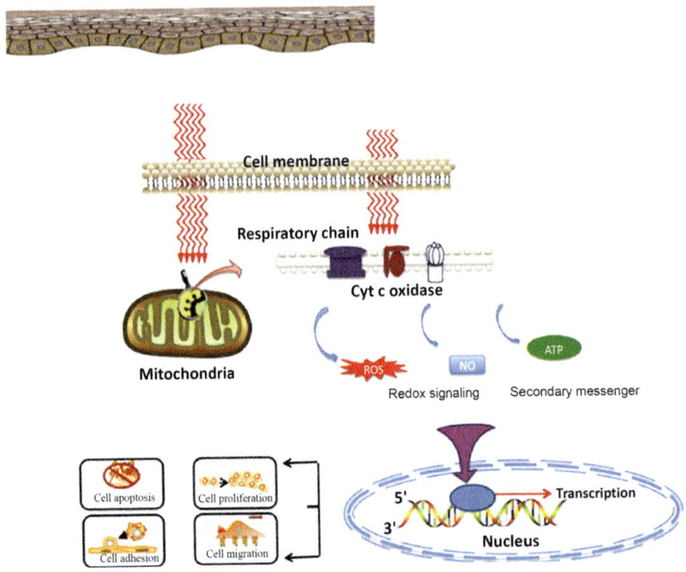

Figure 9.1. *Mechanism of action of LLLT.*

Source: https://www.ncbi.nlm.nih.gov/pmc/articles/PMC4126803/.

The basic biological mechanism underlying the effects of LLLT is believed to occur through the absorption of red and NIR light by mitochondrial chromophores, specifically cytochrome c oxidase (CCO) found in the mitochondria's respiratory chain. It is theorized that this light absorption may result in the release of inhibitory nitric oxide from CCO, leading to increased enzyme activity, electron transport, mitochondrial respiration, and ATP production. Consequently, LLLT may modify the cellular redox state, triggering the activation of multiple intracellular signaling pathways and changing the affinity of transcription factors involved in cell proliferation, survival, tissue repair, and regeneration.

Even though LLLT is now used to treat a wide range of illnesses, there are still two main reasons why it is still a contentious therapy. First, there are questions concerning the basic molecular and cellular processes that convert signals from photons incident on cells to biological effects occurring in the tissue exposed to radiation. Second, there are notable differences in the dosimetry parameters: time of exposure, contact versus non-contact application, repetition schedule, wavelength, irradiance or power density, pulse structure, coherence, polarization, energy, and fluence. Greater dosimetric parameters may cause tissue damage, while lower ones may result in less efficacy from the treatment. This exemplifies the theory behind the biphasic dose response, which has been shown to function in LLLT. There are several published studies on LLLT with unfavorable findings. It might be the result of selecting the wrong light source and dosage. It might also result from improper skin preparation prior to LLLT application, such as failing to remove oily debris and makeup, which can obstruct the light source's penetration, and failing to take skin pigmentation into consideration. The LLLT equipment's performance can be decreased, and improper maintenance can also affect clinical outcomes. It is imperative to take into account that there exists an ideal dosage of light for every specific purpose.

In the absence of considerable heating, laser radiation or non-coherent light can change cellular behavior depending on its wavelength and radiant exposure. Phototherapy uses light that can be either pulsed or continuous wave, with wavelengths ranging from 390 to 1100 nm. Under typical conditions, it employs comparatively low power densities (.04–50 J/cm^2) and fluences (. < 100 mW/cm^2). Wavelengths in the range of 390 nm to 600 nm are used to treat superficial tissue, and longer wavelengths in the range of 600nm to 1100nm, which penetrate further, are used to treat deeper-seated tissues. Wavelengths in the range 700 nm to 750 nm have been found to have limited biochemical activity and are therefore not often used. Various light sources used in LLLT include inert gas lasers and semiconductor laser diodes such as helium neon (HeNe; 633 nm), ruby (694 nm), argon (488 and 514 nm), krypton (521, 530, 568, 647 nm), gallium arsenide (GaAs; > 760 nm, with 904 nm serving as a typical example), and gallium aluminum arsenide (GaAlAs; 612–870 nm). At lower wavelengths, a large variety of LED semiconductors with the elements nitride, phosphide, and indium are accessible. If coherent laser light has any advantages over non-coherent LED light, that is one question that hasn't been definitively answered yet. While some medical professionals use focused lasers in "points" to treat deep tissue lesions, the use of LEDs in dermatology is growing in popularity because relatively large areas of tissue need to be irradiated (Bouzari et al., 2007; Wolfram et al., 2009; Barolet & Boucher, 2010) (Figure 9.2).

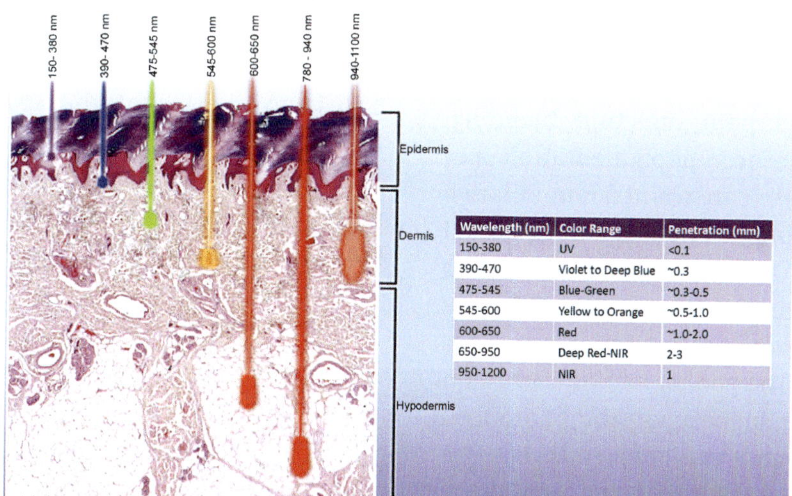

Figure 9.2. *Tissue penetration depths of various wavelengths.*

Source: https://www.ncbi.nlm.nih.gov/pmc/articles/PMC4126803/.

9.2. LLLT for Skin Rejuvenation

The first indications of aging on the skin usually appear in the late 20s and early 30s and include wrinkles, dyspigmentation, telangiectasia, and loss of elasticity. Common histologic and molecular features include decreased collagen content, collagen fiber fragmentation, elastic fiber elastotic degeneration, increased expression of matrix metalloproteinases (MMPs), particularly MMP-1 and

MMP-2, tortuous, and dilated dermal vessels, and epidermis atrophy and disorientation. The aging process of skin is caused by both environmental and chronological factors, but photodamage appears to be the primary cause of these changes.

A number of techniques have been created to address the dermal and epidermal indicators of both chronological and photoaging. The majority of these modalities work on the principle of stimulating collagen biosynthesis and dermal matrix remodeling by excising the epidermis and creating a controlled type of skin wounding. Nowadays, retinoic acid (a vitamin A derivative), chemical peels, dermabrasion, and ablative laser resurfacing using carbon dioxide (CO_2), erbium: yttrium-aluminum-garnet (Er:YAG) lasers, or a combination of these wavelengths, are the most often utilized interventions. But these procedures come with a price: they need a lot of aftercare, a long recovery period, and a risk of complications like persistent erythema, pain, infection, bleeding, oozing, burns, hyper- or hypopigmentation, and scarring. Due to these constraints, non-ablative rejuvenation technologies had to be developed as a substitute for ablative procedures. These alternatives had to be safer, more effective, less invasive, and require less postoperative care and recovery time. The goal of non-ablative skin rejuvenation is to enhance aging and photoaged skin without damaging the epidermis. Intense pulsed light sources (IPL), 532 nm potassium-titanyl-phosphate lasers (KTP), and high-dose 585/595 nm pulsed dye lasers (PDL) can be used to treat irregular pigmentation and telangiectasia. Other IPL sources, such as low-dose 589/595 nm PDLs, 1064 and 1320 nm neodymium:yttrium-aluminum-garnet lasers, (Nd:YAG) 1450 nm diode lasers, and 1540 nm erbium fiber lasers, can also reduce wrinkles and tighten skin by thermally injuring the dermis (photothermolysis).

It has been demonstrated that using LEDs, a novel light source for non-thermal, non-ablative skin rejuvenation, is beneficial for reducing wrinkles and skin laxity. Since the first reports of LLLT effects on increased collagen date back to 1987, this phenomenon is not new. Research conducted by Abergel and colleagues as well as Yu and others reported that both *in vitro* and *in vivo* animal models exposed to low-energy laser irradiation showed an increase in the production of pro-collagen, collagen, basic fibroblast growth factors (bFGF), and fibroblast proliferation. Moreover, it was previously established that LLLT could boost skin vascular perfusion, platelet-derived growth factor (PDGF), transforming growth factor (TGF-β1), and prevent apoptosis. Lee and associates. observed alterations in the status of MMPs and their tissue inhibitors (TIMPs) after examining the histologic and ultrastructural changes after a combination of 830 nm, 55 mW/cm^2, 66 J/cm^2 and 633 nm, 105 mW/cm^2, 126 J/cm2 LED phototherapy. Moreover, after LED phototherapy, mRNA levels of IL-1β, TNF-α, ICAM-1, and connexin 43 (Cx43) were elevated while IL-6 levels were lowered. Ultimately, it was shown that the post-treatment specimens had more collagen.

The purposefully created photothermally-mediated wounds associated with laser treatments are thought to be healed by the pro-inflammatory cytokines IL-1β and TNF-α, and this cascade of wound healing subsequently contributes to new collagen synthesis. Through the non-thermal and atraumatic induction of a subclinical "quasi-wound," LED therapy may be able to initiate this wound healing process without actually causing any thermal damage, which could lead to complications like in some other laser treatments. Since TIMPs block MMP activity, TIMP induction could be an additional explanation for the elevated collagen. Considering all of these findings, it's plausible that early LED therapy-induced MMPs were caused by elevated IL-1β and TNF-α production. To facilitate the biosynthesis of new collagen fibers, this may remove the photodamaged collagen fragments. Subsequently, an increase in TIMPs may shield the recently created collagen from MMP proteolytic degradation. Furthermore, to produce new collagen in a larger area that even includes non-irradiated regions, increased expression of Cx43 may potentially enhance cell-to-cell communication between dermal components, especially the fibroblasts, and enhance the cellular responses to the photobiostimulation effects from LED treatment. A clinical investigation carried out by Weiss et al. 600 patients underwent LED therapy in addition to a thermally based photorejuvenation procedure, and 300 patients received LED therapy alone (590 nm, 0–10 J/cm^2) (Bouzari et al., 2007; Wolfram et al., 2009; Barolet & Boucher, 2010).

90% of patients who underwent LED photorejuvenation alone reported seeing a softening of the skin's texture as well as a reduction in roughness and fine lines, varying from a noticeable reduction to occasionally subtle changes. Furthermore, patients (n = 152) undergoing thermal photorejuvenation laser treatment with or without additional LED photomodulation reported a significant decrease in post-treatment erythema and an overall sense of improved efficacy with the additional LED treatment. The anti-inflammatory properties of LLLT may have contributed to this decrease in post-treatment erythema. 90 patients received eight LED treatments for four weeks in a multicenter clinical trial that used various pulse sequence parameters. With over 90% of patients improving by at least one Fitzpatrick photoaging category and 65% of patients exhibiting a global improvement in facial texture, fine lines, background erythema, and pigmentation, the study's outcome was extremely positive. The outcomes peaked four to six months after the eight treatments were finished. Reduction of MMP-1 and a notable increase in collagen in the papillary dermis were frequent observations. Barolet and associates study is in line with the earlier research as well. The potential of 660 nm, 50 mW/cm, 4 J/cm^2 LED in modulating collagen and MMP-1 was investigated using a 3-D model of tissue-engineered human reconstructed skin. The results showed up-regulation of collagen and down-regulation of MMP-1 *in vitro*. Next, a split-face, single-blinded clinical study was conducted to evaluate the impact of this light treatment on the appearance and texture of skin in people with aged or photoaged skin. After receiving 12 LED treatments, profilometry quantification showed that 87% of the participants reported a decrease in the Fitzpatrick wrinkling severity score, despite the fact that over 90% of the participants had a reduction in rhytid depth and surface roughness.

LLLT helps rejuvenate the skin by boosting collagen production and reducing collagen breakdown. This is achieved through increasing the levels of PDGF and fibroblasts, as well as by decreasing apoptosis, increasing vascular perfusion, bFGF, and TGF-β. Additionally, it decreases IL-6 levels and increases TIMPs, which ultimately leads to a reduction in MMPs and collagen degradation.

9.3. Lllt for Acne

The cause of acne vulgaris is still not fully understood, but it is believed to involve four main factors: follicular hyperconification, increased sebum secretion due to androgenic hormones, colonization of Propionibacterium acnes, and inflammation. *Propionibacterium acnes* plays a critical role by affecting triglycerides and releasing cytokines that lead to inflammatory reactions and changes in keratinization. Treatments for acne vulgaris include topical and oral medications like antibiotics, retinoids, benzoyl peroxide, alpha hydroxy acids, salicylic acid, and azelaic acid. In severe cases, systemic antibiotics, oral retinoids, and hormonal treatments may be necessary. These medications aim to target microcomedone formation, sebum production, *Propionibacterium acnes*, and inflammation. Despite the variety of treatment options available, some patients may not respond well or experience side effects.

It has been suggested that phototherapy, which includes light, lasers, and photodynamic therapy, is a less invasive therapeutic option for treating acne vulgaris than other approaches. Up to 70% of acne cases have been reported to respond well to sun exposure as a treatment. Sunlight therapy for acne is limited by the adverse effects of UVA and UVB radiation, which reduce androgenic hormones in the sebaceous gland. Acne treatment has recently included phototherapy using visible light, primarily blue, red, or a combination of the two. One way that phototherapy for acne works is by having porphyrins, which are endogenous photosensitizers that are produced by *Propionibacterium acnes* as part of its regular metabolism, absorb light, and particularly blue light. Red light is known to penetrate tissues more deeply than blue light. This process results in a photochemical reaction that creates reactive free radicals and Singlet oxygen species, which in turn lead to bacterial destruction. Red light has been shown to alter keratinocyte behavior and impact the sebum secretion of sebaceous glands. Moreover, red light may also work by altering the cytokines produced by macrophages and other cells, which may lessen inflammation.

Red and blue light when used in combination have synergistic effects in treatment of acne. *P. acnes* synthesizes and stores a large amount of porphyrins. Once the porphyrin is exposed to visible light (specifically blue light) it becomes chemically active and transfers to an excited state, resulting in formation of reactive free radicals and singlet oxygen which in turn causes membrane damage in P. acnes. Red light is proposed to exert its effects through reducing the inflammatory process.

Acne vulgaris can be effectively treated with low-level laser therapy (LLLT) in the red to near-infrared spectral range (630–1000 nm) and nonthermal power (less than 200 mW), either alone or in conjunction with other treatment modalities (mostly blue light). One of these studies used 630-nm red spectrum LLLT with a fluence of 12 J/cm^2 twice a week for 12 sessions in conjunction with 2% topical clindamycin and showed a significant reduction in active acne lesions; however, the same study showed no significant effects when an 890 nm laser was used. Additionally, a few studies demonstrated the synergistic benefits of red and blue light therapy for acne. It is suggested that the synergistic effects of mixed light result from the combined action of red and blue light's anti-inflammatory and antibacterial properties. It's also important to note that most studies showed a greater improvement in inflammatory lesions than in comedones (Bouzari et al., 2007; Wolfram et al., 2009; Barolet and Boucher, 2010).

9.4. LLLT for Photoprotection

It is commonly acknowledged that practically all harmful photo-induced effects on human skin occur as a result of exposure to UV radiation (< 400 nm). The degeneration of collagen, the production of free radicals, the inhibition of DNA repair, and the suppression of the immune system are some of the hypothesized processes for UV-induced skin damage. The foundation of current strategies to stop UV-induced damage is reducing the quantity of UV irradiation that gets to the skin, which can be done by wearing sunscreen or avoiding the sun. Sun avoidance can be challenging to practice, though, particularly for those who work outside or engage in outdoor hobbies. However, topical sunscreens' photoprotective efficacy is also limited by factors such as reduced effectiveness after sweating or exposure to water, spectral restrictions, potential toxicity from the nanoparticles present in most sunscreens, user allergies, and compliance.

Recent research suggests that exposure to infrared (IR) light may protect against UV-induced skin damage, primarily by inducing responses to UV irradiation that are protective or reparative. Because UVB and UVA peak around noon and visible and infrared solar wavelengths predominate in the morning in the natural environment, it is likely that mammals already have a built-in mechanism that protects their skin from potentially harmful UV radiation at noon by reacting to morning infrared radiation. On the other hand, counterarguments are also present. For example, Krutmann's research shows that IR-induced disruption of the mitochondrial electron transport chain's electron flow results in insufficient energy production in dermal fibroblasts. Another example comes from Schroeder's report, which claims that IR changes the collagen equilibrium of the dermal extracellular matrix by reducing the de novo synthesis of collagen and increasing the expression of the enzyme MMP-1, which breaks down collagen. As was previously mentioned, depending on the parameters used, the same light source may have opposite effects on the same tissue. These opposing viewpoints are most likely caused by the biphasic effects of light.

Menezes along with others showed that, in the absence of increasing skin temperature, non-coherent near-infrared radiation (NIR) (700–2000 nm) produced a potent cellular defense against solar UV cytotoxicity. It was thought to be a long-lasting (at least 24 hours) and cumulative phenomenon. After doing this research, Frank et al. proposed that by altering the mitochondrial apoptotic pathway, IR irradiation primes cells to withstand UVB-induced damage. It has been demonstrated that IR pre-irradiation of human fibroblasts inhibits UVB activation of caspase –9 and –3, partially releases cytochrome c and Smac/Diablo, and increases anti-apoptotic proteins (Bcl-2 or Bcl-xL) while decreasing pro-apoptotic proteins (Bax). According to the findings, IR prevented UVB-induced apoptosis by altering the Bcl2/Bax balance. This suggests that p53, a gene integrity sensor, is involved in both cell apoptosis and repair processes. Frank et al. conducted a second study. investigated in greater detail how the p53 cell signaling pathway helps to prevent UVB toxicity. It has been demonstrated that the response to IR irradiation is p53 dependent, which implies that IR irradiation primes cells to fend off additional UVB-induced DNA damage and/or repair it. Finally, Applegate et al. supported the IR induction of defense mechanisms who discovered that infrared radiation caused the protective protein ferritin, which is typically involved in skin repair and a scavenger of Fe^{2+} otherwise available for oxidative reactions.

Increased dermal fibroblast procollagen secretion has been shown in an *in vitro* study to decrease the production of collagenase or metalloproteinases (MMP) after non-thermal non-coherent deep red visible LED exposures (660 nm, sequential pulsing mode). In a follow-up *in vivo* pilot study, the effect of this wavelength in three healthy subjects was examined using a minimal erythemal dose (MED) method adapted from sunscreen SPF determination. These results correlated with significant clinical improvement of rhytids *in vivo*. The outcomes demonstrated the effectiveness of LED therapy, resulting in a notable decrease in UVB-induced erythema. To learn more about this phenomenon's *in vivo* components, a follow-up study was conducted. Researchers looked at the effects of non-thermal, non-coherent 660 nm LED pulsed treatments on improving skin resistance before impending

UV damage in a group of subjects with fair, normal skin and in patients with polymorphous light eruption (PLE). The results indicated that there was significant dose-related protection against UVB-induced erythema when LED-based therapy was used before UV exposure. In both the PLE patients and the subjects, 85% of them showed at least one instance of a significant decrease in UVB-induced erythema reaction. Furthermore, a decrease in post-inflammatory hyperpigmentation and an effect similar to sun protection factor SPF-15 were noted. Yu and colleagues conducted an *in vitro* study that showed that exposure to HeNe laser radiation increased the release of nerve growth factor (NGF) from cultured keratinocytes as well as the expression of its gene. NGF is a key paracrine maintenance factor for skin melanocyte survival. It has been demonstrated that NGF can prevent UV-induced apoptosis in melanocytes by increasing the amounts of BCL-2 in the cells. Therefore, another explanation for the photoprotective effects of LLLT could be an increase in NGF production brought on by HeNe laser treatment (Bouzari et al., 2007; Wolfram et al., 2009; Barolet and Boucher, 2010).

9.5. LLLT for Herpes Virus Lesions

Herpes simplex virus (HSV) is a common viral infection that can last a person's entire life. Various physical or emotional stresses, such as fever, UV light exposure, and immune suppression, can trigger virus reactivation and migration through sensory nerves to the skin and mucosa, mainly affecting the lips and perioral area. About 60% of individuals may experience a prodromic stage before developing lesions that progress through different stages until healing occurs. Symptoms such as pain, burning, itching, or tingling at the affected site may accompany the formation of blisters. The immune response to HSV infection involves various cells and mechanisms, including macrophages, Langerhans cells, natural killer cells, lymphocytes, and cytotoxicity.

Acyclovir and valacyclovir are two anti-viral medications that are used to manage recurrent herpes outbreaks; however, there has only been a slight observed reduction in the healing time of lesions. Moreover, the emergence of drug-resistant strains of HSV is becoming increasingly important, particularly in patients with compromised immune systems. New therapeutic approaches are therefore required to reduce the length of recurrent episodes and to significantly lower the associated pain and inflammation.

It has been proposed that LLLT can speed up healing, lessen symptoms, and affect how long it takes for a recurrence to occur instead of the current medications. The frequency of herpes labialis episodes was found to be reduced in 50 patients with recurrent perioral herpes simplex infection (at least once per month for more than 6 months) when LLLT (690 nm, 80 mW/cm^2, 48 J/cm^2) was applied daily for two weeks during recurrence-free periods. Researchers found that patients with recurrent herpes simplex infection experienced significantly longer remission intervals—from 30 to 73 days—in another study using comparable irradiation parameters (647 nm, 50 mW/cm^2, 4.5 J/cm^2). Interestingly, patients with genital infections did not perform as well as those with labial herpes infections. In a murine model, however, radiation had no effect on established HSV latency.

It was suggested that rather than having a direct effect on inactivating the virus, LLLT had an indirect effect on humoral and cellular immune system components involved in antiviral responses, though the exact mechanism of action is still unknown. Inoue and associates examined the effects of tuberculin on the bilateral sites on the backs of guinea pigs that had been sensitized. On one side, they administered a single low-power laser irradiation dose at a fluence of 3.6 J per cm^2, and they contrasted it with non-irradiated contralateral sites. It's interesting to note that after radiation, the tuberculin reaction was inhibited at both the irradiated and contralateral nonirradiated sites. It's important to remember that this phenomenon was seen in the perivascular cellular infiltration when mononuclear cells predominated. Their findings have raised the possibility that LLLT has a systemic inhibitory effect on delayed hypersensitivity reactions. Several researchers have documented the synthesis and expression of cytokines, as well as the activation and proliferation of macrophages and lymphocytes in response to low levels of red and NIR light. It is unknown at this point whether these LLLT effects have any bearing on HSV infection (Bouzari et al., 2007; Wolfram et al., 2009; Barolet and Boucher, 2010).

9.6. LLLT for Vitiligo

Depigmentation of the skin and hair is a characteristic of vitiligo, an acquired pigmentary disorder. Investigations are ongoing to determine the underlying mechanism behind the disappearance of functional melanocytes from the affected skin. Findings, however, indicate that keratinocytes, fibroblasts, melanoblasts, and melanocytes may all be involved in the depigmentation and repigmentation processes of vitiligo, regardless of the pathogenetic mechanism at play. Therefore, one potential course of treatment could involve stimulating these dermal and epidermal cells. Vitiligo has historically not responded well to treatment because of the disease's unclear etiology. Currently available treatments for vitiligo include topical corticosteroids, phototherapy, and photochemotherapy (PUVA), which cause patients to repigment to varied degrees. Researchers discovered in 1982 that low-energy laser irradiation affected the defective biosynthesis of catecholamines in vitiligo and scleroderma, among other dermatological conditions. Subsequently, an investigator from the same group reported that, following 6–8 months of low-energy HeNe laser (632 nm, 25 mW/cm^2) therapy for 18 vitiligo patients, 64% of the patients showed marked repigmentation and the remaining 34% showed some follicular repigmentation. Since then, LLLT has been proposed as a successful substitute therapy for vitiligo patients.

The dysfunction of the sympathetic nerves in the afflicted skin is linked to segmental-type vitiligo, which is comparatively resistant to standard treatments. It was suggested that the HeNe laser might be a viable treatment option for segmental type vitiligo based on earlier reports showing that HeNe laser irradiation improves nerve injury and LLLT causes repigmentation responses. 60% of patients with subsequent treatments showed significant perilesional and perifollicular repigmentation (> 50%) when the HeNe laser light was applied locally (3 J/cm^2, 1.0 mW, 632.8 nm). Melanocyte migration is stimulated by both NGF and bFGF, and deficiencies in these mediators may contribute to the development of vitiligo.

In the same study, it was found that there was a significant increase in the release of bFGF from both keratinocytes and fibroblasts when they were exposed to 0.5–1.5 J cm^2 HeNe laser. There was also a significant increase in the release of NGF from keratinocytes. Furthermore, the medium from keratinocytes exposed to a HeNe laser induced the uptake of [3H]thymidine and the proliferation of melanocytes in culture. Lan et al. showed that the heNe laser (632 nm, 1 J/cm^2, and 10 mW) stimulates the growth of melanocytes by upregulating the expression of phosphorylated cyclic-AMP response element binding protein (CREB), an important regulator of melanocyte growth, and stimulates the proliferation of melanocytes through increased expression of α2β1 integrin. Because ECM molecules regulate the morphology, migration, tyrosinase activity, and proliferation of pigment cells, they are also crucial components of the pigmentation process. Type IV collagen is known to have a complex interaction with melanocytes in the epidermis, including enhancing melanocyte motility. Type IV collagen is found in the basement membrane.

After exposure to HeNe irradiation, there was a noticeable improvement in the attachment of melanocytes to type IV collagen, suggesting that the physiological function of melanocytes can be influenced by HeNe laser irradiation. Additionally, fibronectin, one of the extracellular matrix proteins present in the dermis, was found to have a significant impact on the differentiation and migration of melanoblasts and melanocytes. A study by Gibson et al. in 1983 revealed that the distribution of fibronectin *in vivo* was closely linked to the migration pattern of melanoblasts during the repigmentation process in vitiligo. Furthermore, research by Lan et al. showed that HeNe laser treatment led to a decrease in the attachment of immature melanoblasts to fibronectin, while the attachment of more differentiated melanoblasts increased by 20% after exposure to HeNe laser treatment. Finally, it was observed that the expression of integrin a5b1, which plays a role in pigment cell movement, was enhanced in NCCmelb4 cells (Bouzari et al., 2007; Wolfram et al., 2009; Barolet and Boucher, 2010).

9.7. LLLT for Producing Depigmentation

Most studies carried out for vitiligo show the stimulatory effects of LLLT on pigmentation; however in a previously mentioned study, while testing the effects of blue and red laser for acne treatment, an interesting and unexpected result was found for the first time. Combining both blue (415 +–5 nm, irradiance 40 mW/cm^2, 48 J/cm^2) and red (633 +/–6 nm, 80 mW/cm^2, 96 J/cm^2) light produced an overall decrease in the melanin level. Instrumental measurement results showed that melanin level increased by 6.7 (the median of differences between the melanin level before and after one treatment session) after blue light irradiation without a statistical significance (P >.1), whereas it decreased by 15.5 with statistical significance (P <.005) after red light irradiation. This finding may have some relationship with the laser's brightening effect on the skin tone, which 14 out of 24 patients spontaneously reported after the treatment period. However, as of today, no other studies investigated or reported a similar decrease in melanin levels following red light irradiation. Considering that different parameters are used for vitiligo and acne treatment, different effects of red light on the same tissue might be due to the biphasic effects of LLLT (Bouzari et al., 2007; Wolfram et al., 2009; Barolet and Boucher, 2010).

9.8 LLLT for Hypertrophic Scars and Keloids

Benign skin tumors called keloids and hypertrophic scars are tough to get rid of and typically develop after surgery, trauma, or acne. The two main traits are fibroblastic proliferation and excess collagen deposits; their pathogenesis has been linked to an imbalance between the rates of collagen biosynthesis and degradation, which is imposed on the individual's genetic predisposition. Numerous surgical techniques, such as cryotherapy and excision, non-surgical techniques like pharmacological treatments, mechanical pressure, and silicone gel dressings, and laser therapies like CO_2, pulsed dye, fractional ablative, and non-ablative lasers have been tried with varying degrees of success. Nevertheless, the best way to treat these lesions is still up in the air. Recent research suggests that this process is significantly influenced by dysregulated interleukin (IL)-6 signaling pathways and transforming growth factor beta-I (TGF-βI) expression. As a result, blocking the IL-6 pathway and/or TGF-βI may present a therapeutic target. It was suggested that LLLT be used as an alternative to current treatment options based on reports showing its effects on lowering IL-6 mRNA levels, modulation of PDGF, TGF-β, interleukins like IL-13 and IL-15, MMPs, and all of these factors being linked to aberrant wound healing. The use of LLLT as a prophylactic method to alter the wound healing process to avoid or attenuate the formation of hypertrophic scars or keloids has been investigated by Barolet and Boucher in 3 case studies, where following scar revision by surgery or CO_2 laser ablation on bilateral areas, a single scar was treated daily by the patient at home with NIR – LED 805 nm at 30 mW/cm^2 and 27 J/cm^2. The first patient had pre-auricular linear keloids bilaterally post-face lift procedure and surgical scar revision/excision had been performed. The second patient had hypertrophic scars on the chest bilaterally post-acne when the CO_2 laser was used for resurfacing. The third patient had hypertrophic scars on the back bilaterally post-excision and again the CO_2 laser was used for resurfacing. As a result, significant improvements in the NIR-LED treated vs the control scar were seen in all efficacy measures and moreover, no significant treatment-related adverse effects were reported (Bouzari et al., 2007; Wolfram et al., 2009; Barolet and Boucher, 2010).

9.9. LLLT for Burns

In a clinical study by Weiss et al, 10 patients received LED treatment (590 nm) for acute sunburn using a once-or twice-daily treatment regimen for 3 days, treating only half of the affected anatomic area. Decreased symptoms of burning, redness, swelling, and peeling were reported. One patient received LED treatment twice daily for 3 days only on half of his back, and the other half was left untreated. When compared with the untreated side, decreased MMP-1 was demonstrated on the LED-treated side through immunofluorescence staining. Moreover, RT-PCR gene expression analysis showed a significant decrease in MMP-1 gene expression on the LED-treated side at both 4 and 24 hours post–UV injury compared with the untreated side. Other significant changes were also noted with LED treatment related to inflammation and dermal matrix composition 4 days post–ultraviolet (UV) exposure.

Burns are a major side effect of laser treatment that can be extremely painful for the patient. LED was proposed as a therapeutic approach to promote quicker healing. LED therapy was administered once daily for one week to a group of nine patients who had various second-degree burns from nonablative laser devices. The patients and the doctor reported that the healing process was 50% faster. The same researchers also carried out a pilot study in which they used a computer pattern generator to inflict the same treatment on one test site after a CO_2 laser had damaged another forearm. Every day, a non-stick dressing and Polysporin ointment were changed at both sites; however, one site additionally received LED treatment. Consequently, the LED-treated site showed accelerated reepithelialization in comparison to the untreated control site. Additionally, the same researchers used a computer pattern generator to inflict the same treatment on both test sites in a pilot study in which they used a CO_2 laser to injure one forearm. Every day, a non-stick dressing and Polysporin ointment were changed at both sites; however, one site additionally received LED treatment. Consequently, the LED-treated site showed accelerated reepithelialization in comparison to the untreated control site (Bouzari et al., 2007; Wolfram et al., 2009; Barolet and Boucher, 2010).

9.10. LLLT for Psoriasis

Recently, there has been discussion about using LLLT to treat plaque psoriasis. A recent pilot study examined the effectiveness of using LED irradiation in combination with 830 nm (near infrared) and 630 nm (visible red light) in treating resistant psoriasis. All psoriasis patients who had not responded to traditional therapy were recruited, and for four or five weeks, they received sequential treatment using wavelengths of 830 nm and 630 nm, divided into 2–20-minute sessions separated by 48 hours. The outcomes demonstrated a resolution of psoriasis and no negative side effects (Bouzari et al., 2007; Wolfram et al., 2009; Barolet and Boucher, 2010).

A Closer Look

Lasers and Light Therapies for Skin Rejuvenation

Many technologies are available to treat almost any skin-related concern that patients may have. Non-surgical options for rejuvenation, such as improving the texture and tone of the skin, are provided by lasers and light source treatments. These operations are frequently carried out in the doctor's office as a succession of treatments with little to no discomfort or recovery time. With the use of technology, sun damage can be reversed, including age spots and redness, unwanted broken blood vessels can be removed, and wrinkles and acne scars can be less noticeable on the skin.

Treatments to Address Redness and Unsightly Blood Vessels

Reduction of the appearance of unsightly blood vessels, as in rosacea, telangiectasias, spider veins, and cherry angiomas, is one of the most common indications for laser therapy. Hemangiomas and port wine stains are examples of vascular malformations that are less frequently seen signs. Thankfully, there are several safe and efficient methods available to treat these aesthetic issues. To get the best results, these conditions typically need to be treated in a series.

With a wavelength of 585 or 595 nm, the pulsed dye laser (PDL) is designed specifically for use on blood vessels. It was among the first lasers to be used to treat vascular lesions. This laser is incredibly effective because it strategically targets the oxyhemoglobin absorption peaks. Its shorter wavelength allows it to target the superficial vessels with more energy and frequently results in purpura, which could prolong the healing period following surgery. The PDL can now safely treat structures deeper within the skin thanks to the development of devices that cool the epidermis; however, caution must be used, especially in patients with darker skin types, including those who have tanned skin.

The Neodymium:Yag (Nd:Yag) is a 1064 nm wavelength laser and is also very effective for the treatment of vascular lesions. The Nd:Yag is preferable to the PDL lasers due to the ability to treat deeper vessels and not result in as much purpura. Due to its longer wavelength, it tends to spare the epidermis and is safer in darker skin types. The 1064 nm lasers are safe enough to use for laser sclerotherapy and the ablation of leg spider veins.

Intense pulsed light (IPL) is a third type of laser device. It utilizes a set of replaceable cut-off filters to optimize the treatment of particular lesions. Because of this characteristic, IPL device treatment is highly operator-dependent. IPL is useful for treating rosacea, especially when used in a series of treatments, even though it is not suitable for deeper lesions. In addition to lessening erythema, IPL therapy frequently lessens the brown spot appearance. Because of the large heads, or spot sizes, of the IPL devices, a single treatment can be finished rather quickly.

Treatments to Address Age Spots and Pigment

Solar lentigos and other age spots, as well as facial pigmentation such as melasma, are common complaints among patients undergoing laser therapy. Melanosomes are the target in the majority of pigmented lesions and sun spots. A variety of laser and light treatments, both ablative and non-ablative, are available for the reduction of pigmented lesions.

The intense pulse light (IPL) device is the main non-ablative treatment modality for diffuse epidermal pigmentation. Once more, the IPL tends to be highly operator-dependent because the improvement depends in part on the cut-off filter selection. The 515 nm filter is the most often utilized filter for pigmented lesions. The lesions darken instantly after the treatment and peel off for the following few days. Similar to the majority of laser treatments, this frequently calls for several sessions.

IPL is a very safe and effective modality not only for facial rejuvenation but also for treating sun spots on the back of the hands, neck, and chest. It is crucial to keep in mind that these regions are more vulnerable to thermal damage and have fewer pilosebaceous units than the skin on the face. A skilled operator must carefully regulate the laser's energy and make use of the proper cooling mechanism.

Treatments for Skin Tightening

There are many different laser technologies available for treating skin laxity. These lasers work by targeting water in the skin tissue, which creates a thermal injury in the dermis. This leads to collagen shrinkage and remodeling. The main difference between these lasers is whether they achieve results through ablation (breaking the skin's surface) or not. This difference determines factors like downtime, risk, and how much the skin can be tightened.

Non-Ablative Treatment Modalities

Targeting dermal collagen is how radiofrequency (RF), ultrasonic (US), and infrared (IR) light modalities operate. These technologies avoid cutaneous wounding through epidermal injury while producing thermal effects in the dermis. Skin laxity on the face, neck, or body is one indication of RF/US/IR-based rejuvenation. The response to treatment varies; it frequently takes several treatments to see improvement, and additional sessions may be required to keep the desired effects. These non-ablative technologies have the following advantages: they are totally non-invasive, have no downtime, and can treat most skin surfaces, including the neck, chest, and areas with stretch marks.

In 2004, fractional photothermolysis was first introduced as a new method of skin treatment. Instead of ablating the entire surface of the skin, fractionated lasers create small columns of coagulation through the skin layers, prompting a healing response. This leaves untreated areas of normal skin between the columns, reducing pain during the procedure and speeding up healing time. Non-ablative fractionated lasers heat the skin without ablating it, resulting in minimal impact on the skin surface and minimal downtime similar to a sunburn. These lasers are used for mild acne scarring, mild wrinkling, melasma, and hypomelanosis. Like most lasers, fractionated laser treatments are often done in series to achieve the desired clinical response, unlike traditional resurfacing methods.

Ablative Treatment Modalities Traditional Resurfacing

Dermabrasion was long ago superseded by lasers. Conventional laser resurfacing was considered the best practice until the introduction of fractionated lasers. With the use of an Erbium:YAG or CO_2 water-targeting laser, the entire skin surface was removed. A reaction akin to a second-degree burn occurred; sedation was frequently needed for these procedures, and recovery took several weeks to months. It only affected people with fair skin because it affected the entire surface of the skin. Permanent relative hypopigmentation frequently develops even in these skin types. Fewer patients are opting for traditional resurfacing in light of the latest advancements in fractionated laser technology. 6 Some cases still warrant full surface ablation. For example, wrinkles around the eyes respond particularly well to traditional resurfacing. Instead of needing several fractionated laser treatments, this area's thinner skin can achieve better results with a single treatment and less aggressive resurfacing. Due to swelling, both treatment modalities would necessitate a similar amount of recovery time (roughly one to two weeks).

Fractionated Resurfacing

The latest advancement in laser technology is relative fractionated lasers. By generating fully ablative columns of microthermal injury, they combine the advantages of fractional photothermolysis with the efficacy of CO2 and Erbium:YAG lasers. The cosmetic improvement is more noticeable and can be attained in fewer treatments, but the downtime is greater than with non-ablative counterparts. Because the skin's surface is impacted, one should anticipate brief, pin-point bleeding, which typically goes away in less than a day, to be followed by a severe sunburn-like reaction that lasts for a few days to a week. But after one to two days, patients are free to apply concealer or makeup because a large portion of the skin's surface remains unaltered. Ablative fractionated lasers have outperformed traditional resurfacing in terms of effectiveness for many conditions, including moderate to severe sun damage and wrinkling, moderate to severe textural abnormalities like rhinophyma, moderate to severe acne scars, and traumatic or surgical scars. They also minimize downtime, side effects, and complication risks.

Summary

- Low-level laser (light) therapy (LLLT) is a fast-growing technology used to treat a multitude of conditions that require stimulation of healing, relief of pain and inflammation, and restoration of function.
- Low-level laser therapy (LLLT) was discovered in the late 1960s, but only in recent times has it been widely applied in dermatology.
- The basic biological mechanism behind the effects of LLLT is thought to be through absorption of red and NIR light by mitochondrial chromophores, in particular cytochrome c oxidase (CCO) which is contained in the respiratory chain located within the mitochondria.
- LLLT, phototherapy or photobiomodulation refers to the use of photons at a non-thermal irradiance to alter biological activity. LLLT uses either coherent light sources (lasers) or non-coherent light sources consisting of filtered lamps or light-emitting diodes (LED) or, on occasion, a combination of both.
- The mechanism associated with the cellular photobiostimulation by LLLT is not yet fully understood. From observation, it appears that LLLT has a wide range of effects at the molecular, cellular, and tissue levels.
- Skin starts showing its first signs of aging in the late 20s to early 30s and it usually presents with wrinkles, dyspigmentation, telangiectasia, and loss of elasticity.
- LED which is a novel light source for non-thermal, non-ablative skin rejuvenation has been shown to be effective for improving wrinkles and skin laxity.
- Pathogenesis of acne vulgaris has not yet been clarified, however, the current consensus is that it involves four main events: follicular hyperconification, increased sebum secretion effected by the androgenic hormone secretions, colonization of *Propionibacterium acnes* and inflammation.
- One of the most common virus infections is caused by herpes simplex virus (HSV). HSV is chronic and lasts one's entire life.
- Segmental-type vitiligo is associated with a dysfunction of the sympathetic nerves in the affected skin and it is relatively resistant to conventional therapies.
- Fibroblastic proliferation and excess collagen deposits are the two main characteristics and imbalance between rates of collagen biosynthesis and degradation superimposed on the individual's genetic predisposition and have been implicated in their pathogenesis.

References

1. Abergel, R. P., Lyons, R. F., Castel, J. C., Dwyer, R. M., & Uitto, J. (1987). Bio stimulation of wound healing by lasers: Experimental approaches in animal models and in fibroblast cultures. *Journal of Dermatologic Surgery and Oncology, 13*(2), 127–133.
2. Ablon, G. (2010). Combination 830-nm and 633-nm light-emitting diode phototherapy shows promise in the treatment of recalcitrant psoriasis: Preliminary findings. *Photomedicine and Laser Surgery, 28*(1), 141–146.
3. Airan, L. E., & Hruza, G. (2005). Current lasers in skin resurfacing. *Facial Plastic Surgery Clinics of North America, 13*(1), 127–139.

4. AlGhamdi, K. M., Kumar, A., & Moussa, N. A. (2012). Low-level laser therapy: A useful technique for enhancing the proliferation of various cultured cells. *Lasers in Medical Science, 27*(1), 237–249.

5. Anders, J. J., Borke, R. C., Woolery, S. K., & Van de Merwe, W. P. (1993). Low power laser irradiation alters the rate of regeneration of the rat facial nerve. *Lasers in Surgery and Medicine, 13*(1), 72–82.

6. Applegate, L. A., Scaletta, C., Panizzon, R., Frenk, E., Hohlfeld, P., & Schwarzkopf, S. (2000). Induction of the putative protective protein ferritin by infrared radiation: Implications in skin repair. *International Journal of Molecular Medicine, 5*(3), 247–251.

7. Aziz-Jalali, M. H., Tabaie, S. M., & Djavid, G. E. (2012). Comparison of red and infrared low-level laser therapy in the treatment of acne vulgaris. *Indian Journal of Dermatology, 57*(2), 128–130.

8. Barolet, D. (2008). Light-emitting diodes (LEDs) in dermatology. *Seminars in Cutaneous Medicine and Surgery, 27*(4), 227–238.

9. Barolet, D., & Boucher, A. (2008). LED photoprevention: Reduced MED response following multiple LED exposures. *Lasers in Surgery and Medicine, 40*(2), 106–112.

10. Barolet, D., & Boucher, A. (2010). Prophylactic low-level light therapy for the treatment of hypertrophic scars and keloids: A case series. *Lasers in Surgery and Medicine, 42*(6), 597–601.

11. Barolet, D., Roberge, C. J., Auger, F. A., Boucher, A., & Germain, L. (2009). Regulation of skin collagen metabolism *in vitro* using a pulsed 660 nm LED light source: Clinical correlation with a single-blinded study. *Journal of Investigative Dermatology, 129*(12), 2751–2759.

12. Basford, J. R. (1995). Low intensity laser therapy: Still not an established clinical tool. *Lasers in Surgery and Medicine, 16*(4), 331–342.

13. Bello-Silva, M. S., de Freitas, P. M., Aranha, A. C., Lage-Marques, J. L., Simoes, A., & de Paula Eduardo, C. (2010). Low- and high-intensity lasers in the treatment of herpes simplex virus 1 infection. *Photomedicine and Laser Surgery, 28*(1), 135–139.

14. Ben-Dov, N., Shefer, G., Irintchev, A., Wernig, A., Oron, U., & Halevy, O. (1999). Low-energy laser irradiation affects satellite cell proliferation and differentiation *in vitro*. *Biochimica et Biophysica Acta, 1448*(3), 372–380.

15. Bhat, J., Birch, J., Whitehurst, C., & Lanigan, S. W. (2005). A single-blinded randomised controlled study to determine the efficacy of Omnilux Revive facial treatment in skin rejuvenation. *Lasers in Medical Science, 20*(1), 6–10.

16. Bolton, P., Young, S., & Dyson, M. (1990). Macrophage responsiveness to light therapy: A dose response study. *Laser Therapy, 2*, 101–106.

17. Bouzari, N., Davis, S. C., & Nouri, K. (2007). Laser treatment of keloids and hypertrophic scars. *International Journal of Dermatology, 46*(1), 80–88.

18. Branham, G. H., & Thomas, J. R. (1996). Rejuvenation of the skin surface: Chemical peel and dermabrasion. *Facial Plastic Surgery, 12*(2), 125–133.

19. Calles, C., Schneider, M., Macaluso, F., Benesova, T., Krutmann, J., & Schroeder, P. (2010). Infrared A radiation influences the skin fibroblast transcriptome: Mechanisms and consequences. *Journal of Investigative Dermatology, 130*(6), 1524–1536.

20. Chung, H., Dai, T., Sharma, S. K., Huang, Y. Y., Carroll, J. D., & Hamblin, M. R. (2012). The nuts and bolts of low-level laser (light) therapy. *Annals of Biomedical Engineering, 40*(2), 516–533.

21. Cunliffe, W. J., & Goulden, V. (2000). Phototherapy and acne vulgaris. *British Journal of Dermatology, 142*(5), 855–856.

22. de Paula Eduardo, C., Bezinelli, L. M., de Paula Eduardo, F., et al. (2011). Prevention of recurrent herpes labialis outbreaks through low-intensity laser therapy: A clinical protocol with 3-year follow-up. *Lasers in Medical Science, 16*, 1–6.

23. Dierickx, C. C., & Anderson, R. R. (2005). Visible light treatment of photoaging. *Dermatologic Therapy, 18*(3), 191–208.

24. Frank, S., Oliver, L., Lebreton-De Coster, C., et al. (2004). Infrared radiation affects the mitochondrial pathway of apoptosis in human fibroblasts. *Journal of Investigative Dermatology, 123*(5), 823–831.

25. Funk, J. O., Kruse, A., & Kirchner, H. (1992). Cytokine production after helium-neon laser irradiation in cultures of human peripheral blood mononuclear cells. *Journal of Photochemistry and Photobiology B: Biology, 16*(3, 4), 347–355.

26. Geronemus, R. G., Weiss, R. A., Weiss, M. A., et al. (2003). Non-ablative LED photomodulation light activated fibroblast stimulation clinical trial. *Lasers in Surgery and Medicine, 25*, 22.

27. Ghazizadeh, M., Tosa, M., Shimizu, H., Hyakusoku, H., & Kawanami, O. (2007). Functional implications of the IL-6 signaling pathway in keloid pathogenesis. *Journal of Investigative Dermatology, 127*(1), 98–105.

28. Gibson, W. T., Couchman, J. R., & Weaver, A. C. (1983). Fibronectin distribution during the development of fetal rat skin. *Journal of Investigative Dermatology, 81*(6), 480–485.

29. Goldberg, D. J., & Russell, B. A. (2006). Combination blue (415 nm) and red (633 nm) LED phototherapy in the treatment of mild to severe acne vulgaris. *Journal of Cosmetic Laser Therapy, 8*(2), 71–75.

30. Greco, M., Guida, G., Perlino, E., Marra, E., & Quagliariello, E. (1989). Increase in RNA and protein synthesis by mitochondria irradiated with helium-neon laser. *Biochemical and Biophysical Research Communications, 163*(3), 1428–1434.

31. Gupta, A., Avci, P., Sadasivam, M., et al. (2012). Shining light on nanotechnology to help repair and regeneration. *Biotechnology Advances, 30*(4), 924–940.

32. Hamblin, M. R., & Demidova, T. N. (2006). Mechanisms of low-level light therapy: An introduction. *Proceedings of SPIE, 6140*, 61001–61012.

33. Hardaway, C. A., & Ross, E. V. (2002). Nonablative laser skin remodeling. *Dermatologic Clinics, 20*(1), 97–111. ix.

34. Harris, D. M. (1991). Editorial Comment: Biomolecular mechanisms of laser bio stimulation. *Journal of Clinical Laser Medicine & Surgery, 9*(4), 277–280.

35. Hedley, S. J., Wagner, M., Bielby, S., Smith-Thomas, L., Gawkrodger, D. J., & MacNeil, S. (1997). The influence of extracellular matrix proteins on cutaneous and uveal melanocytes. *Pigment Cell Research, 10*(1, 2), 54–59.

36. Hode, L. (2005). The importance of the coherency. *Photomedicine and Laser Surgery, 23*(4), 431–434.

37. Huang, Y. Y., Chen, A. C., Carroll, J. D., & Hamblin, M. R. (2009). Biphasic dose response in low-level light therapy. *Dose-Response*, *7*(4), 358–383.

38. Huang, Y. Y., Sharma, S. K., Carroll, J., & Hamblin, M. R. (2011). Biphasic dose response in low-level light therapy–An update. *Dose-Response*, *9*(4), 602–618.

39. Ideta, R., Soma, T., Tsunenaga, M., & Ifuku, O. (2002). Cultured human dermal papilla cells secrete a chemotactic factor for melanocytes. *Journal of Dermatological Science*, *28*(1), 48–59.

40. Inoue, K., Nishioka, J., & Hukuda, S. (1989). Altered lymphocyte proliferation by low dosage laser irradiation. *Clinical and Experimental Rheumatology*, *7*(5), 521–523.

41. Inoue, K., Nishioka, J., & Hukuda, S. (1989). Suppressed tuberculin reaction in guinea pigs following laser irradiation. *Lasers in Surgery and Medicine*, *9*(3), 271–275.

42. Karu, T. (1995). Irradiation with He-Ne laser increases ATP level in cells cultivated *in vitro*. *Journal of Photochemistry and Photobiology B: Biology*, *27*(3), 219–223.

43. Karu, T. (1999). Primary and secondary mechanisms of action of visible to near-IR radiation on cells. *Journal of Photochemistry and Photobiology B: Biology*, *49*(1), 1–17.

44. Karu, T. I., & Kolyakov, S. F. (2005). Exact action spectra for cellular responses relevant to phototherapy. *Photomedicine and Laser Surgery*, *23*(4), 355–361.

45. Karu, T. I., Pyatibrat, L. V., & Kalendo, G. S. (2004). Photobiological modulation of cell attachment via cytochrome c oxidase. *Photochemical & Photobiological Sciences*, *3*(2), 211–216.

46. Khullar, S. M., Brodin, P., Barkvoll, P., & Haanaes, H. R. (1996). Preliminary study of low-level laser for treatment of long-standing sensory aberrations in the inferior alveolar nerve. *Journal of Oral and Maxillofacial Surgery*, *54*(1), 2–7. discussion 7, 8.

47. Kimura, E., Kawano, Y., Todo, H., Ikarashi, Y., & Sugibayashi, K. (2012). Measurement of skin permeation/penetration of nanoparticles for their safety evaluation. *Biological & Pharmaceutical Bulletin*, *35*(9), 1476–1486.

48. Kitamura, R., Tsukamoto, K., Harada, K., et al. (2004). Mechanisms underlying the dysfunction of melanocytes in vitiligo epidermis: Role of SCF/KIT protein interactions and the downstream effector, MITF-M. *Journal of Pathology*, *202*(4), 463–475.

49. Kligman, L. H. (1989). Photoaging: Manifestations, prevention, and treatment. *Clinical Geriatrics Medicine*, *5*(1), 235–251.

50. Korner, R., Bahmer, F., & Wigand, R. (1989). The effect of infrared laser rays on herpes simplex virus and the functions of human immunocompetent cells. *Hautarzt*, *40*(6), 350–354.

51. Krutmann, J., & Schroeder, P. (2009). Role of mitochondria in photoaging of human skin: The defective powerhouse model. *Journal of Investigative Dermatology Symposium Proceedings*, *14*(1), 44–49.

52. Kucuk, B. B., Oral, K., Selcuk, N. A., Toklu, T., & Civi, O. G. (2010). The anti-inflammatory effect of low-level laser therapy on experimentally induced inflammation of rabbit temporomandibular joint retro discal tissues. *Journal of Orofacial Pain*, *24*(3), 293–297.

53. Lan, C. C., Wu, C. S., Chiou, M. H., Chiang, T. Y., & Yu, H. S. (2009). Low-energy helium-neon laser induces melanocyte proliferation via interaction with type IV collagen: Visible light as a therapeutic option for vitiligo. *British Journal of Dermatology*, *161*(2), 273–280.

54. Lan, C. C., Wu, C. S., Chiou, M. H., Hsieh, P. C., & Yu, H. S. (2006). Low-energy helium-neon laser induces locomotion of the immature melanoblasts and promotes melanogenesis of the more differentiated melanoblasts: Recapitulation of vitiligo repigmentation *in vitro*. *Journal of Investigative Dermatology, 126*(9), 2119–2126.

55. Landthaler, M., Haina, D., & Waidelich, W. (1983). Treatment of zoster, post-zoster pain, and herpes simplex recidivans in loco with laser light. *Fortschritte der Medizin, 101*(22), 1039–1041.

56. Lane, N. (2006). Cell biology: Power games. *Nature, 443*(7114), 901–903.

57. Lee, A. Y. (2012). Role of keratinocytes in the development of vitiligo. *Annals of Dermatology, 24*(2), 115–125.

58. Lee, S. Y., Park, K. H., Choi, J. W., et al. (2007). A prospective, randomized, placebo-controlled, double-blinded, and split-face clinical study on LED phototherapy for skin rejuvenation: Clinical, profilometric, histologic, ultrastructural, and biochemical evaluations and comparison of three different treatment settings. *Journal of Photochemistry and Photobiology B: Biology, 88*(1), 51–67.

59. Lee, S. Y., You, C. E., & Park, M. Y. (2007). Blue and red-light combination LED phototherapy for acne vulgaris in patients with skin phototype IV. *Lasers in Surgery and Medicine, 39*(2), 180–188.

60. Liu, H., Colavitti, R., & Finkel, T. (2005). Redox-dependent transcriptional regulation. *Circulation Research, 97*(10), 967–974.

61. Liu, W., Wang, D. R., & Cao, Y. L. (2004). TGF-beta: A fibrotic factor in wound scarring and a potential target for anti-scarring gene therapy. *Current Gene Therapy, 4*(1), 123–136.

62. Louw, L. (2007). The keloid phenomenon: Progress toward a solution. *Clinical Anatomy, 20*(1), 3–14.

63. Ma, H. J., Zhu, W. Y., Wang, D. G., Yue, X. Z., & Li, C. R. (2006). Endothelin-1 combined with extracellular matrix proteins promotes the adhesion and chemotaxis of amelanotic melanocytes from human hair follicles *in vitro*. *Cell Biology International, 30*(12), 999–1006.

64. Mandel, A. (1984). Skin repigmentation after laser therapy. *Vestnik Dermatologii i Venerologii, (9)*, 26–29.

65. Mandel, A. S., Haberman, H. F., Pawlowski, D., & Goldstein, E. (1997). Non-PUVA nonsurgical therapies for vitiligo. *Clinical Dermatology, 15*(6), 907–919.

66. Mandel, A., & Dunaeva, L. P. (1982). Effect of laser therapy on blood levels of serotonin and dopamine in scleroderma patients. *Vestnik Dermatologii i Venerologii, (8)*, 13–17.

67. Manteifel, V., Bakeeva, L., & Karu, T. (1997). Ultrastructural changes in chondriome of human lymphocytes after irradiation with He-Ne laser: Appearance of giant mitochondria. *Journal of Photochemistry and Photobiology B: Biology, 38*(1), 25–30.

68. McDaniel, D. H., Newman, J., Geronemus, R., et al. (2003). Non-ablative non-thermal LED photomodulation—a multicenter clinical photoaging trial. *Lasers in Surgery and Medicine, 15*, 22.

69. Menezes, S., Coulomb, B., Lebreton, C., & Dubertret, L. (1998). Non-coherent near infrared radiation protects normal human dermal fibroblasts from solar ultraviolet toxicity. *Journal of Investigative Dermatology, 111*(4), 629–633.

70. Morelli, J. G., Yohn, J. J., Zekman, T., & Norris, D. A. (1993). Melanocyte movement *in vitro*: Role of matrix proteins and integrin receptors. *Journal of Investigative Dermatology, 101*(4), 605–608.

71. Munoz Sanchez, P. J., Capote Femenias, J. L., Diaz Tejeda, A., & Turner, J. (2012). The effect of 670-nm low laser therapy on herpes simplex type 1. *Photomedicine and Laser Surgery, 30*(1), 37–40.

72. Nanni, C. A., & Alster, T. S. (1998). Complications of carbon dioxide laser resurfacing: An evaluation of 500 patients. *Dermatologic Surgery, 24*(3), 315–320.

73. Oron, U. (2011). Light therapy and stem cells: A therapeutic intervention of the future? *Interventional Cardiology, 3*(6), 627–629.

74. Paasch, U., & Haedersdal, M. (2011). Laser systems for ablative fractional resurfacing. *Expert Review of Medical Devices, 8*(1), 67–83.

75. Papageorgiou, P., Katsambas, A., & Chu, A. (2000). Phototherapy with blue (415 nm) and red (660 nm) light in the treatment of acne vulgaris. *British Journal of Dermatology, 142*(5), 973–978.

76. Pastore, D., Greco, M., Petragallo, V. A., & Passarella, S. (1994). Increase in <–H+/e– ratio of the cytochrome c oxidase reaction in mitochondria irradiated with helium-neon laser. *Biochemistry and Molecular Biology International, 34*(4), 817–826.

77. Peacocke, M., Yaar, M., Mansur, C. P., Chao, M. V., & Gilchrest, B. A. (1988). Induction of nerve growth factor receptors on cultured human melanocytes. *Proceedings of the National Academy of Sciences of the United States of America, 85*(14), 5282–5286.

78. Peplow, P. V., Chung, T. Y., Ryan, B., & Baxter, G. D. (2011). Laser photo biomodulation of gene expression and release of growth factors and cytokines from cells in culture: A review of human and animal studies. *Photomedicine and Laser Surgery, 29*(5), 285–304.

79. Perrin, D., Jolivald, J. R., Triki, H., et al. (1997). Effect of laser irradiation on latency of herpes simplex virus in a mouse model. *Pathologie Biologie, 45*(1), 24–27.

80. Posten, W., Wrone, D. A., Dover, J. S., Arndt, K. A., Silapunt, S., & Alam, M. (2005). Low-level laser therapy for wound healing: Mechanism and efficacy. *Dermatologic Surgery, 31*(3), 334–340.

81. Rochkind, S., Rousso, M., Nissan, M., Villarreal, M., Barr-Nea, L., & Rees, D. G. (1989). Systemic effects of low-power laser irradiation on the peripheral and central nervous system, cutaneous wounds, and burns. *Lasers in Surgery and Medicine, 9*(2), 174–182.

82. Ross, E. V. (2005). Optical treatments for acne. *Dermatologic Therapy, 18*(3), 253–266.

83. Rotunda, A. M., Bhupathy, A. R., & Rohrer, T. E. (2004). The new age of acne therapy: Light, lasers, and radiofrequency. *Journal of Cosmetic Laser Therapy, 6*(4), 191–200.

84. Russell, B. A., Kellett, N., & Reilly, L. R. (2005). A study to determine the efficacy of combination LED light therapy (633 nm and 830 nm) in facial skin rejuvenation. *Journal of Cosmetic Laser Therapy, 7*(3–4), 196–200.

85. Sachdev, M., Hameed, S., & Mysore, V. (2011). Nonablative lasers and nonlaser systems in dermatology: Current status. *Indian Journal of Dermatology, Venereology, and Leprology, 77*(3), 380–388.

86. Sadick, N. S. (2008). Handheld LED array device in the treatment of acne vulgaris. *Journal of Drugs in Dermatology, 7*(4), 347–350.

87. Schindl, A., & Neumann, R. (1999). Low-intensity laser therapy is an effective treatment for recurrent herpes simplex infection: Results from a randomized double-blind placebo-controlled study. *Journal of Investigative Dermatology, 113*(2), 221–223.

88. Schindl, A., Heinze, G., Schindl, M., Pernerstorfer-Schon, H., & Schindl, L. (2002). Systemic effects of low-intensity laser irradiation on skin microcirculation in patients with diabetic microangiopathy. *Microvascular Research, 64*(2), 240–246.

89. Schindl, L., Schindl, M., Polo, L., Jori, G., Perl, S., & Schindl, A. (1997). Effects of low-power laser irradiation on differential blood count and body temperature in endotoxin-preimmunized rabbits. *Life Sciences, 60*(19), 1669–1677.

90. Schroeder, P., Calles, C., Benesova, T., Macaluso, F., & Krutmann, J. (2010). Photoprotection beyond ultraviolet radiation: Effective sun protection has to include protection against infrared A radiation-induced skin damage. *Skin Pharmacology and Physiology, 23*(1), 15–17.

91. Seaton, E. D., Mouser, P. E., Charakida, A., Alam, S., Seldon, P. M., & Chu, A. C. (2006). Investigation of the mechanism of action of nonablative pulsed-dye laser therapy in photorejuvenation and inflammatory acne vulgaris. *British Journal of Dermatology, 155*(4), 748–755.

92. Sinha, R. P., & Hader, D. P. (2002). UV-induced DNA damage and repair: A review. *Photochemical & Photobiological Sciences, 1*(4), 225–236.

93. Sriprachya-Anunt, S., Fitzpatrick, R. E., Goldman, M. P., & Smith, S. R. (1997). Infections complicating pulsed carbon dioxide laser resurfacing for photoaged facial skin. *Dermatologic Surgery, 23*(7), 527–535. Discussion 535–526.

94. Takano, N., Kawakami, T., Kawa, Y., et al. (2002). Fibronectin combined with stem cell factor plays an important role in melanocyte proliferation, differentiation, and migration in cultured mouse neural crest cells. *Pigment Cell Research, 15*(3), 192–200.

95. Takema, Y., Yorimoto, Y., Kawai, M., & Imokawa, G. (1994). Age-related changes in the elastic properties and thickness of human facial skin. *British Journal of Dermatology, 131*(5), 641–648.

96. Uitto, J. (2007). IL-6 signaling pathway in keloids: A target for pharmacologic intervention? *Journal of Investigative Dermatology, 127*(1), 6–8.

97. Uitto, J., & Kouba, D. (2000). Cytokine modulation of extracellular matrix gene expression: Relevance to fibrotic skin diseases. *Journal of Dermatological Science, 24*(Suppl 1), S60–69.

98. Weiss, R. A., McDaniel, D. H., & Geronemus, R. G. (2003). Review of nonablative photorejuvenation: Reversal of the aging effects of the sun and environmental damage using laser and light sources. *Seminars in Cutaneous Medicine and Surgery, 22*(2), 93–106.

99. Weiss, R. A., McDaniel, D. H., Geronemus, R. G., & Weiss, M. A. (2005). Clinical trial of a novel nonthermal LED array for reversal of photoaging: Clinical, histologic, and surface profilometric results. *Lasers in Surgery and Medicine, 36*(2), 85–91.

100. Weiss, R. A., McDaniel, D. H., Geronemus, R. G., et al. (2005). Clinical experience with light-emitting diode (LED) photomodulation. *Dermatologic Surgery, 31*(9 Pt 2), 1199–1205.

101. Weiss, R. A., McDaniel, D. H., Geronemus, R., et al. (2004). Non-ablative, non-thermal light emitting diode (LED) phototherapy of photoaged skin. *Lasers in Surgery and Medicine, 16*, 31.

102. Weiss, R. A., Weiss, M. A., Geronemus, R. G., & McDaniel, D. H. (2004). A novel non-thermal non-ablative full panel LED photomodulation device for reversal of photoaging: Digital microscopic and clinical results in various skin types. *Journal of Drugs in Dermatology*, *3*(6), 605–610.

103. Whitley, R. J., Kimberlin, D. W., & Roizman, B. (1998). Herpes simplex viruses. *Clinical Infectious Diseases*, *26*(3), 541–553. quiz 554–545.

104. Wolfram, D., Tzankov, A., Pulzl, P., & Piza-Katzer, H. (2009). Hypertrophic scars and keloids: A review of their pathophysiology, risk factors, and therapeutic management. *Dermatologic Surgery*, *35*(2), 171–181.

105. Wong-Riley, M. T., Liang, H. L., Eells, J. T., et al. (2005). Photobiomodulation directly benefits primary neurons functionally inactivated by toxins: Role of cytochrome c oxidase. *Journal of Biological Chemistry*, *280*(6), 4761–4771.

106. Wu, C. S., Lan, C. C., Chiou, M. H., & Yu, H. S. (2006). Basic fibroblast growth factor promotes melanocyte migration via increased expression of p125(FAK) on melanocytes. *Acta Dermato-Venereologica*, *86*(6), 498–502.

107. Yaar, M., Grossman, K., Eller, M., & Gilchrest, B. A. (1991). Evidence for nerve growth factor-mediated paracrine effects in human epidermis. *Journal of Cell Biology*, *115*(3), 821–828.

108. Yu, H. S. (2000). Treatment of vitiligo vulgaris with helium-neon laser. *MB Derma*, *35*(13–18).

109. Yu, H. S., Chang, K. L., Yu, C. L., Chen, J. W., & Chen, G. S. (1996). Low-energy helium-neon laser irradiation stimulates interleukin-1 alpha and interleukin-8 release from cultured human keratinocytes. *Journal of Investigative Dermatology*, *107*(4), 593–596.

110. Yu, H. S., Wu, C. S., Yu, C. L., Kao, Y. H., & Chiou, M. H. (2003). Helium-neon laser irradiation stimulates migration and proliferation in melanocytes and induces repigmentation in segmental-type vitiligo. *Journal of Investigative Dermatology*, *120*(1), 56–64.

111. Yu, R., Huang, Y., Zhang, X., & Zhou, Y. (2012). Potential role of neurogenic inflammatory factors in the pathogenesis of vitiligo. *Journal of Cutan Medical Surgery*, *16*(4), 230–244.

112. Yu, W., Chi, L. H., Naim, J. O., & Lanzafame, R. J. (1997). Improvement of host response to sepsis by photobiomodulation. *Lasers in Surgery and Medicine*, *21*(3), 262–268.

113. Yu, W., Naim, J. O., & Lanzafame, R. J. (1994). The effect of laser irradiation on the release of bFGF from 3T3 fibroblasts. *Photochemistry and Photobiology*, *59*(2), 167–170.

114. Zhai, S., Yaar, M., Doyle, S. M., & Gilchrest, B. A. (1996). Nerve growth factor rescues pigment cells from ultraviolet-induced apoptosis by upregulating BCL-2 levels. *Experimental Cell Research*, *224*(2), 335–343.

Chapter

ADVANCED TECHNOLOGIES IN DERMATOLOGY

10

Contents

Introduction

Preventive medicine, which aims to prevent disease when possible, and regenerative medicine, which repairs damaged cells, are the two areas of healing that are currently gaining attention in medicine. Over the past few decades, burn, and chronic wound treatments have evolved. The cornerstone of wound treatment remains the early removal of dead necrosis and the closure of the wound with an autologous skin transplant of medium thickness (STSG); however, novel approaches that might yield a more pleasing cosmetic result are still being investigated. This shift is the result of patients' increased awareness and the ensuing demand for novel approaches to wound care and scar healing.

Orientation and Directional Terms

Term	Definition	Illustration
Preventive medicine	Preventive medicine is a medical specialty that aims to prevent disease, disability, and death by promoting, protecting, and maintaining health and well-being.	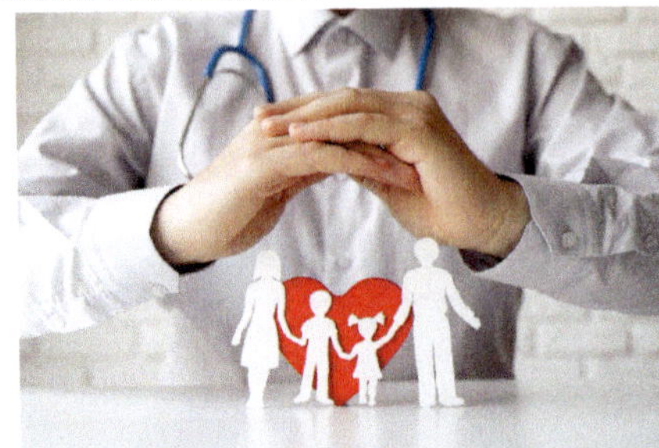
Cell therapy	Cell therapy is a therapy in which viable cells are injected, grafted or implanted into a patient in order to effectuate a medicinal effect, for example, by transplanting T-cells capable of fighting cancer cells via cell-mediated immunity in the course of immunotherapy, or grafting stem cells to regenerate diseased tissues.	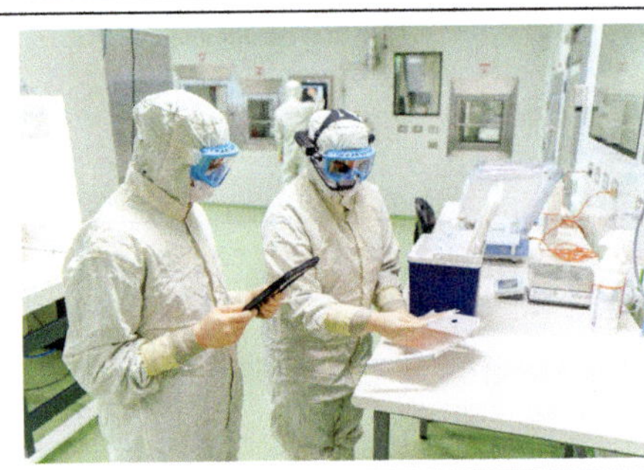
Gram-positive bacteria	Gram-positive bacteria are bacteria that stain blue when treated with a chemical called Gram stain. They are characterized by their thick cell walls, which are made up of peptidoglycans and mucocomplexes.	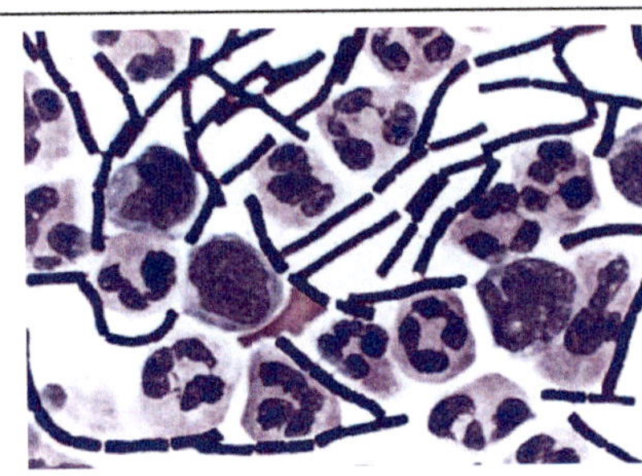
Glycosaminoglycans	Glycosaminoglycans (GAGs), also known as mucopolysaccharides, are long, linear polysaccharides that are negatively charged and made up of repeating disaccharide units. They are found in all mammalian tissues, and are major components of the cell surface and extracellular matrix.	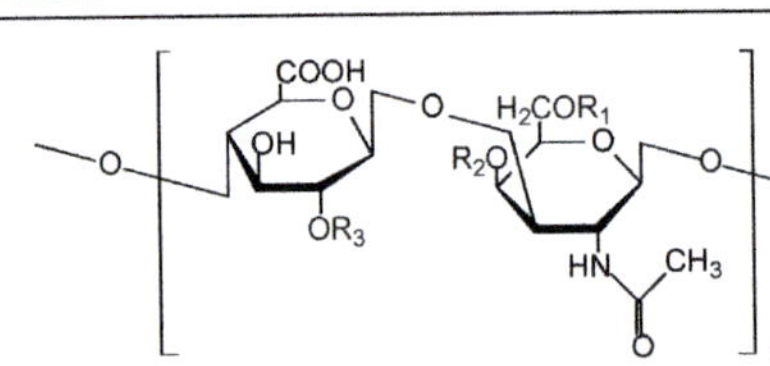
T cells	T cells are one of the important types of white blood cells of the immune system and play a central role in the adaptive immune response. T cells can be distinguished from other lymphocytes by the presence of a T-cell receptor (TCR) on their cell surface.	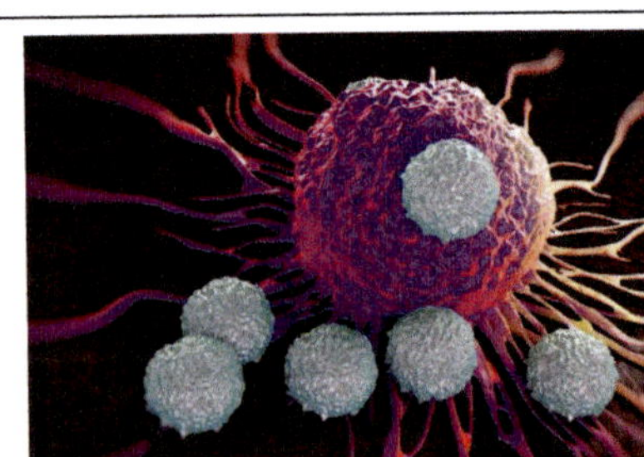

10.1. Cellular Therapies

One intriguing application of translational medicine is the use of cellular therapies to bring patients back to the state of skin completeness. But one should keep in mind that the European Medicines Agency's (EMEA) Commission for Advanced Therapies recognized cell transplants—autologous keratinocytes or stem cells—as a healing product for advanced therapy. This means that the guidelines of Good Practice govern their manufacturing, with all the ramifications. Patients with acquired and hereditary skin diseases are treated with products derived from bioengineering and cultured skin cells. They are particularly helpful in the treatment of long-term surface or deep traumas like burns. Applying autologous cultured cells or skin substitutes made via cellular bioengineering are two techniques for delivering cultured cells to the wound bed. It is possible to transplant keratinocytes because a skin biopsy can yield a significant number of cultured cells in a matter of three to four weeks. The capacity of stem cells to migrate and differentiate the endothelium, thereby promoting revascularization, is one advantage of their use. The injection of stem cells into a long-term wound leads to an increased optimization of microvascular activity. Furthermore, the application of cells influences the local cellular response, which is crucial for the healing of the infected wound's skin integrity. Adipose tissue stem cells have been shown to be capable of regenerating skin layering. In our clinic, every instance of injecting adipose tissue-derived stem cells into the wound bed produced positive results (20 patients). There is a thesis that suggests autologous stem cells from bone marrow or adipose tissue may not be as effective in treating chronic wounds as allogeneic amnion cells. Amniocyte-based skin epidermis transplants behave in a nearly physiological manner, indicating that fibroblasts may be substituted in the stimulation of keratinocyte stratification.

When fibroblasts are seeded over the amnion, they adhere well and remain long. Burn and chronic wounds are recommended candidates for this kind of dressing. As an alternative, the keratinocytes proliferate when seeded over the allogeneic, acellular amnion. Cells that have been seeded can live for up to four weeks. Experience has shown that amnion stem cells double the healing time of wounds. In 2008, keratinocyte culture was introduced to the Center. Since then, roughly 200 patients—mostly those with thermal burns—have had cellular transplants. Roughly 75% of the patients met the requirements for the culture. In over half of the patients who received a cellular transplant, the extent of the wound was between 40 and 79% of the total body surface area (TBSA). As stated by Sood et al. patients undergoing cultured epidermal autografts (CEA) transplants have an average life expectancy of 91%, whereas our results showed an 88% survival rate. It's important to keep in mind that, when it comes to epidermis cells, patient matching is crucial because the main side effects include itching, dermal blisters, and transplant loss. A frequent and long-lasting consequence is the development of a swollen scar. The application of stem cells appears to be one way to lessen scarring. The epidermalcells aid in wound healing up to a maximum depth of IIb. Mansilla and associates along with Rasulov et al. recommend using stem cells to treat deep wounds (Mansilla et al., 2015) (Figure 10.1).

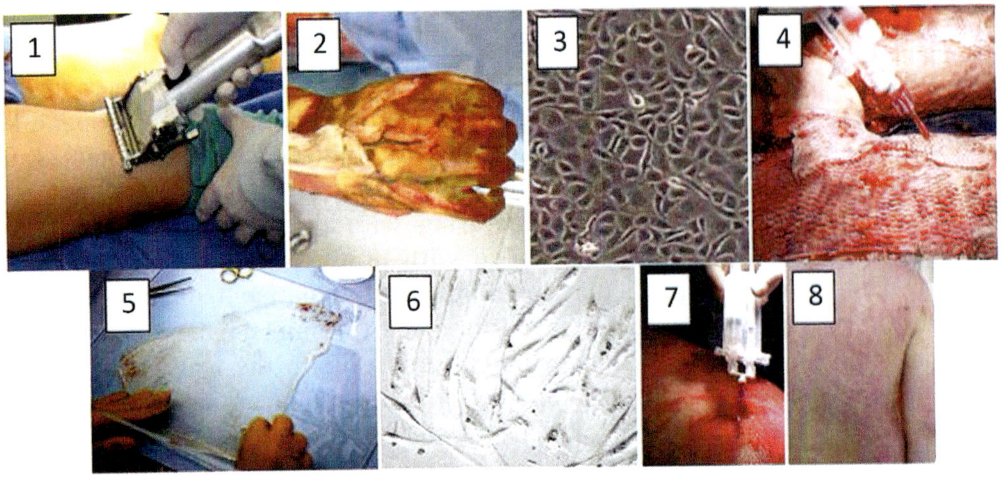

Figure 10.1. *The right choice of the research field for the sourcing of autologous skin for culturing (1) is often problematic due to the limited amount of available research fields (2). The culturing of the epidermis for the transplant (3) and wound before the transplant (4). The source material for the isolation of stem cells (5), stem cell culture (6), the transplant (7) and the final result (8).*

Source: Kitala, D., Klama-Baryła, A., Łabuś, W., Misiuga, M., Nowak, M., and Kawecki, M. (2018). Advanced Technologies in Dermatology. InTech. doi: 10.5772/intechopen.70288.

Clinical trials for RenovaCare's SkinGun™, which applies stem cells in the form of a suspension (fog) to the wound bed, are currently underway. It just takes 90 minutes to isolate, process, and apply the autologous cells. The gun's creators guarantee consumers that the obtained stem cells have up to 97.3% vitality, having won a patent award. With the Harvest® AdiPrep® system, HARVEST TERUMOBCT was able to obtain a cell suspension (containing mesenchymal stem cells) in just four minutes. This company's unique platform makes it possible to convert bone marrow and fatty tissue platelet rich leukocyte concentrate into stem cells with a concentration of 160,000/ml and vitality ranging from 78 to 95%. Therapeutics Cytori, Inc. additionally suggests a device that uses fatty tissue-derived cell fractions (ADRCs) for autologous cell therapy. Although adipose tissue is a valuable source of stem cells, using The Celution® System requires a minimum of 200 g of fatty tissue.

Although Fraser and associates cite 1.5 hours, which is equivalent to the transformation of the framework in our device, our experience shows that the entire sourcing and transformation process takes about 2.5 hours. Because liposuction is a noninvasive procedure and the quantity of sourced stem cells and regenerative cells does not necessitate a protracted cell culturing process, our center uses this system. The CHA Biotech Cha-Station, the PNC's Multi Station (a manual device), and the Medi-Khan's Lipokit from MaxStem all have lower vitality percentages than the 93% obtained using The Celution® System. This system is used in our center to treat chronic wounds because it enables the procedure to be completed the same day the patient is admitted, reducing hospital stay duration and ensuring there are enough hospital beds to accommodate the needs of other burn patients. Patients with non-healing wounds and those who did not respond appropriately to CEA therapy were included in the procedure's subject pool. Application of ADRC cells from The Celution® System has been carried out on 20 patients (ages 18–80) since 2011.

After many months of the wounds not healing, the procedure finally produced good clinic results (final wounds closure), which is a huge success (Kitala et al., 2018) (Figure 10.2).

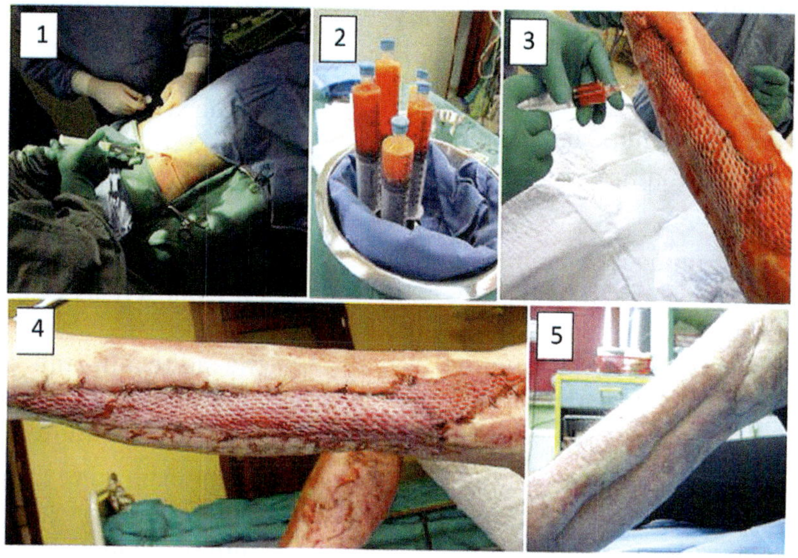

Figure 10.2. *The isolation and application of regenerative cells from fatty tissue: liposuction (1), the sourced lipoaspirate (2), wound bed injection combined with a grated autologous skin cell transplant (3), the healing of the wound 7 days after the procedure (4), the final effect: a functioning, intact limb (5).*

Source: Kitala, D., Klama-Baryła, A., Łabuś, W., Misiuga, M., Nowak, M., & Kawecki, M. (2018). Advanced Technologies in Dermatology. InTech. doi: 10.5772/intechopen.70288.

Patients suffering from burns are eligible for stem cells cultured in a stem cell bank because the largest drawback of the commercially available methods of obtaining stem cells for transplants is the quantity of cells obtained. From a therapeutic success perspective, this is the most effective approach; however, it is considerably more complex from a legal and financial one. It necessitates the production of stem cells in clean rooms in compliance with pharmaceutical law. Our Center has performed amniotic stem cell transplants in a hospital setting that requires additional approval from the Bioethical Commission and the recipient's signed consent form. On the fourth day following the burn, the 30-year-old patient who had a 36% IIb/III thermal wound received the cells. The wounds healed to a very good aesthetic effect in 12 days. It was stated that the procedure cannot be used on a regular basis due to legal regulations. In summary, over the past three decades, cellular engineering has shown promise in treating deep wounds and chronic wounds like diabetic foot and venous ulcers. They appear set to become standard medical procedures. The only thing to consider is which therapy techniques would be best for the particular patient (Kitala et al., 2018).

10.2. The Allogeneic Amnion

Transplanting allogeneic, biostatic amniotic tissue is the best substitute for conventional therapeutic approaches. Amniotic tissue, which is obtained from seronegative donors during pre-planned Cesarean sections, is a thin, partially permeable tissue that makes up the innermost layer of the amnion. The amnion is a five-layer membrane with a thickness of 0 mm to 0 mm, according to histology. Amniotic membrane transplants take place in aseptic settings and are finished with radiation sterilization (Wilshaw et al., 2008).

The clinical reason for amniotic membrane transplants stems from their natural properties, such as

- It being non-immunogenic, mainly an effect of the expression of HLA-G genes in the placenta and amniotic liquid, which are responsible for the immune response during the pregnancy.
- Reducing the risk of infection; it has been proven that the aqueous solution of the amniotic membrane promotes the apoptosis of monocells, such as lymphocytes and macrophages. This effect is proven by the latest research of Alikarami et al., which have proven the limiting effect of mesenchymal amniotic liquid cells on the proliferation of mitogenically active T lymphocytes in the *in vitro* coculturing of T lymphocytes.
- Its anti-inflammatory properties; the antibacterial effect observed during the application of the amniotic membrane in the process of wound healing is a common and documented phenomenon. The antibacterial effect is thought to be due to the presence of lysozyme and progesterone in the amniotic liquid as well as the very exact link between the dressing and the wound. Lysozyme is a protein with the properties of a hydrolytic enzyme which breaks down the peptidoglycan present in the cell wall of the bacteria. Progesterone is bacteriostatic against many Gram (+) bacteria.
- As well as modulating the stroma of the wound; the stromal matrix amnion is rich in extracellular matrix content, such as hyaluronic acid from the embryonic, glycosaminoglycans, various types of collagen and growth factors which promote and modulate the regenerative processes occurring in the wound.
- Stimulating proliferation processes; due to the rich ECM content. The amniotic membrane of the amnion includes laminin, fibronectin, collagen IV, V, and VII, as well as growth factors such as TGF, which greatly facilitates the adhesion and anchoring of the endothelial cells in the stroma and their proliferation.
- Minimizing pain; the painkiller effect is due to the very close link between the amniotic membrane and the wound, thanks to which the exposed, irritated nerve endings are protected.

The clinical applications of using the amniotic membrane are wide-ranging, including its use as a skin substitute for facial burn wounds, hand burn wounds, donor areas, and granulating wounds. An alternative option is the high-quality STSG wound dressing. Amniotic membrane transplants have proven to be effective in treating autoimmune diseases like Lyell's disease. They can also be used in conjunction with biological wound dressings such as allogeneic skin. Aseptically prepared biovital transplants, like allogeneic amniotic membrane transplants, are currently generating significant interest. Intravital transplants of the amniotic membrane have shown promising results in wound treatment due to the amnion cells' secretion of physiological functions.

The Dr Stanisław Sakiel Centre for Burn Treatment in Siemianowice Śląskie, we began the undertaking of biostatic transplants of the amniotic membrane in 2011. The transplants are produced in the Clean Rooms of the Cell Bank in accordance with the Good Manufacturing

Practice (GMP). From August 2011 to March 2017, 245,229 cm^2 transplant cells have been produced. 513 patients have been served by a total of 235,317 cm^2, including 9 patients with the Lyell's Syndrome (Figure 10.3) (Figure 10.4).

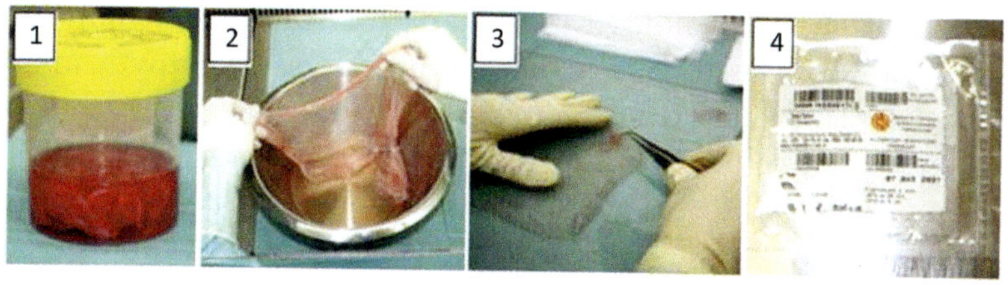

Figure 10.3. *Select stages of production of allogeneic, biostatic transplants of human amnion: (1) the amniotic membrane in a transportation container; (2) rinsing; (3) cutting uneven fragments, measuring the surface; (4) a packaged transplant before sterilization by radiation.*

Source: Kitala, D., Klama-Baryła, A., Łabuś, W., Misiuga, M., Nowak, M., & Kawecki, M. (2018). Advanced Technologies in Dermatology. InTech. doi: 10.5772/intechopen.70288.

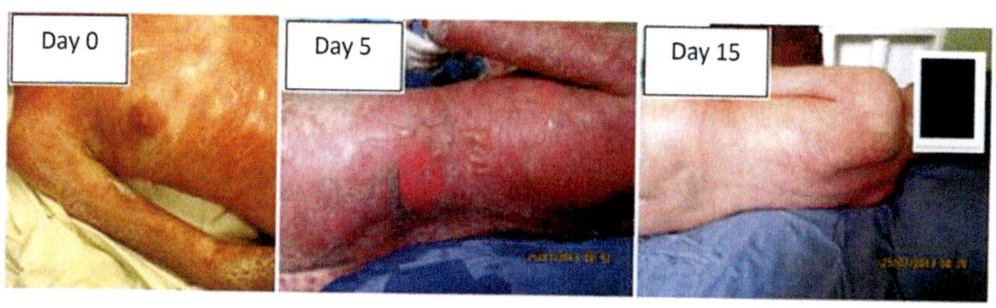

Figure 10.4. *The clinical effect of the therapy of Lyell's effect on days: 0, 5 and 15.*

Source: Kitala, D., Klama-Baryła, A., Łabuś, W., Misiuga, M., Nowak, M., & Kawecki, M. (2018). Advanced Technologies in Dermatology. InTech. doi: 10.5772/intechopen.70288.

Based on the evidence and clinical observations, it can be concluded that the amniotic membrane is an excellent choice for treating shallow burn wounds, particularly those on the face.

10.3. The Allogeneic Skin

The ideal wound dressing is made of allogeneic skin, which is primarily obtained from deceased donors and infrequently from living ones. Its properties include wound protection, healing stimulation, and pain reduction. This explains why it works so well to treat skin conditions like Lyell's disease and Stevens-Johnson's disease. Both superficial and deep burn wounds can be treated with allogeneic skin, particularly in cases where the patient does not have enough skin remaining to cover their wound. Its low toxicity, relative ease of application, ease of gathering, and potential for gathering enough for a large grafting surface are some of its greatest benefits. Allogeneic skin used to cover a surgically cleaned wound keeps the skin from losing water, electrolytes, and proteins in both widespread and deep wounds, while also preventing other cells from becoming dehydrated. Moreover, it inhibits the growth of microorganisms by acting as a barrier against external stimuli. The skin's hypermetabolic reaction to the burn wound lessens as a result of the wound absorbing less heat. An allogeneic skin transplant stimulates the granulation process and wound epithelization in wounds that affect all layers of the skin and therefore have limited potential for regeneration. This creates a stroma that can be used for additional surgical intervention (Kitala et al., 2018).

Allogeneic skin is a beneficial biological dressing for treating medium-depth burn wounds, covering both the epidermis and dermis. It promotes blood vessel growth in the wound bed and stimulates revascularization. This skin closely adheres to the stroma, reducing pain and the need for frequent dressing changes while allowing the epidermis to regenerate undisturbed. In some cases, allogeneic skin is used on wounds previously treated with mesh transplants of autologous skin to minimize stress and prevent infections, as well as create scaffolding for cultured keratinocytes. At the Center of Wound Treatment in Siemianowice Slaskie, allogeneic skin is the standard procedure for severe wounds, providing temporary dressing and protection. It is also used when the depth of a wound is uncertain to prevent further damage. In our clinic, allogeneic skin is used on medium depth wounds to stimulate granulation tissue and aid in wound closure through epithelialization. Initially sourced from multiple organs, allogeneic skin is now sourced from forensic departments, with a higher risk of infection. In 2016, allogeneic skin was transplanted 235 times from about 50 donors. These transplants are prepared in accordance with laws on cell and tissue sourcing, sterilized, tested, and stored before application to burn wounds. The process involves surgical cleaning of the wound, application of the grated skin transplant, and dressing the wound. This process is illustrated in Figure 10.5.

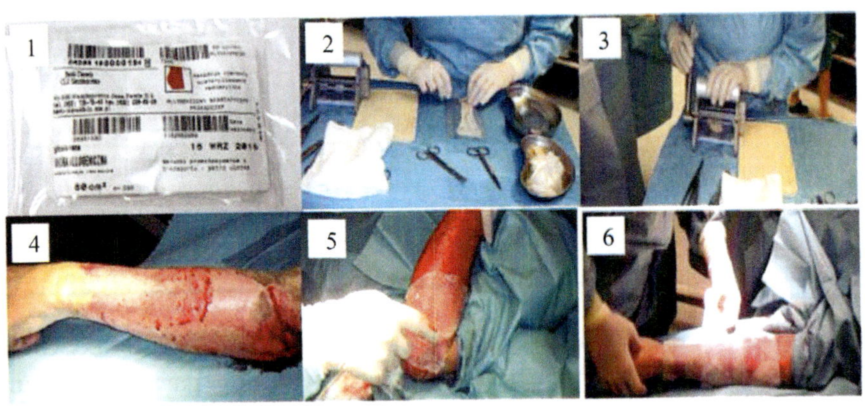

Figure 10.5. *The allogeneic, biostatic transplant (1 and 2), the grating of allogeneic skin (3), an IIB burn wound cleaned from dead tissue (4), the application of an allogeneic skin transplant (5) and the application of an external wound dressing (6).*

Source: Kitala, D., Klama-Baryła, A., Łabuś, W., Misiuga, M., Nowak, M., & Kawecki, M. (2018). Advanced Technologies in Dermatology. InTech. doi: 10.5772/intechopen.70288.

Despite a prior nephrectomy, patients at our center with IIB wounds and some with IIB/III wounds underwent allogeneic skin transplantation, which led to a definitive closure of the wound, stimulated cell growth in the wound bed, revascularized the wound, and started the epithelization process. This removed the need for the patient to undergo a skin transplant of their own. Oliver and colleagues have reported similar outcomes, demonstrating that allogeneic skin influences granulation tissue differentiation and proliferation (Oliver et al.,1991). Allogeneic skin was used as a dressing for other patients with deep skin burn wounds to shield them from bacteria and viruses and stop the loss of water, microelements, and proteins. Thanks to an autologous skin transplant, the dressing served as a source of cytokines and growth factors that promoted cell proliferation and chemotaxation, encouraged tissue grantulation, readyed the stroma for surgery, and created the foundation for the wound's final closure. Additionally, the Center uses allogeneic skin when it is not possible to determine the exact depth of the wound, when there is a demonstrable risk that it will deepen and the transplant will be rejected, and when the patient has a finite number of source beds available for their own skin transplants. Additionally, allogeneic skin is applied to wounds from escharotomies. To sum up, allogeneic skin is a viable substitute for autologous skin grafts (Figure 10.6). With an allogeneic skin transplant, the wound heals completely, removing the need for the donor's own skin, which could cause more problems, discomfort, and scarring. It is important to remember, though, that allogeneic skin can only be used as a band-aid solution. This makes autologous skin transplantation possible and still ranks among the most effective ways to seal a burn wound (Kitala et al., 2018).

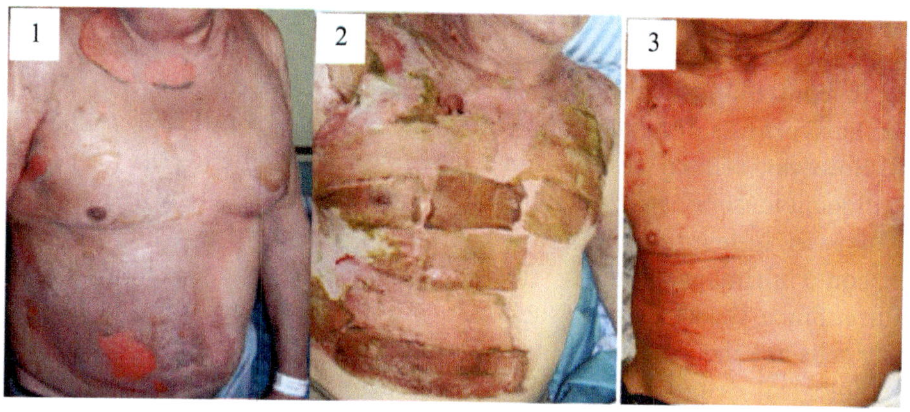

Figure 10.6. *The patient on the day of admission to the Center (1), on the third day after the allogeneic skin transplant (2), on the 16th day from the hospital admission (the day of leaving the Center) (3).*

Source: Kitala, D., Klama-Baryła, A., Łabuś, W., Misiuga, M., Nowak, M., & Kawecki, M. (2018). Advanced Technologies in Dermatology. InTech. doi: 10.5772/intechopen.70288.

10.4. Acellular Collagen Human Skin Matrix (Acellular Dermal Matrix, ADM)

Tissue engineering techniques, such as cell removal, are used to enhance the characteristics and durability of the transplants. The purpose of removing cells from tissues and organs is to create a non-immunogenetic transplant, which may eventually be populated *in vivo* by the patient's own cells. Thus, an empty transplant consists of the components of the extracellular matrix or ECM. It has been demonstrated that the extracellular matrix (ECM) affects cell mitogenesis, chemotaxis, and targeted differentiation. Furthermore, evidence has shown that the extracellular matrix (ECM) stimulates and facilitates positive tissue remodeling in the host. When materials are used appropriately, they can aid in the healing process by facilitating the change from the inflammatory phase to the constructive restructuring of the fractured cells. The interaction between the recipient's body and the biomaterial used has a variety of complex effects, such as immune system reactions and the proliferation and differentiation of stem cells. Furthermore, the colonizing cells of ECM produce and populate a multitude of elements within it. There exists a dynamic mutual relationship between the cells and the extracellular matrix. It has an impact on the cell's differentiation and proliferation as well as their microenvironment. The aforementioned phenomena take place during normal bodily homeostasis, but they are essential for wound healing. Collagen biosynthesis and the synthesis of other extracellular synthesis components were regulated by the ECM cells. These cells play a key role in controlling every step of connective tissue biosynthesis, transformation, and breakdown. However, cellular residue left over from the allogeneic cells' restructuring process may cause an unfavorable immune reaction, which could ultimately lead to the transplant's failure. Since the cellular tissue's proteins and fatty cells are the primary targets of the autoimmunological response, removing cells from the tissue is a promising strategy that could prolong the immune response's induction in the patient's body following transplantation.

The immune-induced inflammation that could impede the transplanted bioprosthesis's biodegradation should be reduced by removing the cellular components. It is important to remember that the immune response is not totally eliminated when cells are extracted from tissue. To remove cells from tissue or organs, there are three basic methods used: chemical, enzymatic, and mechanical. Collagen scaffolding is created by removing cells from human allogeneic skin. This scaffolding can then be de novo seeded with autologous skin cells and inserted into the area that is lacking. The removal of cellular matter from tissues and organs can be achieved through chemical, enzymatic, or mechanical methods. Collagen scaffolding is produced by removing cells from human allogeneic dermis. It can be grafted into the area of skin damage and de novo populated with autologous skin cells. Using human allogeneic, acellular extracellular matrix of the dermis (acellular dermal matrix, or ADM) as a matrix for autologous fibroblasts and keratinocytes that are cultured *in vitro* can be a successful strategy for treating burn wounds. Patients with deep burn wounds containing at least 50% TBSA and those whose autologous skin grafting sites heal poorly are the clinical candidates for this technique. In Siemianowice, Śląskie, the Dr. Stanisław Sakiela Burn Centre started using acellular human skin matrix (ADM) in 2015. Six patients had ADM transplants performed up until March 2017. The patients who were eligible for the procedure had severe burns that had not healed well. They came to the conclusion that using ADM in conjunction with *in vitro* cultured skin cells may be the best course of treatment for burn wounds based on the collected data and clinical observations. To achieve a conclusive scientific outcome, it is necessary to augment the number of cases examined (Kitala et al., 2018).

10.5. Skin Substitutes as Treatment for Chronic Wounds

An alternative to auto- and allogeneic transplants for the treatment of wounds of different origins, such as burn wounds and chronic wounds, is the use of skin substitutes. For skin substitutes to serve as true substitutes, they must fulfill a number of requirements. They shouldn't cause the patient to become immunogenic. They ought to control the wound's proteolytic activity. The primary function of synthetic skin substitutes is to offer a bioresorbtive scaffolding that promotes extracellular matrix deposition and cellular migration. Along with stimulating angiogenesis and fibroblast migration, this scaffolding should also stimulate granulation synthesis, absorb free radicals, and neutralize them. The perfect skin substitutes should be easily accessible and can quickly replicate the different skin layers and functions.

Type of Chronic Wound	Standard of Care
A Arterial 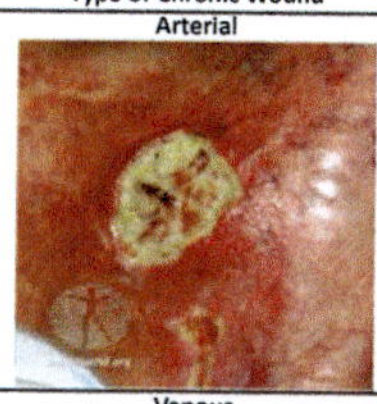	Medical Intervention Arterial Intervention
B Venous 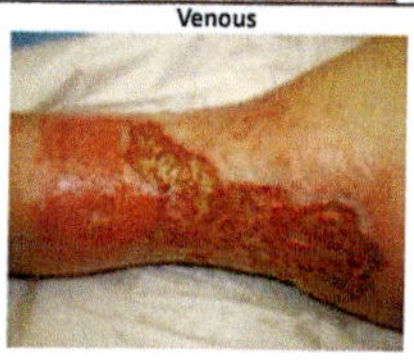	Compression Therapy
C Diabetic Foot Ulcer 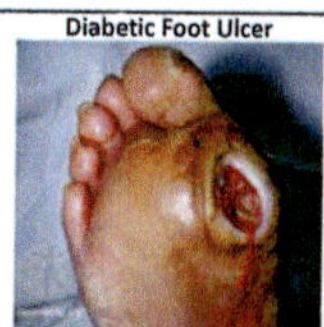	Saline-Moistened Gauze Dressing Debridement Infection Control
D Pressure Ulcer 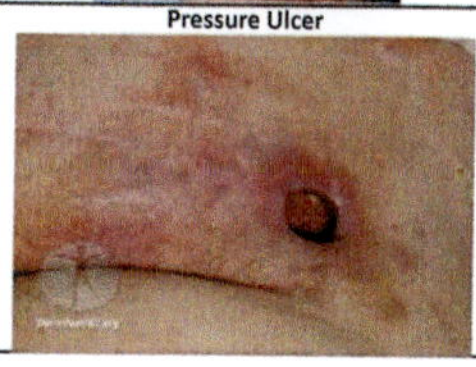	Offloading Infection Control Pain Control

Figure 10.7. *Types of chronic wounds and their standard care. Major types of chronic wounds include arterial, venous, diabetic, and pressure ulcers. The standard care depends on wound etiology.*

Source: Vecin NM and Kirsner RS (2023) Skin substitutes as treatment for chronic wounds: current and future directions. Front. Med. 10:1154567. doi: 10.3389/fmed.2023.1154567.

Anatomical structure and function that are normal are disrupted by a wound. Acute wounds usually heal in 4–6 weeks, but chronic wounds continue to heal even after the initial injury. Persistent injuries impact 2% of the U. S. population, or about 8.2 million Medicare enrollees, who place a heavy financial strain on the healthcare system and use an estimated $28 billion annually. The three most common causes of chronic wounds are changes in the nervous system (diabetic neuropathic ulcers and pressure ulcers), vascular disease (venous or arterial ulcers), or a combination of these (diabetic neuroischemic ulcers). Osteomyelitis, amputation, and sepsis are among the complications associated with chronic wounds. Diabetic foot ulcers (DFUs) are one type of ulcer that can lead to increased mortality, with 5-year mortality rates that are comparable to those of certain cancers. Patients' quality of life is adversely affected by chronic wounds because of pain, odor, decreased mobility, and social isolation. Chronic wounds are frequently accompanied by depression and anxiety, which can further impair immunological and endocrine function (Situm et al., 2016) (Figure 10.7).

If, four weeks after injury, the wound does not heal smaller, advanced therapies like skin substitutes are advised. Skin substitutes are a broad category of goods that cover wounds either permanently or temporarily and aid in their healing via a variety of methods. A stable, frequently biodegradable scaffold that encourages the synthesis of new dermal tissue, prevents infection, allows host cells to proliferate within the scaffold as functional dermal cells rather than scar tissue, delivers or augments production of cytokines and growth factors, and must withstand shearing force are all possible ways that skin substitutes may aid in the healing of wounds.

The practice of skin grafting has a long history, dating back to 2500 BC in India where Susruta, known as the Father of Surgery, developed the "Ancient Indian Method" to treat ulcers and facial deformities. Over time, advancements were made, with autologous skin grafts being the primary method until the 19th century when xenografts were introduced. Skin allograft transplantation followed in the 1870s, with further developments in the use of skin grafts for healing reported by Reverdin. The concept of epithelial cell seeding was introduced in the late 1800s, leading to successful epithelial cell culture in 1975. The first artificial dermal substitute, the Integra Dermal Regeneration Template, was created in the 1980s for burn patients. Composite grafts were introduced in the 1990s, marking the beginning of the term "tissue engineering."

Since then, the field has flourished, and the number of commercially available skin substitutes has reached 76, with more to come, according to data gathered by the federal Agency for Healthcare Research and Quality (AHRQ). The sheer volume of products on the market is overwhelming, so various classification schemes have been devised to group products and help physicians choose the best replacement for their patients. The cellularity of skin substitutes can be used to categorize them (cellular vs. acellular), which skin layer (or layers) the replacement is intended to replace (dermal, epidermal, or both), and whether they come from synthetic or natural sources. The intricacy and redundancy of classification schemes make it difficult to classify skin substitutes into the appropriate groups. Kumar (2008) developed a three-class system for classifying skin substitutes that is both widely used and imperfect. Class I is further subdivided into single layer and bilayer substitutes and consists of impervious, temporary dressing materials. One can use synthetic or naturally occurring single layer substitutes. Class II substitutes are either dermal or epidermal, single-layer, long-lasting skin substitutes. Composite substitutes with both dermal and epidermal layers are known as Class III substitutes (Figure 10.8).

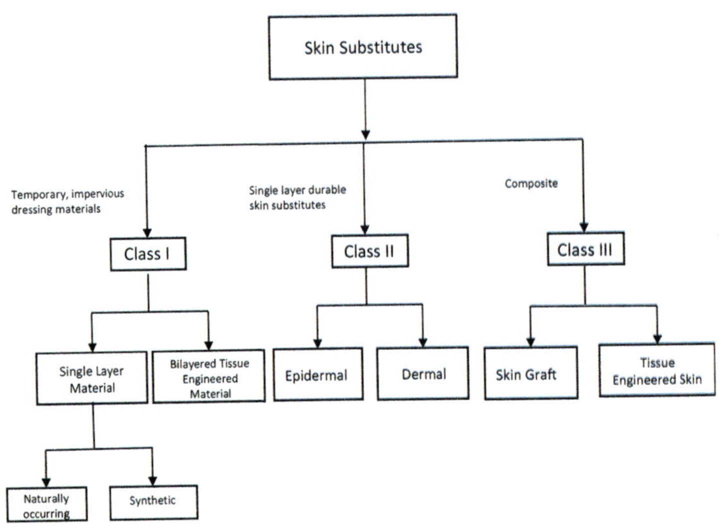

Figure 10.8. *Visual representation of Kumar's classification system. Kumar's classification system is a widely used, imperfect classification system for organizing skin substitutes. The classification system denotes three classes. Class I is comprised of temporary, impervious dressing materials and is further divided into single layer and bilayer substitutes. Single layer substitutes may be naturally occurring or synthetic. Class II substitutes are single layer, durable skin substitutes which are either dermal or epidermal. Class III substitutes are composite substitutes that contain both epidermal and dermal layers.*

Source: Vecin NM and Kirsner RS (2023) Skin substitutes as treatment for chronic wounds: current and future directions. Front. Med. 10:1154567. doi: 10.3389/fmed.2023.1154567.

The US Food and Drug Administration (FDA) is in charge of regulating the entry of novel medications and medical equipment into the U.S. market by analyzing a product's effectiveness and safety as well as the advantages and disadvantages of using it. Human Cells, Tissues, and Cellular and Tissue-Based Products (HCT/Ps), Premarket Approval (PMA), 510(k) Premarket Notification, or Humanitarian Device Exemption (HDE) are the regulatory pathways that usually govern skin substitutes. Depending on its class, a substitute has a different regulatory pathway to follow. There are three classes for medical devices. Devices are categorized into classes based on intended use and potential risks. Class III devices are the highest risk medical devices, such as implantable devices; Class I devices are the lowest risk devices. Skin substitutes fall into one of three classes based on their composition and intended use: Class I, II, or III. Subsequent examination of most Class I and many Class II devices is not necessary. For non-exempt devices, a 510(k) Premarket Notification is needed. Class III devices are those that could potentially pose a serious risk to human health and need PMA, support or sustain human life, or prevent health impairment. The FDA conducts a thorough evaluation of PMAs to make sure there is sufficient scientific data to guarantee a product is both safe and effective. One type of skin substitute made with PMA is the Bilayered Cellular Construct (BLCC, Apligraf®, Organogenesis, Canton, MA). A 510(k) Premarket Notification is a submission to the FDA prior to the product's release in which the manufacturer assesses the product's efficacy and safety by comparing it to a comparable product that is already on the market and for which the safety data is known; this type of product is referred to as a predicate device.

If the new device is found to be Substantially Equivalent (SE) to a predicate device, it will be approved. An HDE is uncommon and is meant for medical devices used to diagnose or treat conditions affecting fewer than 8000 people in the United States. S. every year. Because of their potential to help manage a rare disease, these devices are not subject to the same rigorous evaluation standards. To ensure safety and good tissue practices, skin substitutes containing human cells or tissue, such as Porcine Small Intestine Submucosa (SIS, OASIS®, Smith, and Nephew, Ft Worth, TX), are regulated as HCT/Ps under Title 21 of the Code of Federal Regulations, part 1271 (21 CFR 1271). Products derived from the placenta and those containing amniotic fluid are governed by Public Health Service Act sections 361 and 351. Amniotic products may only be used for homologous use, which is defined as the replacement, augmentation, repair, or reconstruction of a recipient's cells or tissues when applied by implantation, transplantation, infusion, or transfer into a human recipient, as permitted by Section 361 (Vecin and Kirsner, 2023).

10.5.1. Classification

Class I

The temporary, impermeable dressing materials come in single and bilayer forms as class I skin substitutes. Though acellular, they seek to preserve the mechanical characteristics of the skin. They could be artificial or naturally occurring. Amniotic membranes from humans are examples of skin substitutes that exist naturally. Class I skin replacements are useful for preventing infection and dehydration. They support the preservation of a damp atmosphere that promotes wound healing.

Various products derived from the amnion are utilized in the treatment of chronic wounds. Placental membranes have long been known for their ability to regenerate tissue, with the first amniotic membrane transplant taking place in 1910. The placenta is composed of an inner amnion on the fetal side and an outer chorion on the maternal side. The amnion contains epithelial cells that can potentially act as a source of stem cells. Below this is a basement membrane containing collagen, laminins, and fibronectin, as well as fibroblasts within a matrix and a basement membrane for the chorion. The amnion is rich in growth factors and cytokines that play a crucial role in wound healing. Amnion-derived products offer advantages such as pain relief, antibacterial properties, non-immunogenicity, reduced inflammation and scarring, and support for cell migration and proliferation. However, these products can be costly and delicate. Due to a lack of evidence, synthetic Class I substitutes will not be discussed.

Class II

Single-layer, long-lasting skin substitutes are known as class II dressings. They fall into the epidermal and dermal categories further. Epidermal sheets (EpiDex®, Anika Therapeutics, Inc.) are one type of epidermal substitute. Dermal substitutes include SIS and Dermal Skin Substitutes (DSS, Dermagraft®, Organogenesis, Canton, MA, United States) while the former two are available in Bedford, MA, United States, and Freiberg, Germany (BioSeed-S®, BioTissue Technologies AG, Freiberg, Germany). For instance, these skin substitutes were made to replace just one layer of skin.

10.5.1.1. Epidermal

Only the epidermis is replaced by epidermal substitutes, which have an architecture similar to that of the epidermis. The epithelial skin substitutes known as cultured epithelial autografts (CEAs) are made from autologous keratinocytes that are cultured *ex vivo* alongside murine fibroblasts. The keratinocytes from the patient are expanded and multiplied to create a dressing that is several layers thick. The patient's skin or hair follicles may provide the keratinocytes that are cultured to create epidermal substitutes. The isolated keratinocytes of the outer root sheath of anagen hair follicles are the source of EpiDex®, an epidermal equivalent. After being separated, these keratinocytes are cultivated on a sheet that is applied to the injury. The epidermal substitute known as "Laserskin" is made from autologous keratinocytes that are grown on a hyaluronic acid membrane with holes in it to promote cell growth. BioSeed-S® is an epidermal substitute made of fibrin sealant and autologous keratinocytes.

Although epidermal substitutes have shown some promise in the treatment of DFUs and VLUs, their use is fraught with difficulties, making them an unpopular option for treating chronic wounds. The lack of mechanical stability and elasticity that the dermis offers epidermal substitutes is one of their main drawbacks. Because of this, they are delicate, erratic, and difficult to take care of. The fact that these replacements are prone to breaking down, blistering, and leaving scars is a drawback. Furthermore, because CEAs take three to four weeks to construct, this presents a challenge for patients who need an intervention right away. These factors make the epidermal replacements EpiDex®, Laserskin, and BioSeed-S® unavailable for purchase at this time; however, many may be obtained by making direct contact with their manufacturer (Vecin and Kirsner, 2023).

10.5.1.2. Dermal

Compared to epidermal substitutes, dermal substitutes have a number of benefits, including durability and ease of use. They might also reduce the chance of contracture and result in scarring of higher quality. Acellular dermal material is another option that has the benefit of not being immunogenic. Acellular dermal substitutes can be made of synthetic polymers, de-epithelialized cadaveric skin, porcine dermis, or naturally occurring polymers like collagen, elastin, or hyaluronic acid. The price of dermal substitutes is one of their main drawbacks. As human acellular dermal matrices (ADM), Graftjacket® (Wright Medical Technology, Memphis, TN, USA) and DermACELL® (LifeNet Health, Virginia Beach, VA, USA) are subject to 21 CFR Part 1271 Part 361 Human Cells, Tissues, and Cellular and Tissue-based Products (HCT/Ps).

MatriStem MicroMatrix® (ACell Inc., Columbia, MD, United States) is an ADM derived from porcine urinary bladder matrix (UBM). This UBM has U.S. FDA 510(k) Premarket Notification and is indicated for partial and full-thickness wounds, pressure ulcers, VLUs, DFUs, chronic vascular ulcers, tunneled undermined wounds, surgical wounds, traumatic wounds, and draining wounds. AlloPatch® (Musculoskeletal Transplant Foundation Sports Medicine, Edison, NJ, United States) is an open-structure human reticular acellular dermal matrix (HR-ADM) that has been evaluated for its use in DFU treatment. This HR-ADM is regulated under 21 CFR Part 1271 Part 361 Human Cells, Tissues, and Cellular and Tissue-based Products (HCT/Ps). Hyalograft 3D (Anika Therapeutics, Inc., Bedford, MA, United States) is an autologous fibroblast-hyaluronic acid complex dermal substitute.

DSS is a cryopreserved dermal substitute made from human fibroblasts. It is produced by cultivating newborn dermal fibroblasts on a scaffold made of bioabsorbable mesh. The incorporation of fibroblasts onto the scaffold facilitates wound healing through their secretion of multiple growth factors, cytokines, proteins, and collagen. Currently, DSS has U. S. FDA PMA and is recommended for full thickness DFUs that penetrate the dermis and last longer than six weeks, but do not expose any bones, muscles, joints, or tendons. When used in conjunction with SOC and in patients who have a sufficient blood supply, DSS substitutes are recommended.

SIS is an acellular biological extracellular matrix that includes growth factors, glycosaminoglycans, collagen, elastin, and proteoglycans, among other substances that aid in wound healing. Growth factors both promote angiogenesis and lessen the damage caused by matrix metalloproteinases (MMPs). A factor to take into account and possible disadvantages when utilizing porcine SIS replacements is their cultural acceptability. When it's appropriate, facilitating an open dialogue with the patient can help them navigate these obstacles and find alternative treatments. Human Cells, Tissues, and Cellular and Tissue-based Products (HCT/Ps) 21 CFR Part 1271 governs SIS. Type I bovine fibrillar collagen Wound Conforming Matrices (WCM) offer an additional dermal substitute option.

Class III

Composite skin substitutes, which include both dermis and epidermis, make up Class III skin substitutes. They are further subdivided into tissue engineered skin, autografts, allografts, and xenografts. Burn wounds have traditionally been treated with cadaveric skin allografts and xenografts, but tissue-engineered skin substitutes like Biobrane (UDL Laboratories, Inc.), Dermal Regenerative Template (DRT, Integra® Integra LifeSciences, Plainsboro, NJ, United States), and BLCC have also been used., Rockford, IL, USA) have demonstrated effectiveness in treating long-term wounds.

10.5.1.3. Autografts

Healthy skin from a patient is used to create autografts. They can be applied to large or refractory chronic wounds, as well as acute or chronic wounds like burns and traumatic wounds. The use of autografts presents a number of difficulties, such as the creation of a new wound, contracture, and scarring, infection, and bleeding risk, altered or reduced sensation, and, depending on the size of the graft, the requirement and expense of an operating room and hospital stay. Autografts have the benefits of decreased immunogenicity and availability despite these difficulties. Autografts can be split-thick, with only the epidermis and superficial dermis, or full-thick, with both epidermis and full dermis. Allogeneic grafts fail while autologous grafts accept. The term "graft rejection" refers to the process by which donor immune cells reject transplanted host cells because of genetic differences between the donor and recipient. Autografts, however, might not "take," or integrate, into the recipient site. Take happens in three stages: revascularization, inoculation, and plasmatic imbibition. Unlike flaps, autografts are ischemic and pale at first and do not have their own blood supply. Plasmatic imbibition is the process by which oxygen and nutrients are taken up from the underlying wound bed to receive nourishment. The subsequent stage, known as inoculation, is when the graft's capillaries connect with the underlying wound bed to supply blood to the graft. The autograft may look pink at this point. Revascularization of the graft happens last. Failure to advance through these stages may lead to graft failure, which manifests clinically 1–2 weeks after implantation as a black eschar or a pale white color.

One technique has been developed to lessen donor site morbidity and disfigurement, which is the primary challenge associated with autografts. Micro skin tissue columns, or MTSCs, are full-thickness microscopic skin transplants that are less than one millimeter in diameter and are taken from healthy skin. Standard hypodermic needles are used to remove the donor site's skin column. The column is then taken out of the needle using a fluidic device. Spread uniformly across the wound bed are MTSCs. Because of their small size, disfigurement is little to nonexistent even when multiple MTSCs are harvested from the donor site, and donor site morbidity is significantly reduced. Chronic wounds are known to stay in a dysregulated state of inflammation, meaning that either excessive or insufficient inflammation prevents the inflammatory phase from ending. According to recent research, there is a benefit to healing when the inflammatory phase of wound healing is advanced in these stalled wounds. Through reepithelialization and contraction acceleration, epidermal differentiation, increased dermal collagen, and attenuation of the inflammatory response to resolve inflammation, MTSCs facilitate wound healing. An inventive and promising method for autologous skin grafts is offered by MTSCs (Vecin and Kirsner, 2023).

10.5.1.4. Allografts

Allografts of cadaveric skin are made from donated skin that has been cryopreserved or preserved with glycerol and kept in a tissue bank. Patients who receive cadaveric skin allografts are given viable dermis and epidermis. Toprepare the wound bed for a later permanent split-thickness autologous graft, cadaveric skin allografts have been used as temporary biologic dressings in extensive burn injuries. They have also been investigated for use in the treatment of chronic wounds. The allograft serves as a matrix in which granulation tissue is formed. Cadaveric skin allografts have several advantages, such as reduced pain, increased angiogenesis, wound bed preparation for autografting, infection prevention, affordability, and accessibility.A cadaveric cryopreserved human skin allograft (CHSA) product is called Theraskin (LifeNet Health, Virginia Beach, VA, USA), and it's governed by 21 CFR Part 1271 Part 361 Human Cells, Tissues, and Cellular and Tissue-based Products (HCT/Ps). Potential disease transmission, including cytomegalovirus, which has been observed in cadaveric skin allograft transplantation in burn wounds, and the translucency of the grafted skin present challenges in the use of cadaver skin allografts.

Allografts of human skin from living donors are also possible, though they are not frequently employed in the management of chronic wounds. Immunogenicity is a crucial factor to take into account when using human skin allografts, whether they are derived from living donors or preserved cadavers. Close relationship between donor and recipient reduces immunogenicity risk and prolongs graft survival when using living donor skin to treat a wound. Even though cadaveric skin is made up of dead cells, some of these cells may still contain major histocompatibility class II (MHC Class II) molecules, which makes rejection possible. For this reason, processing is essential to avoid immune system stimulation. It is believed that immune cells like dendritic cells, Langerhans cells, T cells, B cells, and NK cells are responsible for immunogenicity. These kinds of resident immune cells are present in all layers of skin. Notably, the epidermis secretes pro-inflammatory cytokines like IL-1 and TNF-α as well as antimicrobial peptides (AMPs), defensins, and damage-associated molecular patterns (DAMPs) and houses $CD8^+$ T cells, Langerhans cells, and dendritic cells, all of which are important for immunity. Known as direct allorecognition, donor dendritic and Langerhans cells from the grafted skin migrate to recipient lymph nodes during allogeneic skin graft transplantation and present donor antigens to recipient T cells.

Recipient T cells and B cells may become activated by donor antigens presented on recipient antigen presenting cells, known as indirect allorecognition. NK cells may also contribute to rejection by killing donor cells via antibody-dependent cellular toxicity. Similar to solid organ transplantation, methods are utilized to prevent skin allograft rejection. However, the use of systemic immunosuppression can increase the risk of infections. Without immune suppression, pretreating the allograft to inhibit immune cell function, such as Langerhans and dendritic cells, can decrease immune reactivity in skin transplantation. Chemical agents or UV irradiation may be used to deplete dendritic cells or hinder antigen presentation. Additionally, oxidative damage can be prevented by pretreatment with antioxidants. Research also suggests modifying grafts through bioengineering to evade the recipient's immune response. These innovative approaches may be advantageous in promoting wound healing with temporary dressings.

10.5.1.5. Xenografts

Like cadaveric allografts, skin xenografts can be used as an initial, temporary treatment to prepare the wound bed for autologous transplantation. Considerations like immunogenicity and disease transmission need to be made when employing xenografts. Usually, strict processing is required to reduce the spread of disease. The xenograft structure may be harmed and denatured by this processing. On the other hand, xenografts offer cheaper costs, infinite supply, and a reduced risk of disease transmission compared to allografts. Fish has recently been used as a xenograft in the treatment of chronic wounds, along with pig and cow. Fish skin grafts have a number of advantages over other xenograft types, including a lower risk of viral transmission and the ability to undergo mild processing without compromising the skin's integrity, which includes healthy levels of collagen, elastin, and Omega-3 polyunsaturated fatty acids that are believed to enhance reepithelialization and microbial defense (Vecin and Kirsner, 2023).

10.5.1.6. Tissue Engineered Skin

The phrase "tissue engineered skin" was first used in the early 1990s to refer to a product made of human skin and bioscaffolds that can replace damaged human skin while preserving its structural integrity and resembling its original function, such as flexibility, barrier function, and ability to stop transepidermal water loss. BLCC and DRT are two instances of composite tissue engineered skin. The primary constraint on this particular subset of composite substitutes is their high production costs. A dermal layer and an overlying silicone layer make up the bilayer regeneration matrix known as DRT. An acellular matrix made of cross-linked bovine collagen and chondroitin-6-sulfate, a kind of glycosaminoglycan, makes up the dermal layer. The epidermis is a thin layer of silicon that sits on top of the dermal layer.

One popular type of composite tissue engineered skin substitute is called BLCC. There are two parts to this bilayer living cellular construct. Keratinocytes make up the epidermal layer, while bovine type I collagen and human neonatal foreskin fibroblasts make up the dermal layer. BLCC possesses U. S. FDA PMA and is recommended for use in conjunction with standard DFU care to treat full-thickness neuropathic DFUs that have lasted longer than three weeks and that have not responded sufficiently to standard therapy. These DFUs extend through the dermis without exposing any muscles, tendons, joints, or bones. Furthermore, it is recommended for use in conjunction with standard therapeutic compression to treat non-infected partial and thickness skin ulcers caused by venous insufficiency lasting longer than one month and not responding well to traditional ulcer therapy. A molecular analysis of BLCC's mode of action in VLUs has been conducted. In randomized controlled trials, BLCC was found to reduce profibrotic TGF-β1 expression, increase TGF-β inhibitor levels, and upregulate matrix metalloproteinases to promote antifibrotic remodeling. Furthermore, an RCT contrasting the healing of venous ulcers treated with BLCC vs. Compression therapy by itself made transcriptome analysis of the wounds treated with various methods possible. Three different transcriptomic patterns, similar to those of an acute healing wound, were observed in BLCC-treated wounds, indicating a change from a non-healing to a healing tissue response.

10.5.2. Evidence for Skin Substitutes

To help clinicians choose which substitute is best for their patients, the authors Vecin and Kirsner (2023). provide RCT data for each of the substitutes in the current section. Since trial quality varies, we offer sample size (n) as a crude proxy for quality.

Class I: Amnion-Derived

The effectiveness of amnion-derived substitutes as a DFU treatment has been assessed by RCTs. These studies showed that amniotic replacements are a useful therapy for DFUs. Serena and associates. (n = 76) discovered that, in comparison to the standard of care, an amniotic membrane kept at a low temperature increased the frequency and likelihood of wound closure in DFUs. An RCT conducted by Snyder and colleagues. (n = 29) discovered that when combined with standard care, a dehydrated human amniotic membrane (dHAM) called AmnioExcel® Amniotic Allograft Membrane (Integra LifeSciences, Plainsboro, NJ, United States) promoted more robust healing than standard care alone. Patients treated with dHAM and total contact cast (n = 13) showed better rates of healing and fewer recurrences than those treated with a total contact cast and standard care when evaluated with concurrent use of the cast. Two trials evaluated the use of a cryopreserved placental membrane containing viable cells (vCPM, Grafix®, Osiris Therapeutics,

Inc., Columbia, MD, United States) for treatment of DFUs ($n = 26$, $n = 97$) and one trial evaluated its use in the treatment of VLUs ($n = 21$). These trials deemed vCPM more effective in treating their respective ulcers than the standard of care. A 2018 RCT ($n = 62$) compared the efficacy of vCPM and DSS, a dermal cellular construct with proven efficacy and effectiveness for DFUs, in the treatment of DFUs. The Osiris sponsored trial's preliminary results indicated that vCPM may have better outcomes for wounds 5 cm or smaller and allows significant cost savings compared to DSS. vCPM, like many placental products, is regulated under 21 CFR Part 1271 Part 361 Human Cells, Tissues, and Cellular and Tissue-based Products (HCT/Ps).

EPIFIX® is a matrix made of dehydrated amnion and chorion membrane (dHACM) that falls under the regulation of 21 CFR Part 1271 Part 361 for Human Cells, Tissues, and Cellular and Tissue-based Products (HCT/Ps). Randomized controlled trials (RCTs) have examined its effectiveness in treating diabetic foot ulcers (DFUs). In a study sponsored by MiMedix (with a sample size of 60–100), dHACM was found to be more effective than standard care with evidence of better outcomes for DFUs and venous leg ulcers (VLUs). The dHACM treated group had a higher rate of complete wound closure and faster healing rates compared to the standard care group. Additionally, the number of grafts used and the associated costs per patient were significantly lower in the dHACM group.To assess their effectiveness in treating DFUs in more detail, Tettelbach et al. An RCT comparing dHACM to the standard of care was carried out on (n = 110), and the findings showed that both dHACM and the standard of care promoted healing. Dehydrated human amniotic chorionic membrane (dHACM) should be administered weekly rather than biweekly for the best outcomes when treating DFUs, according to RCT data (n = 40). Also, dHACM's potential as a VLU treatment was assessed. A comparison was made between dHACM and compression therapy and the standard care of compression alone (n = 109). The outcomes showed that dHACM is beneficial as a treatment adjunct for venous leg ulcers that do not heal (Zelenet al., 2016).

Class II: Epidermal

The epidermal substitutes mentioned here may not be currently available, but they are discussed for their effectiveness and potential availability for direct purchase from the manufacturer.

A randomized controlled trial (n = 77) was conducted in 2003 to compare the effectiveness of epidermal sheets versus mesh grafts in treating chronic leg ulcers. The results indicated that by week 12, the rates of complete closure were comparable between the two groups. However, among patients who did not achieve complete closure by week 12, those receiving epidermal sheets experienced a greater reduction in wound area and continued to heal continuously.

An RCT (n = 225) examined the number of healed ulcers and the time it took for healing in two groups of patients with venous ulcers that did not heal. While compression was the sole component of the standard of care for the other group, one group received treatment with epidermal sheets in addition to compression. There was a statistically significant difference in the healing time of venous leg ulcers when epidermal sheets were used instead of the standard of care.

Treatment for DFUs and VLUs with CEAs has been demonstrated to be safe and effective in clinical trials. Diabetes foot ulcer patients (n = 63) were randomly assigned to one of two treatment arms in a 2012 RCT; treatment arm 1 (n = 31) received gauze soaked in Vaseline, and treatment arm 2 (n = 32) received no treatment at all. Out of the treatment group, 100% experienced complete healing, while only 69% of the control group showed this outcome. When combined with compression rather than by itself, CEAs demonstrated a quicker healing rate for venous leg ulcers.

Class II: Dermal

Patients were randomized into three treatment arms in an RCT (n = 168) to assess the potential of acellular dermal matrices for wound healing: DermACELL® ADM (LifeNet Health, Virginia Beach, VA, USA), GraftJacket® ADM (Wright Medical Technology, Memphis, TN, USA), or standard therapy. GraftJacket® ADM is a freeze-dried version of DermACELL®, an acellular dermal matrix. As a result, it needs time to rehydrate before use. In comparison to standard care, wounds treated with a single application of DermACELL® ADM demonstrated higher rates of wound closure. At no point did GraftJacket® ADM demonstrate higher wound closure rates than standard care. DermACELL® ADM demonstrated improved healing, a longer duration of closure, and a reduction in wound area when compared to standard care and GraftJacket® ADM.

A 2019 RCT (n = 55) revealed that the healing rates of dermal substitutes, SIS, and DSS, were similar in diabetic foot ulcers. There were no discernible differences in wound closure or the percentage of wound area reduction. When SIS is used in addition to compression therapy, VLU healing has been demonstrated to be better than when compression therapy is used alone (n = 120). When treating venous and arterial ulcers that are difficult to heal, it outperformed Hyaloskin, an extracellular matrix that solely contains hyaluronic acid, in terms of healing time, dressing change time, pain, and comfort (n = 54). Additionally, it outperformed moist wound dressings in the healing of VLUs and arterial ulcers (n = 50). Regarding cost-effectiveness, a randomized controlled trial (RCT) revealed that the use of SIS in addition to the standard of care for DFUs leads to better outcomes at a lower cost compared to the standard of care alone.

The ability of UBM to heal wounds was compared to DSS dermal substitute in a 2016 RCT (n = 95) for the treatment of DFUs. Incidence of ulcer closure, ulcer healing rate, wound characteristics, quality of life, cost-effectiveness, and recurrence were among the outcomes examined. According to an interim analysis, UBM improved quality of life and produced healing outcomes comparable to those of DSS at a lower cost.

The effectiveness of HR-ADM in promoting DFU closure was assessed in an RCT (n = 40) in comparison to the collagen-alginate standard dressing. It has been demonstrated that weekly application of HR-ADM is an effective intervention for the treatment of deep flesh ulcers (DFUs). At six weeks, 65% of DFUs treated with HR-ADM healed, compared to 5% treated with standard care, with no difference in adverse events.

RCTs have demonstrated that DSS in addition to standard of care is more effective in treating DFUs than standard of care alone. There was a demonstrated reduction in the incidence of amputation and bone resection (n = 314) when DSS was used as an adjuvant treatment to the standard of care. Its efficacy and safety in the treatment of DFUs were established in an early 2002 trial (n = 46). The results of a 2004 RCT (n = 18) showed that DSS was shown to promote increased healing in conjunction with compression when compared to compression alone, but a larger 2013 RCT (n = 366) found no significant difference in healing rates between the control and treatment groups, suggesting that DSS is not effective in treating venous leg ulcers. The benefit of autologous fibroblast dermis based on hyaluronic acid (AFD, Hyalograft 3D, Anika Therapeutics, Inc. In 2014, a clinical trial (n = 63) was conducted in Bedford, MA, USA, to investigate the use of AFD in treating DFUs. The trial compared the safety and effectiveness of AFD with a non-adherent foam dressing. 84% of patients treated with AFD and 34% of patients treated with a non-adherent foam dressing had complete healing of their ulcers. Furthermore, AFD demonstrated faster healing times than the non-adherent foam dressing (36.4 ± 17.6 vs. 48.4 +/−13.1 days. The frequency of adverse events varied little by group. For dorsal or plantar DFUs, another RCT (n = 180) contrasted AFD with the accepted standard of care. Patients were randomly assigned to receive non-adherent paraffin gauze after AFD or epidermal sheets after AFD. According to the study's findings, both groups' 12-week healing times were comparable, but the treatment group's 50% faster ulcer area reduction was attained. This shows that AFD should be used first, then epidermal sheets. These findings suggest that AFD is a useful intervention for the management of DFUs.

To compare the efficacy of topically applied GAM501 (Ad5PDGF-B/Bovine Type I Collagen Gel) WCM with standard of care in treating DFUs, an RCT with n = 41 was carried out. During a two-week run-in period, patients received standard care, which included changing their gauze dressings every day with saline-moistened gauze.

Patients who had wounds that did not shrink by more than 30% were randomly assigned to receive WCM or to continue with standard care. The RCT's findings showed that WCM did not cause any negative side effects and significantly accelerated wound healing when compared to the standard of care. For DFUs, the WCM offers a therapeutic intervention.

Class III: Allograft

Sanders and associates in 2014 carried out a RCT (n = 23) to evaluate the healing results of DFUs treated with CHSA versus. DFUs given dermal substitutes for DSS. According to the RCT's findings, CHSA is a better healing method than DSS, and DFUs treated with CHSA had a twice-as-higher chance of healing than those treated with DSS.

Although pig skin xenografts are the most common type, recent research has demonstrated the potential benefits of using fish skin xenografts in place of standard care for the treatment of DFUs and VLUs. The outcomes demonstrated that wounds treated with fish skin grafts healed in less than 10% of the expected time and more than 50% faster than the control group. Even though the necessary skin reduction was not achieved in weeks 4–8, the wounds treated with fish skin grafts eventually healed. According to Swiss guidelines, fish skin grafts are the recommended treatment for wounds that do not improve by 40–50% after 4 weeks of standard care, as demonstrated in this study (n = 42). Furthermore, a 2020 study (n = 170) compared the healing outcomes of skin grafts from Atlantic cod fish and dHACM by creating wounds in healthy volunteers that simulated chronic wounds. The results showed that fish skin grafts were superior to dHACM because they caused wounds to heal much more quickly after treatment.

Class IV: Tissue Engineered Skin

Numerous randomized controlled trials (RCTs) have been carried out to evaluate the efficacy, safety, and effectiveness of treating chronic wounds like VLUs and DFUs. DFUs treated with BLCC demonstrated higher rates of wound closure with comparable safety metrics to the standard of care. Treatment with BLCC promotes healing more quickly and in more patients than standard moistened dressings, according to an RCT (n = 31) comparing BLCC to treatment for ischemic wounds. Falanga and associates carried out trials (n = 120, n = 240) to evaluate the efficacy of BLCC versus standard care when used as a treatment for VLUs. The outcomes showed that BLCC is very successful in treating VLUs, particularly those that have persisted for a long time.

An RCT (n = 307) was carried out in 2015 to evaluate the safety and effectiveness of DRT in treating DFUs in comparison to a control group that received offloading, a secondary dressing, and 0.9% sodium chloride gel treatment. The trial's findings demonstrated that the treatment group's rate of wound size reduction per week was higher than that of the control, that patients' quality of life was enhanced, and that DRT was associated with fewer serious adverse events than the control. Complete closure of diabetic foot ulcers was also significantly higher in the treatment group. An RCT from 2021 (n = 36) assessed the effectiveness of DRT by itself versus. NPT combined with DRT helps heal wounds where exposed bone or tendon is present. The time required for skin transplantation and graft removal were among the outcomes evaluated. The results showed that adding NPT to DRT as an adjuvant therapy improved take rate and potentially reduced hospital stays. DRT contains U. S. FDA PMA and is indicated for the repair of scar contractures and post-excisional treatment of life-threatening full-thickness or deep partial thermal injuries when adequate autograft is not available at the time of excision or is not desirable due to the patient's physiological condition (Vecin and Kirsner, 2023).

10.5.3. Future Directions

10.5.3.1. 3D Printing

Every skin substitute that was previously discussed has its own set of drawbacks, including immunogenicity, cost, acceptability in the culture, and risk of disease transmission. New skin substitutes that lessen these difficulties are therefore required. The development of 3D printing in sophisticated tissue engineering in recent years has offered a viable way to address the need for an affordable, effective treatment option. One of the main shortcomings of the skin substitutes that are currently available is that they frequently heal with insufficient pigmentation and are unable to replace skin appendages like glands, vasculature, and hair follicles. These appendages could be produced via 3D printing, offering a practical and realistic alternative. The creation of 3D printed alternatives might even outperform existing healing methods, doing away with the need for autologous grafting.

10.5.3.2. Vascularization

The vascularization of skin substitutes is one area that requires innovation despite the recent advancements made in tissue engineering. The diffusion of nutrients, oxygen, and immune cells into the region of interest depends on vascularization. Large defects can cause problems for the diffusion of nutrients and oxygen, which hinders the proliferation and migration of nutrient-deprived cells that are far from nearby capillaries. The prevascularization approach, in which skin substitutes are vascularized before being applied on the wound bed, is one way to improve vascularization. This can be accomplished by prevascularizing skin substitutes using methods like 3D printing or by using growth factors or stem cells that encourage angiogenesis in the skin substitute. In a murine model, this approach has proven successful. When compared to controls, a bilayer printed graft containing printed endothelial cells demonstrated a 10% increase in wound contraction. Histologically, the printed graft closely resembled normal skin. In tissue engineering, taking vascularity into account while creating skin substitutes offers a promising new direction.

10.5.3.3. Stem Cells

One potential avenue to explore in tissue engineering is the integration of stem cells into skin substitutes. Stem cells have the potential to expedite wound healing, reduce scarring, and regenerate skin appendages that are currently lacking in existing skin substitutes. Studies have shown that stem cells can enhance the production of cytokines and growth factors, which stimulate the creation of new blood vessels and remodeling of the extracellular matrix in wounds. Various types of stem cells, such as bone marrow-derived mesenchymal stem cells, bone marrow-derived endothelial progenitor cells, hematopoietic stem cells, and adipose-derived stromal cells, have been investigated for their ability to aid in wound healing.

Recent research has compared the effectiveness of human neonatal stem cells, amniotic epithelial stem cells, and placenta-derived mesenchymal stem cells in promoting wound healing. These stem cells were differentiated into skin cells and combined with plasma to create a skin substitute, which was then applied to a severe rat burn wound. The results showed promising outcomes in wound healing, including reepithelialization and improved skin structure. Another study in 2019 explored the use of various stem cell types in regenerating the outer layer of skin in wounds. Among the stem cells tested, Wharton's jelly stem cells demonstrated the most potential due to their ability to differentiate into skin cells and low likelihood of being rejected by the immune system.

While the use of stem cells shows promise in advancing wound healing, challenges remain in determining the best source of stem cells, improving processing and application methods, understanding how stem cells transform into skin cells, and considering long-term effects such as immune responses and tumor formation. Further research is necessary to establish stem cell-based skin substitutes as a reliable treatment option for chronic wounds (Vecin and Kirsner, 2023).

10.6. Scars Treatment

An additional class of skin replacements consists of an acellular synthetic polymer matrix. Although there are skin substitutes available on the market, they come with a number of drawbacks, including a reduced ability to promote vascularization, increased scarring, low mechanical resistance, and the potential for immune system rejection. Because synthetic skin substitutes frequently fail to vascularize, cells eventually necrotize and the transplant separates from the wound. Scar formation is a significant drawback to using commercially available skin substitutes as it can result in issues with function, mechanics, and appearance. Scarring frequently results in a pathological process, despite the fact that it is a normal part of wound healing. Since the fibrous tissue in the connective tissue does not naturally contain skin pigment, the fractured skin portion does not heal into a uniform skin tone. Because the connective tissue is devoid of hair follicles, scars in areas with hair growth can present significant aesthetic challenges. The mechanisms of scarring would be revealed, enabling the precise prophylactic and therapeutic actions to be taken. There are several scar treatment techniques available, but none of them is totally successful. Since using a single method causes the illness to relapse quickly, a combined therapeutic approach is typically used, resulting in a good cosmetic outcome.

One of the most effective methods of treating scars is the combined therapeutic approach, which uses cryotherapy either by itself or in conjunction with steroids. Laser therapy is another way to improve the visible aspects of wounds. Because this therapy can be used on a variety of wound types, its efficacy is evaluated in different ways. Corticosteroids usually increase its effects. Another technique, called pressotherapy, involves applying controlled pressure to scars. To achieve this, various compression models, compression apparel, and clips are utilized. Surgical intervention is required when non-surgical scar treatment methods are not effective. The diseased skin tissue fragment is removed, and new, healthy skin—typically from other parts of the patient's body—is placed in its place. Tissue stretchers (expanders) are another surgical technique for burn removal. The application of burn treatment techniques ought to enhance the patient's physical attributes, which in turn impacts their self-worth and standard of living.

More importantly, though, is that the therapy aims to reduce clinical symptoms as much as possible by achieving full joint functionality in the scarred joints and reducing or eliminating pain and burning. Depending on the degree of maturity of the wound, different therapeutic approaches are used during the multiple stages of the wound treatment process. The planning of the surgical procedure itself needs to take scar care into consideration. The reticular layer of the dermis should remain after the necrosis is removed, facilitating quicker wound healing because the scar will adhere to the wound less tightly. The appearance of the cleaned wounds is improved by the early resection of the necrosis using VersaJet. The appearance of the wound at different stages of healing can vary greatly depending on the type of transplant. Closing the incision with a medium-depth autologous transplant yields the best cosmetic results. An *in vitro* transplant of autologous keratinocytes and fibroblasts in the medium density grafted transplant also yields a good cosmetic result. We have seen that skin substitutes that are sold commercially have good cosmetic results (Oasis, Biobrane).

In addition to prevention, wound treatment should aim to create a smooth, even surface without discoloration. Pathological wound formation should be avoided through prompt healing, infection prevention, and scar prevention techniques such as railing and rehabilitation. In the initial stages of treatment, gently massaging the wound with fingers and using silicone gels and ointments is recommended. Silicone helps retain moisture, preventing dryness and discomfort. Applying a protective layer of ointment or gel before dressing the wound creates a slight pressure that aids in healing. Silicone band aids can be applied at night to maintain gentle pressure and prevent drying. Common silicone gels like Dermatix, Veraderm, Medigel, and Cicacare are used along with band aids. Continuous pressure on the wound can be achieved through pressotherapy using flexible fabrics.

The right pressure must be chosen for the therapy to be effective; too little may not work at all, and too much may have unfavorable side effects like chafing, abrasions, skin maceration, sores, or blisters. Pressure clothing, which applies light pressure and is categorized as class I (18–21 mmHg) by the European Standardization Commission, is used in the treatment of severe burn wounds. After the wound has finished healing, wear these clothes for six to 24 months to see any cosmetic benefits, such as the scar's size decreasing, whitening, and flattening. Because the effectiveness of pressure clothing is dependent on size, it must be precisely fitted and exchanged in the event that a change in body size occurs (particularly in children). There are several approaches to treating scars. In our center, laser therapy and surgical treatment are the most often used treatments. One way to correct a wound is to cut them out and sew them together, which will change their direction and release pressure on the skin. The Langer lines must be taken into consideration when cutting the skin. Topical surgical wound healing techniques, like the "Z" method, which involves cutting a "Z" shape, are employed in our center. The center of this cut is located at least 3 cm from the wound's brim and is perpendicular to the closed wound's long axis. This section and the others should have angles ranging from 30 to 90 degrees. The ensuing triangular areas swap positions as the wound brims come together, and the "Z" shape shifts from being perpendicular to parallel to the wound's long axis. Six times a year, this technique was applied.

Surgical wound management also involves the use of adjacent skin. It can be applied to veinless areas because it is stronger and thicker than transplanted skin. These techniques are applied to treat contracted wounds of the eyelid, corpus, and limbs. Depending on the type of laser, wounds at different stages of maturity can be treated with laser therapy. Lasers that stimulate wound healing can be applied at this level. Low energy lasers were used in biostimulation (stimulants). The wavelengths emitted by the lasers used in biostimulation are in the middle of the electromagnetic spectrum, and they can produce radiation up to 5 mW. The primary tools used in biostimulation are lasers, such as the arsen-gala semiconductor diode and the He-Ne laser helium-neon.

When applied at the proper depth, the biostimulation process itself efficiently supplies a predefined quantity of energy, measured in Joules (J). The tissue's structure, blood flow, pH, water content, pigment, melanin, and hemoglobin, as well as the light's wavelength, color, intensity, and length of treatment, all affect how much of the radiation is absorbed and penetrates the tissue. CO_2 laser ablation is used at our center once the scar forms. Radiation with a continuous wavelength of 10,600 nm and a power of 30–100 W is emitted by the CO_2 laser. A CO_2 laser emits radiation that is invisible to the human eye and is absorbed by extracellular and intracellular fluid. Tissue damage is caused by the non-selective absorption of the laser light down to a depth of 0.6 mm. This results in thrombotic necrosis that is 0.4–0.5 mm deep. Thermal damage to the surrounding area of evaporation then forms a reticular layer of skin, which unfortunately can leave a significant scar at the site of the lesion. The evaporation of the damaged tissue is one of the CO_2 laser radiation's beneficial effects on tissue. Adverse skin changes, however, may exacerbate this effect. Because of its shallow tissue penetration and excellent water absorption, this laser is used in scar treatment. Since water makes up the majority of tissues, the laser's beam can cut through both soft tissue and bone. Because of this, lasers are used in other medical specialties like ENT, dermatology, and gynecology where surgery is required. For CO_2 laser ablation techniques to have sufficient and long-lasting effects, three to five repetitions are required. It is necessary to maintain long treatment intervals, giving the patient's tissue four to five weeks to regenerate. Since laser therapy is only applied to 15–25% of the scars during each session, it is crucial to maintain an adequate level of treatment. On average, 96 times a year, these procedures are carried out in the cosmetic surgery department of the center, with 93 of those times involving laser therapy to help with skin fibrosis and scarring (Figure 10.9).

In conclusion, the healing of scars is a gradual process that starts with the resection of the necrosis. Care must be taken to leave a layer of reticularis dermis and to create Langer lines. This is the initial phase of prophylactic treatment aimed at preventing unsightly scar formation. The type of transplant has a significant impact on how scars look; medium depth solid transplants or autologous keratinocyte and fibroblast transplants placed within the scaffolding of reticulated transplants produce the most aesthetically sound scars. As soon as possible, the scar treatment procedure itself should start. Biostimulating lasers can already help with wound healing. The avoidance of scar formation and wound infection is part of the prophylaxis of scars. After the wound has healed, the first line of treatment for scars is pressure therapy with pressure garments, followed by finger massages and the application of silicone gels and ointments. When pathological scars start to form, surgical techniques like the "Z" cut method and the neighboring skin method are used, along with ablative CO_2 laser therapy (Kitala et al., 2018).

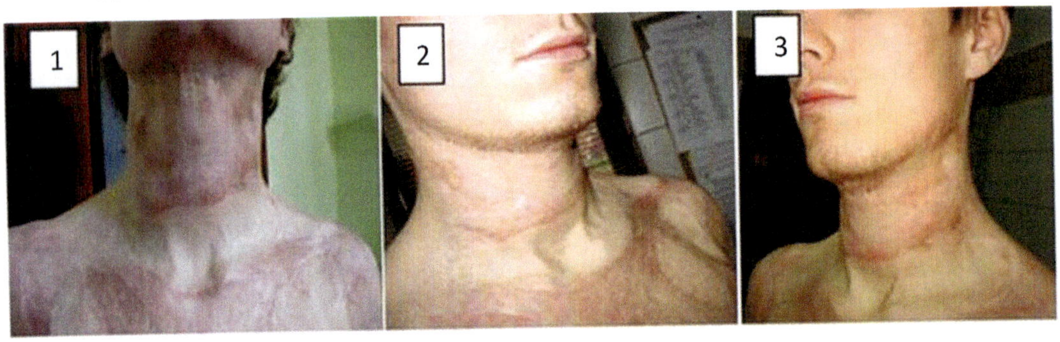

Figure 10.9. *The wound before (1) laser therapy, after the first session (2) after the second session (3).*

Source: Kitala, D., Klama-Baryła, A., Łabuś, W., Misiuga, M., Nowak, M., & Kawecki, M. (2018). Advanced Technologies in Dermatology. InTech. doi: 10.5772/intechopen.70288.

A Closer Look

A Closer Look At Split-Thickness Skin Grafts In Patients With Diabetes

For individuals with diabetes, lower extremity ulcerations remain an expensive and dangerous complication. The World Health Organization projects that 350 million people will have diabetes by 2030, as the disease has become more common over the past 50 years. About 30.3 million Americans, or 9.4% of the US population, according to the Centers for Disease Control and Prevention (CDC), received a diabetes diagnosis in 2015. Diabetes-related problems, mortality, increased disability, and treatment costs continue to rank among the biggest healthcare costs. Roughly 50% of diabetic plantar ulcers progress to a serious infection. Many surgeons choose to amputate in cases of serious infection. Actually, in the US, diabetes is linked to about 83% of all non-traumatic lower-extremity amputations. A lower extremity amputation can cost anywhere from $70,000 to $120,000 in total, taking into account both the initial hospital stay and any follow-up care needed in the three to five years that follow surgery.

The lower extremities experience delayed wound healing for a variety of reasons. These include inadequate vascular supply, poor glycemic control, wound care deficiency, and improper offloading. Wounds should be aggressively and quickly treated to promote healing. This is particularly crucial to avoid the complications that often result in amputation from chronic wounds. An advanced biologic, graft, or flap can help speed up the healing process and lower the risk of additional amputation or tissue loss once the underlying cause of the wound is found and treated.

Advanced skin substitutes based on cells or tissues are widely accessible, but using them is becoming more difficult due to a variety of challenges, such as challenging billing and reimbursement procedures. The use of hundreds of skin substitutes has been restricted due to recent modifications to private insurance policies.

Understanding The Role of Skin Grafts and Flaps for Diabetic Foot Wounds

An autologous skin flap or graft is an additional choice. Depending on the patient's medical comorbidities, circulation, infection status, anatomical location of the wound, and availability of donor sites, the best skin graft or flap may be chosen. For these patients, especially after significant tissue loss, the restoration of healthy intact skin to act as a barrier and prevent further infection is essential.

An autologous split-thickness skin graft is one kind of graft with a high degree of dependability and comparatively low donor site morbidity (STSG). When compared to other topical wound modalitics, skin grafting offers a quicker time to closure with a single treatment; however, there are risks associated with the procedure, such as donor site morbidity and failed graft take.

The choice to use STSG in diabetic patients is debatable. Graft failures may result from improper patient selection and inadequate wound preparation. Additionally, one needs to take into account the patient population's heightened susceptibility to infection, neuropathy, and microvascular disease. Rates rise in patients with additional comorbidities like wound, donor site, and end-stage renal disease.

In wounds where there is exposed bone, tendon, or joint, split-thickness skin grafts should not be performed because there may not be enough vascularity to encourage the growth of granulation tissue. In these regions, wound beds need to be prepared with a dermoconductive product to form a granular bed before an STSG is applied. The viability of an STSG is also decreased by increased shear and pressure. Not only is it critical to optimize the patient and prepare the wound bed, but it's also important to assess the intended graft location and steer clear of directly weight-bearing areas.

Notwithstanding these hazards, STSG is a practical and efficient method for closing diabetic wounds. Skin grafts with split thickness are particularly beneficial for donor sites, partially closed wounds, and open amputation sites. Compared to standard local wound care dressings, STSG allows for faster closure of larger wounds and provides more durable coverage than the scar resulting from secondary closure. According to reports, the use of STSGs by clinicians for primary closure on diabetic foot ulcerations that have been optimized has a success rate of 78% in closing 90% of the wound within eight weeks.

Pertinent Pearls In Technique For Harvesting Split-Thickness Skin Grafts

Autologous skin grafting is said to have originated in India in 3000 BC when doctors used the grafts to cover facial wounds. The grafts should include both the epidermis and a portion of the dermis when obtained from a donor site. Reepithelization is then used to heal the donor site. Aggressive debridement is used to remove biofilm from lower extremity ulcerations and produce a granular bed that is clean and well-vascularized. Negative pressure wound therapy (NPWT) may be used in conjunction with a dermoconductive matrix to help cover exposed bone or tendon and induce granulation tissue. Forming a sufficient tissue bed for the STSG application could take a few weeks. Topical antibiotic powder is a good choice if there is any worry about post-debridement infection. The ipsilateral thigh is usually the donor site. For this procedure, local subcutaneous infiltration of 1% lidocaine combined with epinephrine would be the anesthesia method. To minimize friction, mineral oil must be applied to both the donor site and the dermatome. To harvest the graft at full power and at a 45° angle, one uses a dermatome. Before harvesting, the doctor must measure the donor site to ensure that the width and length are sufficient to cover the wound. It is possible to receive more grafts if needed.

To help with pain and hemostasis, the surgeon infiltrates the donor site using a topical combination of lidocaine and epinephrine. The dressing is made up of non-adherent gauze, such as xeroform, covered in a Tegaderm dressing (3M), which is changed five days after surgery. The STSG is meshed in a 1:1:5 ratio by the surgeon using a Brennen Skin Graft Mesher, and the graft is fastened with 4–0 chromic gut or skin staples. To ensure total coverage, grafts can be cut to fit the irregular shape of the ulceration. Complete contact between the graft and recipient site is crucial for aiding in graft incorporation. For STSGs to be successful, negative pressure wound therapy is incredibly helpful. A mean graft survival rate of 93% was reported by Turissini and colleagues in a 2019 study evaluating the use of NPWT to secure STSGs in complex lower extremity wounds, including diabetic ulcerations and amputation sites. The authors of this study also discovered that patients who underwent NPWT had about 80% lower odds of STSG failure than patients who received bolster dressings as a post-surgical dressing.

Applying NPWT involves setting the system to 75 mmHg, covering the foam with a non-adherent layer, and leaving the NPWT in place for five days. The incorporation of the graft during the healing phase is further improved by immobilization and offloading with a posterior splint or cast to limit motion.

Salient Insights on other Important Aspects of STSG Use in Patients with Diabetes

Hemoglobin A1c (HbA1c) levels do not seem to have a negative effect on split-thickness skin grafts. Research indicates that there is no statistically significant correlation between STSG failure and HbA1c level, although other factors like edema, infection, and congestive heart failure (CHF) may play a role.

One of the main reasons graft failure occurs is infection, which emphasizes the significance of controlling any underlying infection and minimizing biofilm. To avoid infection, surgeons need to place STSGs on a wound bed that is well-vascularized and has low bacterial counts. Comorbid conditions like end-stage renal disease (ESRD) and peripheral vascular disease (PVD) have a detrimental effect on an STSG's viability, even though there is no direct link between HbA1c and STSG failure.

Offloading is crucial for preventing ulcerations from coming back. Offloading with STSG can also lessen the formation of hematomas, seromas, and shearing beneath the graft. Through "plasmatic imbibition," which distributes nutrition from the recipient site, proper offloading will enable the graft to integrate.

Split-thickness skin grafts have various uses. They can be used as a primary treatment for diabetic wounds, a secondary option, as well as a supplement to a treatment that was partially accepted or unsuccessful. They can also aid in the healing of the donor site for other plastic surgery procedures. STSGs are particularly effective in treating burns. Using STSG for main closure on properly managed diabetic foot ulcers can be highly effective and may be more cost-effective than other similar treatments.

Yammine and Assi reported in a 2019 meta-analysis on the use of STSG for diabetic ulcerations that 85.5% of the ulcers healed in an average of five weeks, with a recurrence rate of 40.2%, an infection rate of 40.4%, and a re-grafting rate of 12.1%. The investigators discovered that the morbidity rate at the donor site was a mere 1.75%.

Anecdotal or retrospective reviews make up a large portion of the current literature on STSGs for diabetic ulcerations. Therefore, additional prospective studies are required to demonstrate the usefulness of these grafts.

Summary

- The current trend in medicine is focused on two aspects of healing: on preventive medicine, preventing disease when possible and regenerative medicine, regenerating fractured cells.
- Cellular therapies used to return the patient to the stage of skin completeness are an attractive area of translational medicine.
- The preparation which is an optimal alternative for traditional treatment methods is a transplant of allogeneic, biostatic amniotic tissue.
- The clinical scope of the use of the amniotic membrane may include its application as a skin substitute on facial burn wounds, hand burn wounds, on donor areas and granulating wounds.
- To improve the properties and the longevity of the transplants, tissue engineering methods such as cell removal are used. The reason for the removal of cells from tissues/organs is the obtaining of a non-immunogenetic transplant, which could be populated *in vivo* by the patient's own cells after the transplantation is completed.
- The use of skin substitutes is an alternative to auto-and allogeneic transplants in the treatment of wounds of various provenance, including burn wounds and chronic wounds.
- Class I skin substitutes are comprised of single and bilayer temporary, impervious dressing material. They aim to maintain the mechanical traits of the skin but are acellular.
- Class II dressings are single layer durable skin substitutes. They can be further categorized as epidermal or dermal.
- Despite current advances made in tissue engineering, one area in need of innovation is the vascularization of skin substitutes. Vascularization is essential for the diffusion of nutrients, oxygen, and immune reactors into the area of interest.
- Stem cells have been shown to promote the secretion of cytokines and growth factors that stimulate angiogenesis and extracellular matrix (ECM) remodeling in the wound bed.

References

1. Alikarami, F., Yari, F., Amirizadeh, N., Nikougoftar, M., & Jalili, M. A. (2015). The immunosuppressive activity of amniotic membrane mesenchymal stem cells on T lymphocytes. *Avicenna Journal of Medical Biotechnology*, *7*(3), 90–96.
2. Aronowitz, J. A., & Ellenhorn, J. D. (2013). Adipose stromal vascular fraction isolation: A head-to-head comparison of four commercial cell separation systems. *Plastic and Reconstructive Surgery*, *132*(6), 932e–939e. DOI: 10.1097/PRS.0b013e3182a80652.
3. Atiyeh, B. S., & Costagliola, M. (2007). Cultured epithelial autograft (CEA) in burn treatment: Three decades later. *Burns*, *33*(4), 405–413. https://doi.org/10.1016/j.burns.2006.11.002.
4. Atiyeh, B., Masellis, A., & Conte, C. (2009). Optimizing burn treatment in developing low- and middle-income countries with limited health care resources (part 1). *Annals of Burns and Fire Disasters*, *22*(3), 121–125.
5. Bargues, L., Prat, M., Leclerc, T., Bey, E., & Lataillade, J. J. (2011). Present and future of cell therapy in burns. *Pathologie-Biologie*, *59*(3), e49–e56.
6. Barling, P. M., John, M. J., Walsh, J. R., & Niall, H. D. (1985). The isolation and characterization

of lysozyme from human foetal membranes: A comparison with the enzyme from other sources. *Comparative Biochemistry and Physiology Part B, 81*(2), 509–513.

7. Blais, M., Parenteau-Bareil, R., Cadau, S., & Berthod, F. (2013). Concise review: Tissue-engineered skin and nerve regeneration in burn treatment. *Stem Cells Translational Medicine, 2*(7), 545–551.

8. Borzęcki, A., & Cielica, W. (2000). Zastosowanie lasera CO_2 w praktyce dermatologicznej. *Borgis–Nowa Medycyna, 11*, 1–14.

9. Celis, P. (2010). CAT—The new committee for advanced therapies at the European Medicines Agency. *Bundesgesundheitsblatt, Gesundheitsforschung, Gesundheitsschutz, 53*(1), 9–13.

10. Cleland, H., Wasiak, J., Dobson, H., Paul, M., Pratt, G., Paul, E., Herson, M., & Akbarzadeh, S. (2014). Clinical application and viability of cryopreserved cadaveric skin allografts in severe burn: A retrospective analysis. *Burns, 40*(1), 61–66. https://doi.org/10.1016/j.burns.2013.05.006.

11. Danner, S., Kremer, M., Petschnik, A. E., Nagel, S., Zhang, Z., Hopfner, U., Reckhenrich, A. K., Weber, C., Schenck, T. L., Becker, T., Kruse, C., Machens, H. G., & Egaña, J. T. (2012). The use of human sweat gland-derived stem cells for enhancing vascularization during dermal regeneration. *The Journal of Investigative Dermatology, 132*(6), 1707–1716.

12. Debels, H., Hamdi, M., Abberton, K., & Morrison, W. (2015). Dermal matrices and bioengineered skin substitutes: A critical review of current options. *Plastic and Reconstructive Surgery Global Open, 3*(1), e284. https://doi.org/10.1097/GOX.0000000000000219.

13. Di Domenico, L., Landsman, A. R., Emch, K. J., & Landsman, A. (2011). A prospective comparison of diabetic foot ulcers treated with either cryopreserved skin allograft or bioengineered skin substitute. *Wounds, 23*(7), 184–189.

14. DiDomenico, L. A., Orgill, D. P., Galiano, R. D., Serena, T. E., Carter, M. J., Kaufman, J. P., Young, N. J., & Zelen, C. M. (2016). Aseptically processed placental membrane improves healing of diabetic foot ulcerations: Prospective, randomized clinical trial. *Plastic and Reconstructive Surgery-Global Open, 4*(10), e1095. DOI: 10.1097/GOX.0000000000001095.

15. Dumville, J. C., Keogh, S. J., Liu, Z., Stubbs, N., Walker, R. M., & Fortnam, M. (2015). Alginate dressings for treating pressure ulcers. *Cochrane Database of Systematic Reviews, 3*, CD011277.

16. Fletcher, J. L., Caterson, E. J., Hale, R. G., Cancio, L. C., Renz, E. M., & Chan, R. K. (2013). Characterization of skin allograft use in thermal injury. *Journal of Burn Care & Research, 34*(1), 168–175. DOI: 10.1097/BCR.0b013e318270000f.

17. Flores-Espinosa, P., Pineda-Torres, M., Vega-Sánchez, R., Estrada-Gutiérrez, G., Espejel-Nuñez, A., Flores-Pliego, A., Maida-Claros, R., Paredes-Vivas, Y., Morales-Méndez, I., Sosa-González, I., Chávez-Mendoza, A., & Zaga-Clavellina, V. (2014). Progesterone elicits an inhibitory effect upon LPS-induced innate immune response in pre-labor human amniotic epithelium. *American Journal of Reproductive Immunology, 71*(1), 61–72. DOI: 10.1111/aji.12163.

18. Fraser, J. K., Hicok, K. C., Shanahan, R., Zhu, M., Miller, S., & Arm, D. M. (2014). The Celution® system: Automated processing of adipose-derived regenerative cells in a functionally closed system. *Advances in Wound Care, 3*(1), 38–45.

19. Gierek, M., Kawecki, M., Mikuś, K., Glik, J., Klama-Baryła, A., Hoff-Lenczewska, D., & Nowak, M. (2012). The treatment of burn wounds with human amniotic membrane dressings in the

Centre for Burns in Siemianowice Śląskie—Own experience. *Journal of Orthopaedics Trauma Surgery and Related Research, 3*(29), 75–83.

20. Gierek, M., Kawecki, M., Mikuś, K., Glik, J., Klama-Baryła, A., Hoff-Lenczewska, D., & Nowak, M. (2012). Use of amniotic membrane in treatment of burns. *Journal of Orthopaedics Trauma Surgery and Related Research, 3*(29), 70–75.

21. Gould, L. J. (2016). Topical collagen-based biomaterials for chronic wounds: Rationale and clinical application. *Advances in Wound Care, 1*(5), 19–31. https://doi.org/10.1089/wound.2014.0595.

22. Grauss, R. W., Hazekamp, M. G., van Vliet, S., Gittenberger-de Groot, A. C., & DeRuiter, M. C. (2003). Decellularization of rat aortic valve allografts reduces leaflet destruction and extracellular matrix remodeling. *The Journal of Thoracic and Cardiovascular Surgery, 126*(6), 2003–2010. https://doi.org/10.1016/S0022.

23. Greenwood, J. E., Clausen, J., & Kavanagh, S. (2009). Experience with Biobrane: Uses and caveats for success. *Eplasty, 9*, e25.

24. Halim, A. S., Khoo, T. L., & Mohd, S. J. (2010). Biologic and synthetic skin substitutes: An overview. *Indian Journal of Plastic Surgery, 43*(Suppl), S23–S28. DOI: 10.4103/0970-0358.70712.

25. Hartmann-Fritsch, F., Hosper, N., Luginbühl, J., Biedermann, T., Reichmann, E., & Meuli, M. (2013). Human amniotic fluid-derived cells can competently substitute dermal fibroblasts in a tissue-engineered dermo-epidermal skin analog. *Pediatric Surgery International, 29*(1), 61–69.

26. He, H., Li, W., Chen, S. Y., Zhang, S., Chen, Y. T., Hayashida, Y., Zhu, Y. T., & Tseng, S. C. (2008). Suppression of activation and induction of apoptosis in RAW264.7 cells by amniotic membrane extract. *Investigative Ophthalmology & Visual Science, 49*(10), 4468–4475. DOI: 10.1167/iovs.08-1781.

27. Hodde, J. P., Badylak, S. F., Brightman, A. O., & Voytik-Harbin, S. L. (1996). Glycosaminoglycan content of small intestinal submucosa: A bioscaffold for tissue replacement. *Tissue Engineering, 2*(3), 209–217.

28. Hodde, J. P., Record, R. D., Liang, H. A., & Badylak, S. F. (2001). Vascular endothelial growth factor in porcine-derived extracellular matrix. *Endothelium, 8*(1), 11–24.

29. Hoff-Lenczewska, D., Klama-Baryła, A., Kawecki, M., Łabuś, W., Glik, J., Maj, M., Gola, J., Mazurek, U., & Sieroń, A. L. (2012). The use of modern technologies of cell and tissue engineering in burn treatment. *Acta Biochimica Polonica, 59*(supplement 1), 17–22.

30. Horner, C. W. M., Atkins, J., Simpson, L., Philp, B., Shelley, O., & Dziewulski, P. (2011). Estimating the usage of allograft in the treatment of major burns. *Burns, 37*(4), 590–593. https://doi.org/10.1016/j.burns.2010.12.006.

31. Hubik, D. J., Wasiak, J., Paul, E., & Cleland, H. (2011). Biobrane: A retrospective analysis of outcomes at a specialist adult burns centre. *Burns, 37*(4), 594–600.

32. Jeong, J. H. (2010). Adipose stem cells and skin repair. *Current Stem Cell Research & Therapy, 5*(2), 137–140.

33. Kagan, R. J., Peck, M. D., Ahrenholz, D. H., Hickerson, W. L., Holmes, J. IV, Korentager, R., Kraatz, J., Pollock, K., & Kotoski, G. (2013). Surgical management of the burn wound and use of skin

substitutes: An expert panel white paper. *Journal of Burn Care & Research, 34*(2), e60–e79. https://doi.org/10.1097/BCR.0b013e31827039a6.

34. Kawecki, K., Pawlik-Kanpik, D., Glik, J., & Misuga, M. (2016). Oparzenia. Blizny jako problem w chirurgii oparzeń. In A. Dziki (Ed.), *Przegląd Piśmiennictwa Chirurgicznego 2015* (pp. 1–8). Warszawa: Fundacja Polski Przegląd Chirurgiczny.

35. Kawecki, M., Glik, J., Kitala, D., & Misiuga, M. (2017). Oparzenia [Burns]. In A. Dziki (Ed.), *Przegląd Piśmiennictwa Chirurgicznego* (1st ed., pp. 192–196). Łódź: Stowarzyszenie Popierania Rozwoju Proktologii.

36. Kawecki, M., Hoff-Lenczewska, D., Klama-Baryła, A., & Glik, J. (2013). Oparzenia. In Dziki (Ed.), *Przegląd Piśmiennictwa Chirurgicznego*. Fundacja Polski Przegląd Chirurgiczny.

37. Kawecki, M., Łabuś, W., Klama-Baryla, A., Kitala, D., Kraut, M., Glik, J., Misiuga, M., Nowak, M., Bielecki, T., & Kasperczyk, A. (Forthcoming). A review of decellurization methods caused by an urgent need for quality control of cell-free extracellular matrix scaffolds and their role in regenerative medicine. *Journal of Biomedical Materials Research—Part B: Applied Biomaterials.* https://doi.org/10.1002/jbm.b.33865.

38. Kim, S. W., Zhang, H. Z., Guo, L., Kim, J. M., & Kim, M. H. (2012). Amniotic mesenchymal stem cells enhance wound healing in diabetic NOD/SCID mice through high angiogenic and engraftment capabilities. *PLoS One, 7*(7), e41105.

39. Kitala, D., Kawecki, M., Klama-Baryła, A., Łabuś, W., Kraut, M., Glik, J., Ryszkiel, I., Kawecki, M. P., & Nowak, M. (2016). Allogeneic vs. autologous skin grafts in the therapy of patients with burn injuries: A retrospective, open-label clinical study with pair matching. *Advances in Clinical and Experimental Medicine, 25*(5), 923–929. https://doi.org/10.17219/acem/61961.

40. Kitala, D., Klama-Baryła, A., Kawecki, M., Kraut, M., Łabuś, W., Glik, J., Ples, M., Tomanek, E., & Nowak, M. (2016). Infections in the tissue material and their impact on the loss of transplants in the laboratory of *in vitro* cell and tissue culture with tissue bank in the years 2011–2015. *Cell and Tissue Banking, 17*(66), 1–8. https://doi.org/10.1007/s10561-016-9597-y.

41. Kitala, D., Klama-Baryła, A., Łabuś, W., Misiuga, M., Nowak, M., & Kawecki, M. (2018). *Advanced Technologies in Dermatology*. InTech.

42. Klama-Baryła, A., Kraut, M., Łabuś, W., Maj, M., Kawecki, M., Nowak, M., Glik, J., Cichowski, A., Szydło, A., Lesiak, M., Anioł, J., & Sieroń, A. L. (2011). Application of platelet leukocyte gel in *in vitro* cultured autologous keratinocyte grafts. *Journal of Orthopaedics Trauma Surgery and Related Research, 2*(22), 77–86.

43. Kurkus, B., & Kuliński, W. (2005). Laseroterapia w medycynie fizykalnej. *Borgis–Balneologia Polska, 3*(4), 76–83.

44. Lal, S., Barrow, R. E., Wolf, S. E., Chinkes, D. L., Hart, D. W., Heggers, J. P., & Herndon, D. N. (2000). Biobrane improves wound healing in burned children without increased risk of infection. *Shock, 14*(3), 314–318.

45. Lloyd, E. C., Michener, M., & Williams, M. S. (2013). Outpatient burns: Prevention and care. *American Family Physician, 85*(9), 25–32.

46. Londono, R., & Badylak, S. F. (2015). Biologic scaffolds for regenerative medicine: Mechanisms of *in vivo* remodeling. *Annals of Biomedical Engineering, 43*(3), 577–592. https://doi.org/10.1007/s10439-014-1103-8.

47. Macedo, J. L., & Santos, J. B. (2007). Predictive factors of mortality in burn patients. *Revista do Instituto de Medicina Tropical de São Paulo, 49*(6), 365–370.

48. Mahmoudi-Rad, M., Abolhasani, E., Moravvej, H., Mahmoudi-Rad, N., & Mirdamadi, Y. (2013). Acellular amniotic membrane: An appropriate scaffold for fibroblast proliferation. *Clinical and Experimental Dermatology, 38*(6), 646–651.

49. Mansilla, E., Marín, G. H., Berges, M., Scafatti, S., Rivas, J., Núñez, A., Menvielle, M., Lamonega, R., Gardiner, C., Drago, H., Sturla, F., Portas, M., Bossi, S., Castuma, M. V., Luengas, S. P., Roque, G., Martire, K., Tau, J. M., & Orlandi, G. (2015). Cadaveric bone marrow mesenchymal stem cells: First experience treating a patient with large severe burns. *Burns & Trauma, 3*(1), 1–9. DOI: 10.1186/s41038-015-0018-4.

50. Misiuga, M., Glik, J., Kawecki, M., et al. (2016). The effect of hyperbaric oxygen therapy on burn wounds covered with skin allografts. *Journal of Orthopaedics Trauma Surgery and Related Research, 1*(38), 17–27.

51. Miturska, R., & Borzęcki, A. (2009). Papilloma condylomatoides okolic narządów płciowych i odbytu leczona laserem CO_2. *Dermatologia Estetyczna, 11*(6), 481–485.

52. Moore, M., Samsell, B., Wallis, G., Triplett, S., Chen, S., Linthurst Jones, A., et al. (2015). Decellularization of human dermis using non-denaturing anionic detergent and endonuclease: A review. *Cell and Tissue Banking, 16*, 249–259.

53. MS, H., Rennert, R. C., McArdle, A., Chung, M. T., Walmsley, G. G., Longaker, M. T., & Lorenz, H. P. (2014). The role of stem cells during scarless skin wound healing. *Advances in Wound Care, 3*(4), 304–314. DOI: 10.1089/wound.2013.0471.

54. Nihsen, E. S., Johnson, C. E., & Hiles, M. C. (2008). Bioactivity of small intestinal submucosa and oxidized regenerated cellulose/collagen. *Advances in Skin & Wound Care, 21*(10), 479–486.

55. O'Meara, S., Martyn-St James, M., & Adderley, U. J. (2015). Alginate dressings for venous leg ulcers. *Cochrane Database of Systematic Reviews, 19*, CD010182.

56. Ogliari, K. S., Marinowic, D., Brum, D. E., & Loth, F. (2014). Stem cells in dermatology. *Anais Brasileiros de Dermatologia, 89*(2), 286–292.

57. Oliver, A. M., Kaawach, W., Mithoff, E. W., Watt, A., Abramovich, D. R., & Rayner, C. R. (1991). The differentiation and proliferation of newly formed epidermis on wounds treated with cultured epithelial allografts. *British Journal of Dermatology, 125*(2), 147–154.

58. Ott, H. C., Matthiesen, T. S., Goh, S. K., Black, L. D., Kren, S. M., Netoff, T. I., & Taylor, D. A. (2008). Perfusion-decellularized matrix: Using nature's platform to engineer a bioartificial heart. *Nature Medicine, 14*(2), 213–221. https://doi.org/10.1038/nm1684.

59. Pellegrini, G., Ranno, R., Stracuzzi, G., Bondanza, S., Guerra, L., & Zambruno, G. (1999). The control of epidermal stem cells (holoclones) in the treatment of massive full-thickness burns with autologous keratinocytes cultured on fibrin. *Transplantation, 68*, 868–879.

60. Petrof, G., Abdul-Wahab, A., & McGrath, J. A. (2014). Cell therapy in dermatology. *Cold Spring Harbor Perspectives in Medicine, 4*(6), a015156.

61. Philandrianos, C., Andrac-Meyer, L., Mordon, S., Feuerstein, J. M., Sabatier, F., Veran, J., Magalon, G., & Casanova, D. (2012). Comparison of five dermal substitutes in full-thickness skin wound healing in a porcine model. *Burns, 38*(9), 820–829.

62. Rasulov, M. F., Vasilchenkov, A. V., Onishchenko, N. A., Krasheninnikov, M. E., Kravchenko, V. I., Gorshenin, T. L., Pidtsan, R. E., & Potapov, I. V. (2005). First experience of the use of bone marrow mesenchymal stem cells for the treatment of a patient with deep skin burns. *Bulletin of Experimental Biology and Medicine, 139*(1), 141–144.

63. Rogers, A. D. (2013). Indications for cadaver skin in burns and complex wound care. *Wound Healing Southern Africa, 6*(2), 54–55.

64. Schmidt, C., & Baier, J. M. (2000). Acellular vascular tissues: Natural biomaterials for tissue engineering. *Biomaterials, 21*(22), 2215–2231.

65. Selig, H. F., Lumenta, D. B., Giretzlehner, M., Jeschke, M. G., Upton, D., & Kamolz, L. P. (2012). The properties of an "ideal" burn wound dressing—What do we need in daily clinical practice? Results of a worldwide online survey among burn care specialists. *Burns, 38*(7), 960–966. https://doi.org/10.1016/j.burns.2012.04.007.

66. Shen, Y. M., Hu, X. H., Mi, H. R., Yu, D. N., Qin, F. J., Chen, H., Wang, H., & Zhang, G. A. (2011). Early treatment of high-voltage electric burn wound in the limbs. *Zhonghua Shao Shang Za Zhi, 27*(3), 173–177.

67. Shi, L., & Ronfard, V. (2013). Biochemical and biomechanical characterization of porcine small intestinal submucosa (SIS): A mini review. *International Journal of Burns and Trauma, 3*(4), 173–179.

68. Shi, L., Ramsay, S., Ermis, R., & Carson, D. (2012). *In vitro* and *in vivo* studies on matrix metalloproteinases interacting with small intestine submucosa wound matrix. *International Wound Journal, 9*(1), 44–53.

69. Singh, V., Devgan, L., Bhat, S., & Miler, S. M. (2007). The pathogenesis of burn wound conversion. *Annals of Plastic Surgery, 59*(1), 109–115. https://doi.org/10.1097/01.sap.0000252065.90759.e6.

70. Situm, M., Kolic, M., & Spoljar, S. (2016). Quality of life and psychological aspects in patients with chronic leg ulcer. *Acta Med Croatica, 70*, 61–63.

71. Sood, R., Roggy, D., Zieger, M., Balledux, J., Chaudhari, S., Koumanis, D. J., Mir, H. S., Cohen, A., Knipe, C., Gabehart, K., & Coleman, J. J. (2010). Cultured epithelial autografts for coverage of large burn wounds in eighty-eight patients: The Indiana University experience. *Journal of Burn Care & Research, 31*(4), 559–568.

72. Sorg, H., Betzler, C., Rennekampff, H. O., & Vogt, P. M. (2012). Burns. *Unfallchirurg, 115*(7), 635–648.

73. Stocka, A., Huryń, A., Królicki, A., Orzechowska, B., & Maleszka, R. (2010). Laseroterapia ablacyjna w leczeniu skórnej manifestacji stwardnienia guzowatego-opis przypadku. *Dermatologia Estetyczna, 12*(6), 367–372.

74. Strom, S. C., & Gramignoli, R. (2016). Human amnion epithelial cells expressing HLA-G as novel cell-based treatment for liver disease. *Human Immunology, 77*(9), 734–739. DOI: 10.1016/j.humimm.2016.07.002.

75. Sullivan, D. C., Mirmalek-Sani, S. H., Deegan, D. B., Baptista, P. M., Aboushwareb, T., Atala, A., & Yoo, J. J. (2012). Decellularization methods of porcine kidneys for whole organ engineering using a high-throughput system. *Biomaterials, 33*(31), 7756–7764. https://doi.org/10.1016/j.biomaterials.2012.07.023.

76. Sumide, T., Nishida, K., Yamato, M., Ide, T., Hayashida, Y., Watanabe, K., Yang, J., Kohno, C., Kikuchi, A., Maeda, N., Watanabe, H., Okano, T., & Tano, Y. (2006). Functional human corneal endothelial cell sheets harvested from temperature-responsive culture surfaces. *The FASEB Journal, 20*(2), 392–394.

77. Taghiabadi, E., Nasri, S., Shafieyan, S., Jalili Firoozinezhad, S., & Aghdami, N. (2015). Fabrication and characterization of spongy denuded amniotic membrane-based scaffold for tissue engineering. *Cell Journal, 16*(4), 476–487. DOI: 10.22074/cellj.2015.493.

78. Troy, J., Karlnoski, R., Downes, K., Brown, K. S., Cruse, C. W., Smith, D. J., & Payne, W. G. (2013). The use of EZ Derm® in partial-thickness burns: An institutional review of 157 patients. *Eplasty, 13*, e14.

79. Vecin, N. M., & Kirsner, R. S. (2023). Skin substitutes as treatment for chronic wounds: Current and future directions. *Frontiers in Medicine, 10*, 1154567.

80. Whitaker, I. S., Prowse, S., & Potokar, T. S. (2008). A critical evaluation of the use of Biobrane as a biologic skin substitute: A versatile tool for the plastic and reconstructive surgeon. *Annals of Plastic Surgery, 60*(3), 333–337.

81. Wilshaw, S. P., Kearney, J., Fisher, J., & Ingham, E. (2008). Biocompatibility and potential of acellular human amniotic membrane to support the attachment and proliferation of allogeneic cells. *Tissue Engineering. Part A, 14*(4), 463–472.

82. Wójcicka, P., Gadomska-Krasny, J., & Zawodny, J. P. (2010). Zastosowanie laserów w medycynie estetycznej J: Fotoodmładzanie w terapii przebarwień oraz rozszerzonych naczyń Krwionośnych–cz. 1. *OPM, 12*, 46–49.

83. Zaulyanov, L., & Kirsner, R. S. (2007). A review of a bi-layered living cell treatment (Apligraf®) in the treatment of venous leg ulcers and diabetic foot ulcers. *Clinical Interventions in Aging, 2*(1), 93–98.

84. Zelen, C. M., Serena, T. E., Gould, L., Le, L., Carter, M. J., Keller, J., et al. (2016). Treatment of chronic diabetic lower extremity ulcers with advanced therapies: A prospective, randomised, controlled, multi-centre comparative study examining clinical efficacy and cost. *International Wound Journal, 13*, 272–282. https://doi.org/10.1111/iwj.12566.

85. Zhang, T., Yam, G. H., Riau, A. K., Poh, R., Allen, J. C., Peh, G. S., Beuerman, R. W., Tan, D. T., & Mehta, J. S. (2013). The effect of amniotic membrane de-epithelialization method on its biological properties and ability to promote limbal epithelial cell culture. *Investigative Ophthalmology & Visual Science, 54*(4), 3072–3081. DOI: 10.1167/iovs.12-10805.

86. Zhao, J. H., Diao, J. S., Xia, W. S., Pan, Y., & Han, Y. (2012). Clinical application of full-face, whole, full-thickness skin grafting: A case report. *Journal of Plastic, Reconstructive & Aesthetic Surgery, 65*(11), 1576–1579. https://doi.org/10.1016/j.bjps.2012.04.002.

87. Zidan, S. M., & Eleowa, S. A. (2014). Banking and use of glycerol preserved full-thickness skin allograft harvested from body contouring procedures. *Burns, 40*(4), 641–647. https://doi.org/10.1016/j.burns.2013.08.039.

INDEX

I

K

L

M

N

O

P

R

Printed and bound by CPI Group (UK) Ltd, Croydon, CR0 4YY
18/09/2026
14965061-0002